Lower Your Iron Intake,
Raise Your Health Quotient

A leading Finnish study indicates that high iron levels raise the risk of heart disease, and that low iron levels protect against it. The iron theory was advanced eleven years ago in the groundbreaking research of Dr. Jerome L. Sullivan, Director of Clinical Laboratories at the Veterans Affairs Medical Center in Charleston, South Carolina. Recent clinical evidence further supports Dr. Sullivan's theory about the role of dietary iron in the development of heart disease, cancer, diabetes, arthritis and in the aging process. Excess dietary iron may be hazardous to your health! In the first book to address these revolutionary findings, *THE IRON COUNTER* offers you the facts and figures you need to monitor your iron intake, decrease your risk of heart disease, and safeguard your health.

LOOK FOR
THE SODIUM COUNTER

Coming Soon from Pocket Books

Books by Annette B. Natow and Jo-Ann Heslin

The Cholesterol Counter
The Diabetes Carbohydrate and Calorie Counter
The Fat Attack Plan
The Fat Counter
The Iron Counter
Megadoses
No-Nonsense Nutrition for Kids
The Pocket Encyclopedia of Nutrition
The Pregnancy Nutrition Counter
The Sodium Counter

Published by POCKET BOOKS

T·H·E
IRON
COUNTER

Annette B. Natow, Ph.D., R.D., and Jo-Ann Heslin, M.A., R.D.

FOREWORD BY
JEROME L. SULLIVAN, M.D., PH.D.

POCKET BOOKS

New York   London   Toronto   Sydney   Tokyo   Singapore

An *Original* Publication of POCKET BOOKS

POCKET BOOKS, a division of Simon & Schuster Inc.
1230 Avenue of the Americas, New York, NY 10020

ISBN: 0-671-78324-6

First Pocket Books printing April 1993

10 9 8 7 6 5 4 3 2

POCKET and colophon are registered trademarks of
Simon & Schuster Inc.

Printed in the U.S.A.

To our families, who support us through every project: Harry, Allen, Irene, Sarah, Meryl, Laura, Marty, George, Emily, Steven, Joe, Kristen and Karen.

ACKNOWLEDGMENTS

Without the tireless cooperation of Steven and Stephen, *The Iron Counter* would never have been completed. Our thanks to Drs. Martin Lefkowitz and Irene E. Rosenberg for reviewing the material. A special thanks to our editor, Sally Peters, and our agent, Nancy Trichter.

———————

"Iron is another element essential to body structure."

"There is not so much leeway on the iron, but an allowance adequate . . . is covered by the small contributions of many foods."

MARY SWARTZ ROSE, PH.D.
Feeding the Family
The Macmillan Company, 1919

CONTENTS

SOURCES OF DATA

Values in this counter have been obtained from the Composition of Foods, United States Department of Agriculture, Agricultural Handbooks: No. 8-1, Dairy and Egg Products; No. 8-2, Spices and Herbs; No. 8-3, Baby Foods; No. 8-4, Fats and Oils; No. 8-5, Poultry Products; No. 8-6, Soups, Sauces and Gravies; No. 8-7, Sausages and Luncheon Meats; No. 8-8, Breakfast Cereals; No. 8-9, Fruits and Fruit Juices; No. 8-10, Pork Products; No. 8-11, Vegetables and Vegetable Products; No. 8-12, Nut and Seed Products; No. 8-13, Beef Products; No. 8-14, Beverages; No. 8-15, Finfish and Shellfish Products; No. 8-16, Legumes and Legume Products; No. 8-17, Lamb, Veal and Game Products; No. 8-18, Baked Products; No. 8-19, Snacks and Sweets; No. 8-20, Cereal Grains and Pasta; No. 8-21, Fast Foods; Supplements 1989, 1990.

Nutritive Value of Foods, United States Department of Agriculture, Home and Garden Bulletin No. 72.

J. Davies and J. Dickerson, *Nutrient Content of Food Portions* (Cambridge, UK: The Royal Society of Chemistry, 1991).

G. A. Leveille, M. E. Zabik, and K. J. Morgan, *Nutrients in Foods* (Cambridge, MA: The Nutrition Guild, 1983).

Souci, Fachmann, and Kraut, *Food Composition and Nutrition Tables* (Stuttgart: Wissenschaftliche Verlagsgesellschaft MbH, 1989).

Information from food labels, manufacturers and processors. The values are based on research conducted prior to 1992. Manufacturers' ingredients are subject to change, so current values may vary from those listed in this book.

FOREWORD

Doctors today may be violating the fundamental principle of medical practice—"First, do no harm"—by giving their patients too much stored iron. Current medical textbooks tell your doctor not only to correct iron deficiency anemia by giving iron supplements, but to go much further and give enough to build up *stored* iron. Adding hundreds of milligrams to iron stores is, I believe, a dangerous practice that may increase your risk of heart attack and serious diseases. The role of iron in the development of heart disease and other serious disorders is not yet conclusively proven, but in my judgment, what we *do* know now puts the burden of proof squarely on those who believe that stored iron is beneficial. We simply cannot wait for final proof of danger.

There is in fact general agreement on some key points. First, everyone agrees that stored iron can promote injury to body tissues. The only remaining controversy concerns how much stored iron is too much. Second, we know that the "condition" of iron depletion is, in itself, completely harmless. "Iron depletion" means having no stored iron at all, but not being anemic. Many women go through their entire reproductive life in a state of complete iron depletion and still outlive men! Common sense tells us that if stored iron can hurt, and having none of it is harmless, we should do without.

Even if stored iron had no important role in causing heart disease, it can endanger your life in other ways. Abundant stored iron can also cause fatal delays in the diagnosis of potentially curable cancers. Many forms of cancer first come to medical attention because of iron deficiency anemia caused by chronic mild bleeding from the gastrointestinal tract. Having hundreds of milligrams of iron in storage means that months, or even years, may be needed before the constant slight bleeding from the tumor produces iron deficiency anemia. The stored iron load recommended in current medical textbooks can actually delay the diagnosis of potentially curable cancers. Delay in the diagnosis of such cancers can give them time to grow and become inoperable. A patient with iron depletion quickly becomes anemic from such tumors, giving the doctor a lifesaving early warning of cancer. The conventional screening test for gastrointestinal cancers is the fecal occult blood test. With iron depletion, the indication of anemia can give a much earlier warning than the conventional screening test. It also sounds the alarm at the time you need it, not months or years later when you finally get around to having a fecal occult blood test.

Jo-Ann Heslin and Annette Natow's *The Iron Counter* gives you and your doctor an easily accessible tool for helping to control your iron storage level by eating low-iron foods. Your doctor should help you keep stored iron at a level that will do no harm. Find out what your iron storage level is by having the doctor measure your serum ferritin. If it is low, your doctor must find out why. But if you have iron in storage, you and your doctor should take steps to get it down to a safe level. *The Iron Counter* is an important contribution to help you control the iron in your diet.

Jerome L. Sullivan, M.D., Ph.D.
Charleston, South Carolina

INTRODUCTION

If you take a daily iron supplement you may be doing yourself more harm than good. For years iron supplements have been routinely recommended for all sorts of medical problems because iron has always been thought of as healthy. But in the past few years research has started to show that there may be a downside to iron. We may be getting too much of a "good thing." It is becoming increasingly clear that "normal" iron levels play a vital role in promoting heart disease and cancer and may be as important as, if not more important than, cholesterol. It may be time to limit your iron intake, just as you have cut down fat and salt.

All the answers aren't in yet, but researchers are saying that it's time to take a careful look at iron. While it is true that we need some iron to build strong bodies and good blood, too much may not be healthy. And too much iron may be a lot less than we think. Let's take a closer look.

Doctors have known for a long time that young women are protected from heart disease. Men under the age of 45 are almost four times more likely to suffer from heart disease than women under the age of 45. Over age 45, men and women have an equal chance of developing heart disease.

Why are young women protected? What happens to women as they age that increases their risk of heart disease?

To understand the answers to these questions you will have to change the way you think about heart disease. Serum cholesterol levels and dietary fat don't completely explain why young women are less likely to develop heart disease. While young women have somewhat lower choles-terol levels than young men, the differences are small and probably not enough to account for the dramatically lower risk of heart disease in young women.

Young women make more estrogen than men do. Is it estrogen that protects them from heart disease? The answer is probably "no." Research shows that young women who undergo a hysterectomy—in which the uterus is removed but the ovaries are left behind (the ovaries produce estrogen)—end up with a greatly *increased* risk of heart disease. They still produce estrogen, but they have the heart disease risk of a postmenopausal woman. What else do these women have in common with postmenopausal women? These women no longer menstruate.

Most women under the age of 45 do one thing that men never do. Young women menstruate. This means that young women lose blood from their bodies once a month. When you lose blood, you lose iron. And it turns out that when you look at the amount of iron stored in a young woman's body and compare it to that of a young man of the same age, women have less iron in their bodies than men do. It is not until women reach menopause that they begin to have the same level of iron as men. In fact, men under the age of 45 have almost four times as much iron in their bodies as do women under age 45. Sound familiar? Men under age 45 have almost four times the risk of heart disease as women under age 45. This is pretty strong evidence that the body's iron level plays a role in heart disease. Let's look at some more evidence.

What about exercise? Regular exercise of a certain intensity decreases the risk of heart disease. Well, strenuous exercise is also associated with iron loss from the body.

What about aspirin? Doctors recommend that people at risk for heart disease take aspirin every day. Well, regular aspirin use is associated with iron loss from the body.

What about fish-oil supplements? Doctors are also advising people at risk for heart disease to take fish-oil supplements to decrease their risk. Well, regular consumption of fish oils is also associated with iron loss. Even cholestyramine, a medication that lowers cholesterol levels in the blood, can cause the body to lose iron.

What does iron do to promote heart disease and possibly even cancer? No one knows for sure, but the evidence seems to suggest that the presence of iron in body cells causes the formation of particles called oxygen radicals. Oxygen radicals, also called free radicals, are unstable particles that easily damage cells. They break down cell membranes and oxidize fat, making it rancid, similar to when cooking-fat spoils.

Finally, the most convincing evidence linking iron to heart disease comes from a study done in Finland in 1992. In this study, scientists measured body iron stores in almost 2,000 men and discovered that the higher their level of body iron, the greater their risk of heart disease. For each 1 percent increase in the amount of ferritin (storage iron), the risk of heart attack increased by more than 4 percent.

There is also evidence that high iron stores are associated with an increased risk of cancer. One large study done in 1988 showed that a high iron level in men was associated with an increased risk of cancers of the lung, colon, bladder and esophagus. Researchers suspect that exposing the intestines to dietary iron may increase the risk for colon/rectal cancer. A study now being conducted by the American Medical Center (AMC) Cancer Research Center in Denver is investigating a possible link between iron and breast cancer in women.

Now that we are beginning to understand the dangers of high iron levels, how do we redefine how much iron is needed for good health and how much is too much?

DO YOU NEED IRON?

Yes, iron is an essential mineral found in every cell in the body. But it is present in very tiny amounts. The total amount of iron in a man is only about three fourths of a teaspoon

(3.8 grams); in a woman, even less, about one half of a teaspoon (2.3 grams)!

Where is iron found in the body?

Most of the iron in the body is part of:

Hemoglobin, the red pigment in blood cells that carries oxygen from the lungs through the bloodstream to body tissues.

Myoglobin, the red pigment in muscles that carries and stores oxygen for use during muscle contractions.

Heart Damage After a Heart Attack and Brain Damage After a Stroke

Too much iron increases the damage to body tissues right after a heart attack or stroke.

Liver Disease

Too much iron damages the liver, reducing its ability to function and ultimately leading to liver cancer.

Diabetes

Iron overload puts people at higher risk for diabetes.

Rheumatoid Arthritis and Other Inflammations

Excess iron aggravates the inflammation process.

Parkinson's Disease and Alzheimer's Disease

Excess iron increases oxidation (damage) in the brain.

Drug Poisoning

Excess iron intensifies body damage from certain herbicides and anti-cancer drugs.

A small amount of the body's iron is found in:

Enzymes, substances necessary for the body to function. Some enzymes do not contain iron but need it to make them work, to build new cells and to make other vital substances.

The rest of the body's iron is stored. And too much stored iron can result in serious health problems.

Stored iron is bound to a protein called ferritin. A small amount of ferritin circulates in the blood and the rest can be found in the liver, spleen and bone marrow. Incorporation of iron into ferritin increases when iron stores are high and decreases during iron deficiency. It is estimated that 1 microgram (mcg) of ferritin in the blood represents about 8 milligrams (mg) of stored iron. A serum (blood) ferritin test is a good measure of iron stores. During iron deficiency, the blood (or serum) ferritin level is far less than 10 mcg per liter in women and 20 mcg per liter in men. In severe iron overload, the ferritin level ranges from 1,000 mcg to 10,000 mcg per liter of serum.

We no longer know what a "normal" ferritin level is. It's possible that so-called normal stores may actually injure the body.

Let's review.

Yes, you do need iron to make:

> hemoglobin
> myoglobin
> enzymes
> enzymes work

Too much iron can be harmful because it can cause or complicate:

> cancer
> heart disease
> heart damage after a heart attack
> brain damage after a stroke

liver disease
diabetes
rheumatoid arthritis
inflammation
Parkinson's disease
Alzheimer's disease
drug poisoning

Too much iron can be a serious health threat.

How Much Iron Is Enough?

In 1989, the National Research Council gave the following Recommended Dietary Allowances (RDA) of iron for healthy adults.

Females:	Ages 19 to 50	15 mg/day
	Over 50	10 mg/day
	Pregnant	30 mg/day
	Lactating	15 mg/day
Men:	Over age 19	10 mg/day

Men lose an average of 1 mg of iron a day. Women lose 1.5 mg a day, because of their monthly menstrual flow. Women with heavy menstrual flow can lose more than 1.5 mg of iron a day. On the other hand, using birth control pills reduces the monthly iron loss. The RDAs provide enough iron to replace these losses and maintain adequate body stores.

After menopause, because there is no iron lost through menstruation, the recommendation for daily iron intake for older women is the same as that for adult men.

It is very possible that the RDAs listed above are too high.

During Pregnancy

Pregnancy increases the need for iron. A pregnant woman's expanding blood supply requires extra iron. Additionally, iron is used to build the placenta and support the baby's growth. The placenta eagerly accepts iron, delivering large quantities to the developing baby even if it means depriving the mother's body of iron.

The total iron used during pregnancy averages 1,000 mg (1 gram). This is more than the amount of iron most women have stored. That's why women need additional iron during pregnancy. Their stores and normal iron intake during pregnancy are not enough to see them through nine months.

There is little need for extra iron during the first trimester (three months). During the later stages of pregnancy, the need for iron increases. The body responds by absorbing iron more efficiently. In spite of this, the RDA for iron during pregnancy is doubled, to 30 mg, to make sure that there will be enough. Because this increased amount of iron cannot be met by the usual diet in this country, daily iron supplements are almost always recommended. However, many of the supplements used contain *double* the amount of iron needed.

For Children

Birth to 6 months	6 mg/day
6 months to 1 year	10 mg/day
Children 1 to 10	10 mg/day
Boys 11 to 18	12 mg/day
Girls 11 to 18	15 mg/day

Full-term babies are born with enough stored iron to meet their needs for the first three months. Iron deficiency, when it occurs, is not usually seen until around the age of four months, when the iron stores have been used up. This is more likely to occur when a baby is prematurely switched to regular milk from formula or breast milk, both of which have inadequate iron for a young infant.

Regular milk is a poor source of iron and may cause blood loss from the intestines in young infants, resulting in iron loss. When young children drink so much milk that they eat very little other food, they may also develop iron deficiency.

During periods of rapid growth, extra iron is needed to

support growth, maintain normal blood levels and provide for adequate stores. Adolescence is a time of accelerated growth, weight gain and body maturation; therefore, iron needs are high.

At ages 10 to 17, the growth spurt in boys is coupled with increasing hemoglobin levels as they mature sexually. An additional 2 mg of iron per day is needed during this time. Sometime after the age of 10, girls also have a growth spurt which, when coupled with the start of menstruation, calls for an additional 5 mg of iron per day.

Are You Iron Overloaded?

Usually the body carefully balances its supply of iron. The amount of iron absorbed is closely linked to the body's iron needs. A small amount of iron is normally lost on a daily basis in stools, bile, sweat, urine and discarded cells from the intestines and skin. Any kind of blood loss (including menstruation) increases the amount of iron lost.

To balance daily iron loss, healthy adult males and menopausal women need to absorb about 1 mg of iron per day. Healthy young females need to absorb 1.5 mg per day to balance the extra iron lost in menstruation. When the need for iron goes up, iron absorption increases. This happens during pregnancy, in growing children and when there is an iron deficiency. Iron absorption can also be increased even though there is no increased need for iron. This occurs when healthy people take excess iron supplements or follow diets extremely high in iron.

THE MYTH OF IRON DEFICIENCY ANEMIA

Iron deficiency may be a major problem in some parts of the world, but it is not a major problem in the United States or other developed countries. Surveys show that only a small percentage of Americans are iron deficient.

Even among children in low-income families, a group considered vulnerable to iron deficiency, more than 90 percent have adequate iron stores. There has been a striking decline in the prevalence of anemia in infants and children over the past years. This is due to the use of iron-fortified cereals, breads and other foods, and iron-fortified formula, recommended by the American Academy of Pediatrics for any child not breastfed.

Experts estimate that there has also been a substantial decline in the incidence of anemia in young women. The National Health and Nutrition Examination Survey (1976–1980) found the following prevalence of iron deficiency in men and women:

> Men: 0.6% were deficient in ages 20 to 44
> 1.9% were deficient in ages 45 to 64
> Women: 9.6% were deficient in ages 20 to 44
> 4.8% were deficient in ages 45 to 64

While people who are iron deficient may benefit from increased iron, what about the majority of Americans who are not iron deficient?

Don't be fooled by advertisements that tell you that you can't get enough iron, or that iron is healthy and harmless. The vast majority of Americans don't have "iron-poor blood" and are not tired because of iron deficiency. Most of us don't need iron supplements.

Unfortunately, many Americans have been fooled by the ads that say they do. Nationwide surveys show that 35 to 60 percent of Americans use over-the-counter vitamin and mineral supplements, and many of these supplements contain large amounts of iron.

Older people frequently use supplements in the hope that the supplement will keep them healthy. But older adults are not likely to be iron deficient. In fact, studies show that between the ages of 50 and 70 iron stores actually increase.

Many people self-medicate with iron, considering it a tonic that will help them feel better and give them more energy. Others mistakenly believe that they are taking the iron under the direction of a doctor. They may have asked their doctor whether they ought to be taking a supplement and were told that "they could take one if they wanted to." They then conclude that the doctor has actually recommended the iron supplement.

Still others, especially women, take iron by habit or even tradition. They may have been advised to take iron years earlier because of a need and continue to take it long after the need has passed. Others may have seen an older family member use iron supplements and so they do the same.

Some people take iron supplements without even thinking about it or realizing it. Many over-the-counter multivitamin/mineral tablets contain the full RDA for iron. The problem is compounded when these vitamin/mineral supplements are taken with an additional iron tablet. This can be even more of a problem for the 10 percent of the population who are carriers of an iron-overloading gene, since it is easier for them to accumulate unsafe levels of iron. (See Appendix 2 for a discussion of hemochromatosis, a disorder of individuals with two iron-overloading genes.)

Iron used to be considered a cheap, safe dietary supplement. But besides being unnecessary, iron supplements can lead to harmfully high iron stores in healthy people. In addition, iron supplements often have undesirable side effects. They cause constipation, diarrhea and stomach irritation in 25 percent of the people who use them.

Finally, having iron supplements in the house can pose a danger to young children. The Center for Disease Control reports thousands of cases of poisoning each year when children accidentally take too many iron supplements. Iron is the single most frequent cause of poisoning death in children. The American Association of Poison Control Centers reported that the number of deaths in children caused by iron supplements more than doubled in 1991. Because of these tragedies, some experts have advocated a mandatory warning label on iron supplements.

How Do I Determine If I Am Iron Deficient?

Symptoms alone do not indicate iron deficiency. A blood test that checks your serum ferritin level will determine if you are iron deficient. You are iron deficient only if your serum ferritin level is below 10 mcg (micrograms) per liter, in women, or below 20 mcg per liter, in men. See Appendix 1 for more information on the common tests used to determine iron deficiency.

Iron deficiency can occur when:

iron is lost from the body, usually as blood iron stores are used up
dietary intake of iron is low
absorbed iron cannot balance lost iron

Infants, adolescents, and women during the childbearing years are at greatest risk for iron deficiency. Iron deficiency is *rarely* found in adult men or in women after menopause. Normally, iron stores increase in these individuals.

Iron deficiency and anemia are not the same, although iron deficiency may lead to anemia. You can be iron deficient, with reduced iron stores, and still not have anemia. Stored iron may be almost entirely depleted before anemia develops.

Iron deficiency is caused by reduced iron stores.

Iron deficiency anemia produces small, pale red blood cells.

The small, light-colored, anemic, red blood cells that result from iron deficiency anemia can't carry enough oxygen to other body cells. Weakness, fatigue, headaches and loss of interest are some of the obvious signs of iron deficiency anemia.

Some other signs of iron deficiency anemia are subtle and may not be easily recognized. They include a reduced ability to work, exercise and learn, and a poor tolerance of the cold, with difficulty keeping warm. Iron deficiency is also associated with decreased resistance to infections.

Iron deficiency increases the risk of lead poisoning. Children who are iron deficient absorb more lead. This is compounded by the fact that iron-deficient children often have *pica,* the craving for and eating of nonfood substances. Because of the pica, they are more likely to eat dirt, paint chips and other lead-contaminated substances. That is why high blood levels of lead are seen most often in children who are iron deficient.

GREENSICKNESS

Since early times there have been descriptions of young women with pale, greenish skin who were also weak and tired. We now know that this condition, once called "greensickness" or chlorosis (from a Greek word meaning "green"), is actually iron deficiency anemia.

In the seventeenth century, Thomas Sydenham (famous for introducing the use of opium into medicine) suggested using a "steel tonic" to treat chlorosis. He made his tonic by soaking steel filings in wine. The mixture was then strained and made into a syrup. Sydenham's tonic helped women with greensickness, but he did not know why it worked.

It wasn't until 1747 that an Italian researcher proved that there was iron in blood by showing that particles from dried, powdered blood could be lifted with a magnet. Later researchers showed that giving iron supplements would increase the level of iron compounds in the blood and cure chlorosis. By 1832, iron tablets were widely used to treat iron deficiency anemia.

CONTROLLING IRON INTAKE

Nearly one half of the iron in the American diet comes from grains, pasta, rice and other cereals even though we get only about one quarter of our calories from these foods. More than 25 percent of the iron comes from meat, poultry and fish. The remainder comes from other foods.

The typical American consumes about 6 mg (milligrams) of iron in 1,000 calories of food. Of this, about 10 to 15 percent of the iron is absorbed. This means that, for most people, for every 1,000 calories consumed only 1 mg of iron is absorbed.

Iron is found in two forms in food:

Heme iron: 40 percent of the iron in meats, poultry and fish is made up of heme iron. Heme iron is better absorbed but makes up a small part of the iron in food.

Nonheme iron: the only kind of iron found in vegetables, fruits and grains. Nonheme iron makes up the remaining 60 percent of the iron found in meat, fish and poultry. Nonheme iron is more poorly absorbed.

Nonheme Iron Absorption

Very little of the nonheme iron in foods is absorbed by the body. However, you can increase the absorption of nonheme iron by eating certain foods. On the other hand, there are several foods and medicines that decrease the absorption of nonheme iron.

Nonheme iron absorption is:

Increased by	Decreased by
MFP factor	EDTA
Vitamin C	Antacids
Food acids	Phosphates
Sugars	Tannins
Calcium	Egg yolk
Alcohol	Oxalic acid
	Tetracycline
	Cholestyramine
	Phytic acid
	Large amounts of iron

MFP (Meat, Fish, Poultry) *factor.* Meat, fish and poultry naturally contain MFP, an unknown factor that automatically **increases the absorption of nonheme iron.** This means that when you eat a steak at dinner, you more efficiently absorb the nonheme iron in the dinner roll, green beans and baked potato you have along with it.

Vitamin C. Eating a food or drinking a juice high in vitamin C (ascorbic acid) **increases the absorption of nonheme iron.** Having a sliced tomato or drinking orange juice at lunch will increase the amount of iron absorbed from the meal.

Food acids. Citric acid and malic acid found in fruits and many other foods and also used as an additive in canned vegetables, margarines, jellies, preserves, candies and sherbet **increases nonheme iron absorption.**

Sugars. Like vitamin C and citric and malic acids, sugars convert nonheme iron to a more soluble form, **so more is absorbed.**

Calcium. A mineral found mainly in milk and cheese, calcium **helps nonheme iron absorption.**

Alcohol. A glass of wine or any other alcohol-containing drink may increase the acidity of the stomach and intestines, **making nonheme iron more absorbable.**

EDTA (ethylenediaminetetraacetic acid). This common food additive used in fruit drinks, beer, vegetable juices, margarines, salad dressings, mayonnaise and processed fruits and vegetables **reduces nonheme iron absorption.**

Antacids. Heavy use of antacids will neutralize stomach acid, **reducing nonheme iron absorption.**

Phosphates. These are phosphorus-containing substances found in foods. They can **combine with nonheme iron, preventing its absorption.**

Tannins. The astringent-tasting substances found in coffee and tea will **interfere with the absorption of nonheme iron.**

Egg yolk. Phosvitin, in egg yolk, will **reduce iron absorption** unless a vitamin C–containing food is eaten at the same time.

Oxalic acid. When large amounts of spinach or rhubarb

are eaten, the oxalic acid they contain **combines with non-heme iron, reducing its absorption.**

Tetracycline. Antibiotics in this family **combine with non-heme iron, reducing absorption.**

Cholestyramine. This cholesterol-lowering drug **reduces nonheme iron absorption.**

Phytic Acid. Found in bran, whole-grain cereals, peas, beans, soybeans and soybean products, phytic acid can **bind nonheme iron, preventing its absorption.** This is an important issue as more people regularly eat more beans and grains.

Large amounts of iron. The **more iron eaten at one time, the less iron is absorbed.**

FIBER FOODS HIGH IN PHYTIC ACID

Almonds	Oats	Walnuts
Barley	Peanuts	Wheat bran
Brazil nuts	Pinto beans	Wheat germ
Brown rice	Rye	White beans
Corn	Sesame seeds	Whole wheat
Cornmeal	Soy	Wild rice
Cowpeas	Soybeans	
Lentils	Split peas	

FOODS HIGH IN VITAMIN C

Bok choy	Grapefruit juice	Strawberries
Broccoli	Green pepper	Tomato juice
Brussels sprouts	Mango	Tomatoes
Cabbage	Orange juice	Turnip greens
Cantaloupe	Oranges	Watermelon
Cauliflower	Papaya	
Grapefruit	Parsley	

Rating Your Iron Intake

1. Do you regularly eat more than 3 ounces of meat a day?   YES   NO
2. Do you regularly eat highly fortified cereals?   YES   NO
3. Do you regularly take large doses of vitamin C?   YES   NO
4. Do you rarely drink coffee and tea with meals?   YES   NO
5. Do you regularly drink alcoholic beverages with meals?   YES   NO
6. Do you rarely eat whole grain breads?   YES   NO
7. Do you usually eat processed foods that are low in fiber?   YES   NO
8. Do you usually cook in iron pots?   YES   NO
9. Do you regularly take multivitamin/mineral supplements?   YES   NO
10. Do you regularly take iron supplements?   YES   NO
11. Do you rarely (never) donate blood?   YES   NO
12. Do you exercise less than one hour a week or rarely play organized sports (softball, tennis, etc.)?   YES   NO

Too many "yes" answers signal that you may be storing more iron than is healthy.

Read the following suggestions to discover ways to lower your iron intake. Aim for fewer "yes" answers the next time you rate your iron intake. Rate your iron intake once in a while to make sure your health habits are on track.

Getting Less Iron

The evidence is beginning to show that it may be healthier to eat less iron and reduce iron stores. This can be done by:

Eating less meat
Eating more whole-grain bread

Eating fewer highly fortified cereals
Eating high-fiber foods
Choosing the best beverages
Eating more fruits and vegetables
Eating more lowfat dairy foods
Using non-iron cookware
Avoiding excessive amounts of vitamin C
Avoiding supplements that contain iron
Increasing exercise
Donating blood

Eating Less Meat

Meat is a major contributor to the iron in your diet. The heme iron, which is plentiful in meat, is very easily absorbed. Experts estimate that heme iron is absorbed five to ten times faster than the nonheme iron in food plants. In fact, as mentioned earlier, there is a substance in meat (MFP factor) that increases the absorption of nonheme iron from other foods eaten at the same time.

People who eat for good health may have already decided to eat less red meat and more chicken and fish. That's good, because it turns out that poultry and fish usually have less iron than red meat. In fact white-meat poultry and fish have only one half the iron found in the same size serving of red meat. Dark-meat poultry has slightly more iron but still one-third less than red meat. For example, a three-ounce portions of flank steak contains 3 mg iron, a three-ounce portion of chicken breast contains 1 mg, and a three-ounce serving of salmon contains 1 mg.

Portion size is important. You don't have to avoid meat, just eat less of it. Three ounces is enough for one serving. A three-ounce portion of boneless meat, fish or poultry is about the same size as a deck of playing cards. Use this as your guide when eating at home or in a restaurant.

Enrichment is the addition of iron and three B vitamins—thiamin (B_1), riboflavin (B_2) and niacin—to grains in amounts equal to the amount present in the natural whole grains before they were refined. The policy of enriching flour and other grains began in the early 1940s, and this is the reason breads and cereals supply so much iron. All refined grains shipped from one state to another must be enriched. Thirty-eight states have enrichment laws; flour and grains sold within these states must be enriched. The National Millers Association estimates that 95 percent of all flour is enriched.

STANDARDS FOR IRON ENRICHMENT

FOOD	MG PER POUND
Enriched flour	20
Enriched self-rising flour	20
Enriched bread, rolls, buns, white	12.5
Enriched cornmeal and grits	13–26
Enriched self-rising cornmeal	13–26
Enriched rice	13–26
Enriched macaroni and noodle products	13–16.5

Source: United States Department of Agriculture

Eating More Whole-Grain Bread

Eating whole wheat, rye, pumpernickel and other breads that contain whole grains is a healthy way to go. You get all the vitamins and fiber in the whole grain plus phytates that reduce iron absorption.

Most breads are made with leavening agents, such as baking powder and yeast, that help the bread rise. While these leavening agents make the bread light they also break down the phytate in grains, so that more iron is absorbed. You get less iron from unleavened breads and crackers like pita bread and matzo.

Eating Less Highly Fortified Cereals

All ready-to-eat cereals are enriched with iron and vitamins to the levels that were present in the original grains. But some are also fortified, so they have even greater than whole-grain amounts of iron and vitamins. They usually provide 25 percent of the USRDA in a one-ounce serving, about one bowl.

Some ready-to-eat cereals are even more highly fortified than that. In some cereals so much iron and vitamins are added that one ounce provides 50 percent or more of the USRDA. Total, Product 19 and Just Right are three of these highly fortified cereals. In 1973 the FDA required that these cereals be labeled "multivitamin and iron supplements."

Highy fortified cereals should really be considered as supplements, not cereals. This is particularly important because many children, especially teens, eat much more than one bowl at a time.

Choose unenriched, unfortified, whole-grain cereals like regular oatmeal and farina whenever you can.

Eat Foods High in Fiber

Fiber binds with iron in the intestines, stopping it from being absorbed. To get the most fiber from fiber-rich foods like grains, beans, fruits and vegetables, it is best to have them close to their original state. That means eating an apple instead of applesauce or eating an apple instead of drinking apple juice. Applesauce has less fiber than an apple, and apple juice has even less.

Eat potatoes with their peel, unblanched nuts (with their brown papery skin), and whole fruits and vegetables. Eat brown rice instead of white, and whole grains instead of their refined relatives. Peanuts, seeds, peas, beans, corn, barley, artichokes, dried fruits, dates, figs, berries, mangoes, pears, plantains, eggplant, broccoli, Brussels sprouts, spinach, and squash are all high in fiber.

Choose the Best Beverages

Both coffee and tea contain iron-binding substances that interfere with iron absorption. Drinking coffee or tea with meals or soon after will reduce the amount of iron that is absorbed during the meal. When milk is added to coffee or tea, the iron-binding substances bind instead to the calcium in the milk. So adding milk to coffee or tea increases absorption of more of the iron in the meal. Regular tea and coffee contain caffeine, so it is best not to drink more than two to three cups a day. Decaffeinated coffee or tea and herbal teas are believed to contain iron binding substances too.

Vitamin C–containing juices like orange, grapefruit or tomato will increase iron absorption. Drinking these juices at mealtime causes more iron to be absorbed.

Eating More Fruits and Vegetables

Most fruits and vegetables have very little iron. Spinach, dried fruits, lentils and beans, however, are exceptions. But these fruits and vegetables also contain substances that interfere with the absorption of the iron that they contain.

Eating More Lowfat Dairy Foods

Dairy foods contain very little iron. Choose lowfat dairy foods because they are rich in protein, vitamins and other minerals while being low in fat.

Using Non-Iron Cookware

Foods cooked in iron pans contain more iron than if they had been cooked in glass, aluminum or stainless steel. This is especially true when you cook acid foods, like tomato, for a long time. A study showed that a three-and-a-half-ounce serving of spaghetti sauce cooked in a glass pan contained 3 milligrams of iron, but when cooked in an iron pan, the sauce had over 87 milligrams of iron. A similar study showed that scrambled eggs cooked in an iron pan contained three times more iron than eggs cooked in a non-iron pan. Cooking and/or storing foods in iron cooking pans can substantially increase the amount of iron in those foods.

Avoiding Excessive Amounts of Vitamin C

Vitamin C increases iron absorption. In fact some iron supplements include vitamin C in their formula to enhance absorption of the iron. While vitamin C is essential, it may be a good idea to avoid taking vitamin C–rich foods at mealtime since they may cause excess absorption of iron. It's also wise not to routinely take large amounts of vitamin C supplements.

Avoiding Supplements That Contain Iron

Nationwide surveys show that 35 to 60 percent of Americans use vitamin and mineral supplements. They spend about 3.3 billion dollars a year on them. In a survey of over 13,000 adults and children, 25 percent of the 3,400 different supplements consumed contained iron. The average amount of iron in supplements is often several tmes the RDA.

Iron supplements should be reserved for use during times when there is a deficiency determined by a blood test. For a list of iron-containing supplements see Part III.

Increasing Exercise

Exercise has been shown to cause iron loss in several ways: sweating, bleeding in the intestines and breakdown of red blood cells. Heavy sweating during prolonged exercise can by itself result in a loss of almost one milligram of iron a day.

Studies show that athletes have lower than average iron stores. Regular strenuous exercise has been shown to interfere with the normal increase in iron absorption which occurs when the body's iron stores are depleted.

Donating Blood

Donating blood has always been a wonderful way to help others who need blood. Now, according to experts, it is also a way to help yourself by reducing unhealthy excess iron stores in your body. Periodic blood donations have been recommended as a way to achieve a healthy iron balance. This is something to discuss with your doctor to see whether donating blood is something you should do.

* * *

Now let's look at a typical day to see where iron comes from in the foods you choose. On Sample Day Number 1, over 41 milligrams of iron were eaten. This is far more than the average adult needs. On Sample Day Number 2 some of the choices have been changed to reduce the iron intake for the day. You can see how easy this is.

IRON COUNTING
SAMPLE DAY NUMBER 1

Breakfast	IRON (MG)	CALORIES
Orange juice (½ cup)	tr	52
Total Cereal (1 ounce)	18	100
Lowfat milk (½ cup)	tr	51
Raisin bran muffin	5	220
Coffee	tr	4
& Lowfat milk (2 tbsp)	tr	13
Lunch		
Black bean soup (1 cup)	5	218
Chicken fillet sandwich	5	515
Tossed salad (½ cup)	tr	15
Mineral water	tr	0
Snack		
Blueberry nonfat yogurt (4.4 oz)	0	60
Dinner		
Pot roast, chuck (4 oz)	4	376
Peas, frozen (½ cup)	1	63
Minute Long Grain & Wild Rice (½ cup)	2	149
Waldorf salad (½ cup)	tr	79
Date nut bread (1 slice)	1	92
Diet cola (12 ounces)	tr	2
TV Snack		
Borden's Vanilla Fat-free Ice Cream (½ cup)	0	90
Total	41	2099

This is too much iron for one day—41 milligrams. Now you can see how easy it is to eat too much.

IRON COUNTING
SAMPLE DAY NUMBER 2
A SAMPLE DAY OF LOWER IRON FOOD CHOICES

Breakfast	IRON (MG)	CALORIES
Orange juice (½ cup)	tr	52
Kellogg's Corn Flakes (1 ounce)	2	100
Lowfat milk (½ cup)	tr	51
Raisin bread (1 slice)	2	142
Honey (2 tsp)	tr	43
Coffee	tr	4
& Lowfat milk (2 tbsp)	0	13
Lunch		
Cream of mushroom soup (1 cup)	1	203
Ham sandwich with cheese	3	353
Potato salad (½ cup)	1	179
Mineral water	tr	0
Snack		
Blueberry nonfat yogurt (4.4 oz)	0	60
Dinner		
½ Chicken breast with skin, roasted	1	193
Minute Rice (⅔ cup)	1	141
Peas, frozen (½ cup)	1	63
Waldorf salad (½ cup)	0	79
Whole wheat dinner roll, 1 oz	1	75
Butter (1 pat)	tr	36
Date nut bread (1 slice)	1	92
Tea &	tr	2
Sugar (1 tsp)	0	15
TV Snack		
Borden's Vanilla Fat-free Ice Cream (1 cup)	0	180
Total	14	2076

Wise food choices! A much healthier intake of iron for the day. Choosing chicken instead of chuck beef pot roast means there is less iron in the meal. Bean soups have more iron than other vegetable soups. Other helpful changes are the whole wheat roll, the tea with dinner and substituting a breakfast cereal with less added iron.

Now it's your turn to count your iron. Use the following sample worksheet to note everything you ate today, then look up the iron in each food you have eaten to see how much iron you have eaten. While you're at it jot down the calories, too!

Aim for:

    10 milligrams of iron a day for a man
    15 milligrams of iron a day for a woman
    10 milligrams of iron a day for a postmenopausal
       woman

Did you eat too much iron today? If you did, start right now to make lower iron food choices.

IRON COUNTING:
A SAMPLE WORKSHEET

FOOD	AMOUNT	IRON (MG)	CALORIES
Breakfast			
Snack			
Lunch			
Snack			
Dinner			
Snack			

Total
Iron mg: ____

Total
Calories: ____

USING YOUR IRON COUNTER

This book lists the iron and calorie content of over 9,000 foods. For the first time, information about iron values is at your fingertips. Now you will find it easy to avoid eating too much iron. Before *The Iron Counter* it was impossible to compare so many foods at one time. When you want to pick a cereal with less iron, look in the cereal category, beginning on page 62. Fresh foods like meat, chicken, fish and cheese do not usually have a label. The same goes for take-out foods like potato salad, coleslaw, ice cream or bakery items. How can you tell how much iron there is in a burger or taco that you enjoy at the local fast-food restaurant? *The Iron Counter* lists them all!

The Iron Counter is divided into three main sections. Part I, Brand-Name and Generic Foods, lists foods alphabetically. For each group, you will find brand-name foods listed in alphabetical order, then an alphabetical listing of generic foods. Large categories are divided into subcategories—canned, fresh, frozen, ready-to-use—to make it easier to find what you are looking for.

If you want to know how much iron is in the hamburger you are having for lunch, look under HAMBURGER, where you will find all kinds of hamburgers listed. Or, if you are making a hamburger at home, look under ROLL, where you will find the hamburger roll listed alphabetically, and under BEEF, where you will find a cooked chopped-beef patty. For foods like FRENCH TOAST, BACON or BREAD, simply look for the specific food alphabetically in the complete listing. For example, FRENCH TOAST is found on page 143, listed alphabetically between FRENCH BEANS and FROG'S LEGS. One slice has 1 milligram of iron.

If you are eating at home, simply look up the individual foods you are eating and total the iron for the meal. For example, your dinner may consist of:

	IRON (MG)
Rib lamb chop, broiled (3 oz)	2
Green Giant Broccoli Cuts (½ cup)	0
Ore Ida Cheddar Browns (3 oz)	1
Pepperidge Farm Dinner Roll	1
Strawberry frozen yogurt	0
Sunshine Almond Crescents (2 cookies)	tr
Coffee, regular	tr
Glass of white wine	tr
TOTAL IRON FOR THE MEAL:	4

Many food categories have a take-out subcategory. Items found in the take-out subcategory will help you estimate the iron and calories in similar restaurant or take-out menu items when you are eating out. For example, if you order spaghetti and meatballs, look under PASTA DISHES on page 205.

Most foods are listed alphabetically. But in some cases foods are grouped by category. For example, all pasta dishes—like spaghetti and meatballs, lasagna and fettucini—are found under the category PASTA DISHES.

Other group categories include:

DINNERS   Page 123
   Includes all frozen dinners by brand name

ICE CREAM AND FROZEN DESSERTS   Page 162
   Includes all dairy and nondairy ice cream
   and frozen novelties except ices and
   sherbet

LIQUOR/LIQUEUR   Page 172
   Includes all alcoholic beverages except
   wine or beer

LUNCHEON MEATS/COLD CUTS   Page 174
   Includes all sandwich meats except
   chicken, ham and turkey

Part II, Restaurant, Take-Out and Fast-Food Chains, contains an alphabetical listing of 22 popular chains. Fast foods are listed alphabetically under the chain's name, for example, BURGER KING, TACO BELL and WENDY'S. The listing for Burger King begins on page 340.

We have tried to include all foods for which iron values are known. There will be some foods, however, that are not listed in *The Iron Counter* because the iron values are not available for that particular food.

When you can't locate your favorite brand, look at other similar foods. You will probably find a brand food, a generic product or a home recipe that is like your favorite food. For example: You find that your favorite brand of waffles is not listed. Look at the different waffles listed on page 321. From these entries you can quickly determine that blueberry waffles have from 2 to 4 milligrams of iron in a serving. You can then assume that your favorite brand has a comparable amount.

With *The Iron Counter* as your guide, you will never again wonder how much iron is in food. You will always be able to tell if a food is high in iron, moderate in iron or low in iron.

Part III, Vitamin and Mineral Supplements, will help you find out the amount of iron in common supplements.

Discrepancies in figures are due to rounding, product reformulation and reevaluation.

DEFINITIONS

as prep (as prepared): refers to food that has been prepared according to package directions

cooked: refers to food cooked without the addition of fat (oil, butter, margarine, etc.); steaming, poaching, broiling and dry roasting are examples of this type of preparation

home recipe: describes homemade dishes; those included can be used as guide to the iron and calorie values of similar products you may prepare or take-out food you buy ready-to-eat

lean and fat: describes meat with some fat on its edges that is not cut away before cooking or poultry prepared with skin and fat as purchased

lean only: lean portion, trimmed of all visible fat

shelf-stable: refers to prepared products found on the supermarket shelf that are ready to be heated and do not require refrigeration

take-out: describes prepared dishes that you purchase ready-to-eat; those included serve as a guide to the iron and calorie values of similar products you may purchase

trace (tr): value used when a food contains less than one calorie or less than one milligram (mg) of iron

ABBREVIATIONS

avg	=	average
diam	=	diameter
frzn	=	frozen
g	=	gram
gal	=	gallon
lb	=	pound
lg	=	large
med	=	medium
mg	=	milligram
oz	=	ounce
pkg	=	package
pt	=	pint
prep	=	prepared
qt	=	quart
reg	=	regular
serv	=	serving
sm	=	small
sq	=	square
tbsp	=	tablespoon
tr	=	trace
tsp	=	teaspoon
w/	=	with
w/o	=	without
"	=	inch
<	=	less than

EQUIVALENT MEASURES

1 tablespoon	=	3 teaspoons
4 tablespoons	=	¼ cup
8 tablespoons	=	½ cup
12 tablespoons	=	¾ cup
16 tablespoons	=	1 cup
1000 milligrams	=	1 gram
28 grams	=	1 ounce

LIQUID MEASUREMENTS

2 tablespoons	=	1 ounce
¼ cup	=	2 ounces
½ cup	=	4 ounces
¾ cup	=	6 ounces
1 cup	=	8 ounces
2 cups	=	1 pint
4 cups	=	1 quart

DRY MEASUREMENTS

16 ounces	=	1 pound
12 ounces	=	¾ pound
8 ounces	=	½ pound
4 ounces	=	¼ pound

ALL IRON VALUES OF FOODS ARE GIVEN IN MILLIGRAMS (MG)

PART I
Brand-Name and Generic Foods

FOOD	PORTION	CALORIES	IRON
ABALONE			
fresh, fried	3 oz	161	3
raw	3 oz	89	3
ACEROLA			
FRESH			
acerola	1	2	tr
JUICE			
juice	1 cup	51	1
ADZUKI BEANS			
CANNED			
sweetened	1 cup	702	3
DRIED			
cooked	1 cup	294	5
READY-TO-USE			
yokan, sliced	3¼" slice	112	1
AKEE			
fresh	3.5 oz	223	3
ALE			
(see BEER AND ALE, MALT)			
ALFALFA			
sprouts	1 cup	40	tr
sprouts	1 tbsp	1	tr
ALLSPICE			
ground	1 tsp	5	tr

FOOD	PORTION	CALORIES	IRON

ALMONDS

FOOD	PORTION	CALORIES	IRON
Almond Butter (Erewhon)	1 tbsp	90	1
Almonds (Planters)	1 oz	170	1
Blanched Slivered (Dole)	1 oz	170	1
Blanched Whole (Dole)	1 oz	170	1
Chopped Natural (Dole)	1 oz	170	1
Honey Roasted (Planters)	1 oz	170	1
Sliced (Planters)	1 oz	170	1
Sliced Natural (Dole)	1 oz	170	1
Slivered (Planters)	1 oz	170	1
Whole Natural (Dole)	1 oz	170	1
almond butter honey & cinnamon	1 tbsp	96	1
almond butter w/ salt	1 tbsp	101	1
almond butter w/o salt	1 tbsp	101	1
almond meal	1 oz	116	2
almond paste	1 oz	127	1
dried, blanched	1 oz	166	1
dried, unblanched	1 oz	167	1
dry roasted, unblanched	1 oz	167	1
dry roasted, unblanched, salted	1 oz	167	1
oil roasted, blanched	1 oz	174	2
oil roasted, blanched, salted	1 oz	174	2
oil roasted, unblanched	1 oz	176	1
toasted, unblanched	1 oz	167	1

AMARANTH
(*see also* CEREAL, COOKIES)

FOOD	PORTION	CALORIES	IRON
Amaranth Cereal w/ Bananas (Health Valley)	½ cup	110	1
Amaranth Crunch w/ Raisins (Health Valley)	¼ cup	110	tr

FOOD	PORTION	CALORIES	IRON
Amaranth Flakes 100% Organic (Health Valley)	½ cup	90	2
Fast Menu Amaranth w/ Garden Vegetables (Health Valley)	7.5 oz	140	5
cooked	½ cup	59	1
uncooked	½ cup	366	7

ANCHOVY

CANNED			
in oil	1 can (1.6 oz)	95	2
in oil	5	42	1
FRESH			
raw	3 oz	62	3

ANISE

seed	1 tsp	7	1

ANTELOPE

roasted	3 oz	127	3.6

APPLE

CANNED			
Applesauce			
100% Gravenstein Sweetened (S&W)	½ cup	90	1
Cinnamon (Tree Top)	½ cup	80	tr
Natural (Tree Top)	½ cup	60	tr
Original (Tree Top)	½ cup	80	tr
sweetened	½ cup	97	tr
unsweetened	½ cup	53	tr
Sliced, sweetened	1 cup	136	tr

FOOD	PORTION	CALORIES	IRON
DRIED			
cooked w/ sugar	½ cup	116	tr
cooked w/o sugar	½ cup	172	tr
rings	10	155	1
FRESH			
apple	1	81	tr
w/o skin, sliced	1 cup	62	tr
w/o skin, sliced & cooked	1 cup	91	tr
w/o skin, sliced & microwaved	1 cup	96	tr
FROZEN			
Apple Fritters (Mrs. Paul's)	2	270	tr
sliced w/o sugar	½ cup	41	tr
JUICE			
Bruce Lite	½ cup	88	tr
Juice & More	8 oz	120	tr
Kern's Cinnamon Nectar	6 oz	110	tr
S&W 100% Unsweetened	6 oz	85	1
Tree Top	6 oz	90	1
Tree Top Cider	6 oz	90	1
Tree Top Cider, frzn, as prep	6 oz	90	1
Tree Top, frzn, as prep	6 oz	90	1
Tree Top Unfiltered	6 oz	90	1
Tree Top Unfiltered, frzn, as prep	6 oz	90	1
Tree Top w/ Vitamin C	6 oz	90	1
apple	1 cup	116	1
frzn, as prep	1 cup	111	1
frzn, not prep	6 oz	349	2

APRICOTS

FOOD	PORTION	CALORIES	IRON
CANNED			
Halves Diet (S&W)	½ cup	35	tr

FOOD	PORTION	CALORIES	IRON
Halves Unpeeled in Heavy Syrup (S&W)	½ cup	110	tr
Halves Unsweetened (S&W)	½ cup	35	tr
Whole Peeled Diet (S&W)	½ cup	28	1
Whole Peeled in Heavy Syrup (S&W)	½ cup	100	tr
heavy syrup w/ skin	3 halves	70	tr
juice pack w/ skin	3 halves	40	tr
light syrup w/ skin	3 halves	54	tr
water pack w/ skin	3 halves	22	tr
water pack w/o skin	4 halves	20	tr
DRIED			
halves	10	83	2
halves, cooked w/o sugar	½ cup	106	2
FRESH			
apricots	3	51	1
FROZEN			
sweetened	½ cup	119	1
JUICE			
Kern's Nectar	6 oz	100	1
Libby's Nectar	6 oz	110	tr
S&W Nectar	6 oz	35	1
nectar	1 cup	141	1

ARROWHEAD

fresh, boiled	1 med (¾ oz)	9	tr

ARROWROOT

flour	1 cup	457	tr

FOOD	PORTION	CALORIES	IRON

ARTICHOKE

CANNED

FOOD	PORTION	CALORIES	IRON
Hearts Marinated (S&W)	½ cup	225	1

FRESH

FOOD	PORTION	CALORIES	IRON
boiled	1 med (4 oz)	60	2
hearts, cooked	½ cup	42	1
jerusalem, raw, sliced	½ cup	57	3

FROZEN

FOOD	PORTION	CALORIES	IRON
Hearts Deluxe (Birds Eye)	½ cup	30	1
cooked	1 pkg (9 oz)	108	1

ASPARAGUS

CANNED

FOOD	PORTION	CALORIES	IRON
Points Water Pack (S&W)	½ cup	17	1
Spears Colossal Fancy (S&W)	½ cup	20	tr
Spears Fancy (S&W)	½ cup	18	tr
spears	½ cup	24	2

FRESH

FOOD	PORTION	CALORIES	IRON
cooked	½ cup	22	1
cooked	4 spears	14	tr
raw	½ cup	16	1
raw	4 spears	14	1

FROZEN

FOOD	PORTION	CALORIES	IRON
Big Valley	2.7 oz	23	1
Cut (Birds Eye)	½ cup	23	1
Harvest Fresh Cuts (Green Giant)	½ cup	25	1
Spears (Birds Eye)	½ cup	25	1
cooked	1 pkg (10 oz)	82	2
cooked	4 spears	17	tr

FOOD	PORTION	CALORIES	IRON
AVOCADO			
FRESH			
avocado	1	324	2
puree	1 cup	370	2
BACON			
(*see also* BACON SUBSTITUTES)			
Oscar Mayer Center Cut, cooked	1 slice	24	tr
Oscar Mayer, cooked	1 slice	35	tr
Oscar Mayer Lower Salt, cooked	1 strip	33	tr
Oscar Mayer Thick Sliced, cooked	1 slice	58	tr
breakfast strips beef, cooked	3 strips (1.2 oz)	153	1
cooked	3 strips	109	tr
gammon, lean & fat, grilled	4.2 oz	274	2
grilled	2 slices (1.7 oz)	86	tr
BACON SUBSTITUTES			
Bac-Os	2 tsp	25	tr
Louis Rich Turkey Bacon, cooked	1 slice	32	tr
Oscar Mayer Bacon Bits	.25 oz	20	tr
bacon substitute	1 strip	25	tr
BAGEL			
FRESH			
cinnamon raisin	1 (3½")	194	3
cinnamon raisin, toasted	1 (3½")	194	3
egg	1 (3½")	197	3
egg, toasted	1 (3½")	197	3
oat bran	1 (3½")	181	2
oat bran, toasted	1 (3½")	181	2

FOOD	PORTION	CALORIES	IRON
onion	1 (3½")	195	3
plain	1 (3½")	195	3
plain, toasted	1 (3½")	195	3
poppy seed	1 (3½")	195	3
FROZEN			
Cinnamon & Raisin (Sara Lee)	1 (3 oz)	240	3
Cinnamon 'n Raisin (Lender's)	1	200	1
Cinnamon Raisin (Sara Lee)	1 (2.5 oz)	200	2
Egg (Lender's)	1	150	1
Egg (Sara Lee)	1 (2.5 oz)	200	3
Egg (Sara Lee)	1 (3 oz)	250	4
Ham & Cheese on a Bagel (Great Starts)	3 oz	240	2
Oat Bran (Sara Lee)	1 (2.5 oz)	180	2
Oat Bran (Sara Lee)	1 (3 oz)	220	3
Onion (Lender's)	1	160	1
Onion (Sara Lee)	1 (2.5 oz)	190	4
Onion (Sara Lee)	1 (3 oz)	230	4
Plain (Lender's)	1	150	1
Plain (Sara Lee)	1 (2.5 oz)	190	3
Plain (Sara Lee)	1 (3 oz)	230	3
Poppy Seed (Sara Lee)	1 (2.5 oz)	190	3
Poppy Seed (Sara Lee)	1 (3 oz)	230	4
Sesame Seed (Sara Lee)	1 (2.5 oz)	190	1
Sesame Seed (Sara Lee)	1 (3 oz)	240	1

BAKING POWDER

FOOD	PORTION	CALORIES	IRON
Clabber Girl	1 tsp	0	tr
baking powder	1 tsp	2	1
low sodium	1 tsp	5	tr

FOOD	PORTION	CALORIES	IRON

BAKING SODA

FOOD	PORTION	CALORIES	IRON
Arm & Hammer	1 tsp	0	tr
baking soda	1 tsp	0	0

BALSAM PEAR

FOOD	PORTION	CALORIES	IRON
leafy tips, cooked	½ cup	10	tr
leafy tips, raw	½ cup	7	tr
pods, cooked	½ cup	12	tr

BAMBOO SHOOTS

FOOD	PORTION	CALORIES	IRON
CANNED			
La Choy	¼ cup	6	tr
sliced	1 cup	25	tr
FRESH			
cooked	½ cup	15	tr
raw	½ cup	21	tr

BANANA

FOOD	PORTION	CALORIES	IRON
DRIED			
powder	1 tbsp	21	tr
FRESH			
banana	1	105	tr
mashed	1 cup	207	1

BARLEY

FOOD	PORTION	CALORIES	IRON
Quaker Medium Pearled	¼ cup	172	1
Quaker Quick Pearled	¼ cup	172	1
Scotch Medium Pearled	¼ cup	172	1
Scotch Quick pearled	¼ cup	172	1
pearled, cooked	½ cup	97	1
pearled, uncooked	½ cup	352	3

FOOD	PORTION	CALORIES	IRON

BASIL
ground	1 tsp	4	1

BASS

FRESH
freshwater, raw	3 oz	97	1
sea, cooked	3 oz	105	tr
sea, raw	3 oz	82	tr
striped, baked	3 oz	105	1

BAY LEAF
crumbled	1 tsp	2	tr

BEAN SPROUTS
  (*see also individual bean names*)

CANNED
La Choy	⅔ cup	8	tr

BEANS
  (*see also individual bean names*)

Baked Beans (Brick Oven)	½ cup	160	3
Baked Beans (Van Camp's)	1 cup	260	4
Barbecue Beans (Campbell)	½ can (7⅞ oz)	210	3
Barbecue Beans Texas Style (S&W)	½ cup	135	2
Beanee Weenee (Van Camp's)	1 cup	326	4
Big John's Beans 'n Fixin's (Hunt's)	4 oz	170	2
Boston Baked (Health Valley)	7.5 oz	190	4
Boston Baked No Salt Added (Health Valley)	7.5 oz	190	4
Brown Sugar Beans (Van Camp's)	1 cup	290	3

FOOD	PORTION	CALORIES	IRON
Chili (Gebhardt)	4 oz	115	2
Deluxe Baked Beans (Van Camp's)	1 cup	320	4
Fast Menu Honey Baked Organic Beans w/ Tofu Wieners (Health Valley)	7.5 oz	150	5
Home Style Beans (Campbell)	½ can (8 oz)	220	4
Hot Chili Beans (Campbell)	½ can (7.75 oz)	180	4
Maple Sugar Beans (S&W)	½ cup	150	3
Mexican Style Chili Beans (Van Camp's)	1 cup	210	4
Mixed Bean Salad Marinated (S&W)	½ cup	90	1
Old Fashioned Beans in Molasses & Brown Sugar Sauce (Campbell)	½ can (8 oz)	230	4
Pork & Beans (Hunt's)	4 oz	135	2
Pork & Beans (Van Camp's)	1 cup	216	4
Pork 'n Beans (S&W)	½ cup	130	1
Pork & Beans in Tomato Sauce (Campbell)	½ can (8 oz)	200	3
Pork & Beans in Tomato Sauce (Green Giant)	½ cup	90	1
Refried (Casa Fiesta)	3.5 oz	110	2
Refried (Gebhardt)	4 oz	100	2
Refried (Rosarita)	4 oz	100	2
Refried Jalapeno (Gebhardt)	4 oz	115	2
Refried Spicy (Rosarita)	4 oz	100	2
Refried Vegetarian (Rosarita)	4 oz	100	2
Refried w/ Bacon (Rosarita)	4 oz	110	3
Refried w/ Green Chilies (Rosarita)	4 oz	90	2
Refried w/ Nacho Cheese (Rosarita)	4 oz	110	3
Refried w/ Onions (Rosarita)	4 oz	110	3

FOOD	PORTION	CALORIES	IRON
Smokey Ranch Beans (S&W)	½ cup	130	3
Three Bean Salad (Green Giant)	½ cup	70	tr
Vegetarian Beans (Campbell)	½ can (7.75 oz)	170	4
Vegetarian Beans w/ Miso (Health Valley)	7.5 oz	180	3
Vegetarian Style (Van Camp's)	1 cup	206	4
baked beans plain	½ cup	118	tr
baked beans vegetarian	½ cup	118	tr
baked beans w/ beef	½ cup	161	2
baked beans w/ franks	½ cup	182	2
baked beans w/ pork	½ cup	133	2
baked beans w/ pork & sweet sauce	½ cup	140	2
baked beans w/ pork & tomato sauce	½ cup	123	4
refried beans	½ cup	134	2
TAKE-OUT baked beans	½ cup	190	3
barbecue beans	3.5 oz	120	2
four-bean salad	3.5 oz	100	1
refried beans	½ cup	43	1
three-bean salad	¾ cup	230	3

BEAR

simmered	3 oz	220	9

BEAVER

roasted	3 oz	140	9
simmered	3 oz	141	7

FOOD	PORTION	CALORIES	IRON

BEEF
(*see also* BEEF DISHES, VEAL)

FRESH

FOOD	PORTION	CALORIES	IRON
Fillet (Double J)	3.5 oz	130	4
NY Strip (Double J)	3.5 oz	133	4
Rib Eye (Double J)	3.5 oz	134	4
Top Butt (Double J)	3.5 oz	136	4
bottom round lean & fat trim 0", Choice, braised	3 oz	193	3
bottom round lean & fat, trim 0", Choice, roasted	3 oz	172	3
bottom round lean & fat, trim 0", Select, braised	3 oz	171	3
bottom round lean & fat, trim 0", Select, roasted	3 oz	150	3
bottom round lean & fat, trim ¼", Choice, braised	3 oz	241	3
bottom round lean & fat, trim ¼", Choice, roasted	3 oz	221	2
bottom round lean & fat, trim ¼", Select, braised	3 oz	220	3
bottom round lean & fat, trim ¼", Select, roasted	3 oz	199	2
brisket flat half, lean & fat, trim 0", braised	3 oz	183	2
brisket flat half, lean & fat, trim ¼", braised	3 oz	309	2
brisket point half, lean & fat, trim 0", braised	3 oz	304	2
brisket point half, lean & fat, trim ¼", braised	3 oz	343	2
brisket whole, lean & fat, trim 0", braised	3 oz	247	2

FOOD	PORTION	CALORIES	IRON
brisket whole, lean & fat, trim ¼", braised	3 oz	327	2
chuck arm pot roast, lean & fat, trim 0", braised	3 oz	238	3
chuck arm pot roast, lean & fat, trim ¼", braised	3 oz	282	3
chuck blade roast, lean & fat, trim 0", braised	3 oz	284	3
chuck blade roast, lean & fat, trim ¼", braised	3 oz	293	3
corned beef brisket, cooked	3 oz	213	2
eye of round, lean & fat, trim 0", Choice, roasted	3 oz	153	2
eye of round, lean & fat, trim 0", Select, roasted	3 oz	137	2
eye of round, lean & fat, trim ¼", Choice, roasted	3 oz	205	2
eye of round, lean & fat, trim ¼", Select, roasted	3 oz	184	2
flank, lean & fat, trim 0", braised	3 oz	192	2
flank, lean & fat, trim ¼", braised	3 oz	224	3
ground, extra lean, broiled medium	3 oz	217	2
ground, extra lean, broiled well done	3 oz	225	2
ground, extra lean, fried medium	3 oz	216	2
ground, extra lean, fried well done	3 oz	224	2
ground, extra lean, raw	4 oz	265	2
ground, lean, broiled medium	3 oz	231	2
ground, lean, broiled well done	3 oz	238	2
ground, regular, broiled medium	3 oz	246	2
ground, regular, broiled well done	3 oz	248	2
porterhouse steak, lean & fat, trim ¼", Choice, broiled	3 oz	260	2

FOOD	PORTION	CALORIES	IRON
porterhouse steak, lean only, trim ¼", Choice, broiled	3 oz	185	3
rib eye small end, lean & fat, trim 0", Choice, broiled	3 oz	261	2
rib large end, lean & fat, trim 0", roasted	3 oz	300	2
rib large end, lean & fat, trim ¼", broiled	3 oz	295	2
rib large end, lean & fat, trim ¼", roasted	3 oz	310	2
rib small end, lean & fat, trim 0", broiled	3 oz	252	2
rib small end, lean & fat, trim ¼", broiled	3 oz	285	2
rib small end, lean & fat, trim ¼", roasted	3 oz	295	2
rib whole, lean & fat, trim ¼", Choice, broiled	3 oz	306	2
rib whole, lean & fat, trim ¼", Choice, roasted	3 oz	320	2
rib whole, lean & fat, trim ¼", Prime, roasted	3 oz	348	2
rib whole, lean & fat, trim ¼", Select, broiled	3 oz	274	2
rib whole, lean & fat, trim ¼", Select, roasted	3 oz	286	2
shank crosscut, lean & fat, trim ¼", Choice, simmered	3 oz	224	3
short loin top loin, lean & fat, trim 0", Choice, broiled	1 steak (5.4 oz)	353	4
short loin top loin, lean & fat, trim 0", Choice, broiled	3 oz	193	2
short loin top loin, lean & fat, trim 0", Select, broiled	1 steak (5.4 oz)	309	4
short loin top loin, lean & fat, trim ¼", Choice, broiled	1 steak (6.3 oz)	536	4

FOOD	PORTION	CALORIES	IRON
short loin top loin, lean & fat, trim ¼", Choice, broiled	3 oz	253	2
short loin top loin, lean & fat, trim ¼", Prime, broiled	1 steak (6.3 oz)	582	4
short loin top loin, lean & fat, trim ¼", Select, broiled	1 steak (6.3 oz)	473	4
short loin top loin, lean only, trim 0", Choice, broiled	1 steak (5.2 oz)	311	4
short loin top loin, lean only, trim ¼", Choice, broiled	1 steak (5.2 oz)	314	4
short ribs, lean & fat, Choice, braised	3 oz	400	2
t-bone steak, lean & fat, trim ¼", Choice, broiled	3 oz	253	2
t-bone steak, lean only, trim ¼", Choice, broiled	3 oz	182	3
tenderloin, lean & fat, trim 0", Choice, broiled	3 oz	208	3
tenderloin, lean & fat, trim 0", Select, broiled	3 oz	194	3
tenderloin, lean & fat, trim ¼", Choice, broiled	3 oz	259	3
tenderloin, lean & fat, trim ¼", Choice, roasted	3 oz	288	3
tenderloin, lean & fat, trim ¼", Prime, broiled	3 oz	270	3
tenderloin, lean & fat, trim ¼", Select, roasted	3 oz	275	3
tenderloin, lean only, trim 0", Select broiled	3 oz	170	3
tenderloin, lean only, trim ¼", Choice, broiled	3 oz	188	3
tenderloin, lean only, trim ¼", Select, broiled	3 oz	169	3
tip round, lean & fat, trim 0", Choice, roasted	3 oz	170	2

FOOD	PORTION	CALORIES	IRON
tip round, lean & fat, trim 0", Select, roasted	3 oz	158	2
tip round, lean & fat, trim ¼", Choice, roasted	3 oz	210	2
tip round, lean & fat, trim ¼", Prime, roasted	3 oz	233	2
tip round, lean & fat, trim ¼", Select, roasted	3 oz	191	2
top round, lean & fat, trim 0", Choice, braised	3 oz	184	3
top round, lean & fat, trim 0", Select, braised	3 oz	170	3
top round, lean & fat, trim ¼", Choice, braised	3 oz	221	3
top round, lean & fat, trim ¼", Choice, broiled	3 oz	190	2
top round, lean & fat, trim ¼", Choice, fried	3 oz	235	2
top round, lean & fat, trim ¼", Prime, broiled	3 oz	195	2
top round, lean & fat, trim ¼", Select, braised	3 oz	199	3
top round, lean & fat, trim ¼", Select, broiled	3 oz	175	2
top sirloin, lean & fat, trim 0", Choice, broiled	3 oz	194	3
top sirloin, lean & fat, trim 0", Select, broiled	3 oz	166	3
top sirloin, lean & fat, trim ¼", Choice, broiled	3 oz	228	3
top sirloin, lean & fat, trim ¼", Choice, fried	3 oz	277	3
top sirloin, lean & fat, trim ¼", Select, broiled	3 oz	208	3
tripe, raw	4 oz	111	2

FOOD	PORTION	CALORIES	IRON
FROZEN			
patties, broiled medium	3 oz	240	2
READY-TO-USE			
Roast Beef (Oscar Mayer)	1 slice (.4 oz)	14	tr

BEEF DISHES

FOOD	PORTION	CALORIES	IRON
CANNED			
Beef Stew (Healthy Choice)	½ can (7.5 oz)	140	2
Beef Stew (Wolf Brand)	1 cup	179	2
Manwich Mexican, as prep	1 sandwich	310	4
Sloppy Joe, as prep (Manwich)	1 sandwich	310	4
MIX			
Hamburger Helper			
Beef Noodle, as prep	1 cup	330	1
Beef Romanoff, as prep	1 cup	350	4
Beef Taco, as prep	1 cup	330	3
Cheddar 'n Bacon, as prep	1 cup	380	3
Cheeseburger Macaroni, as prep	1 cup	370	3
Cheesy Italian, as prep	1 cup	370	3
Chili Macaroni, as prep	1 cup	330	3
Hamburger Hash, as prep	1 cup	320	3
Hamburger Pizza Dish, as prep	1 cup	360	4
Hamburger Stew, as prep	1 cup	300	3
Lasagne, as prep	1 cup	340	3
Meat Loaf, as prep	5 oz	360	4
Nacho Cheese, as prep	1 cup	360	3
Pizzabake, as prep	⅙ pkg (4.5 oz)	320	3
Potatoes au Gratin, as prep	1 cup	350	3
Potatoes Stroganoff, as prep	1 cup	330	3
Rice Oriental, as prep	1 cup	340	3

FOOD	PORTION	CALORIES	IRON
Sloppy Joe Bake, as prep	5 oz	340	3
Spaghetti, as prep	1 cup	340	4
Stroganoff, as prep	1 cup	390	3
Tacobake, as prep	⅙ pkg (5.75 oz)	320	4
Zesty Italian, as prep	1 cup	340	4
Lipton Microeasy Hearty Beef Stew	¼ pkg	71	tr
Lipton Microeasy Homestyle Meatloaf	¼ pkg	87	1
Manwich Seasoning Mix, as prep	1 sandwich	320	4
SHELF-STABLE Beef Stew (Healthy Choice)	7.5-oz cup	140	2
TAKE-OUT bubble & squeak	5 oz	186	1
cornish pasty	1 (8 oz)	847	4
kebab indian	1 (5.4 oz)	553	5
kheena	6.7 oz	781	5
koftas	5	280	2
roast beef sandwich plain	1	346	4
roast beef sandwich w/ cheese	1	402	5
roast beef submarine sandwich w/ tomato, lettuce & mayonnaise	1	411	3
samosa	2 (4 oz)	652	1
shepherd's pie	6 oz	196	2
steak & kidney pie w/ top crust	1 slice (5 oz)	400	4
steak sandwich w/ tomato, lettuce, salt & mayonnaise	1	459	5
stew	6 oz	208	2
stew w/ vegetables	1 cup	220	3
stroganoff	¾ cup	260	2

FOOD	PORTION	CALORIES	IRON
swiss steak	4.6 oz	214	3
toad-in-the-hole	1 (4.7 oz)	383	1

BEEFALO

roasted	3 oz	160	3

BEER AND ALE

ale, brown	10 oz	77	tr
ale, pale	10 oz	88	tr
beer, light	12-oz can	100	tr
beer, regular	12-oz can	146	tr
lager	10 oz	80	0
stout	10 oz	102	tr

BEETS

CANNED			
Diced Tender (S&W)	½ cup	40	tr
Julienne French Style (S&W)	½ cup	40	tr
Pickled Whole Extra Small (S&W)	½ cup	70	tr
Pickled w/ Red Wine Vinegar Sliced (S&W)	½ cup	70	1
Sliced Small Premium (S&W)	½ cup	40	tr
Sliced Water Pack (S&W)	½ cup	35	tr
Whole Small (S&W)	½ cup	40	tr
harvard	½ cup	89	tr
pickled	½ cup	75	tr
sliced	½ cup	27	2
FRESH			
cooked	½ cup	26	1
greens, cooked	½ cup	20	1

FOOD	PORTION	CALORIES	IRON
greens, raw	½ cup	4	1
greens, raw, chopped	½ cup	4	1
raw, sliced	½ cup	30	1

BEVERAGES
(see BEER AND ALE, COFFEE, COFFEE SUBSTITUTES, DRINK MIXERS, FRUIT DRINKS, LIQUOR/LIQUEUR, MALT, MINERAL WATER/BOTTLED WATER, SODA, TEA/HERBAL TEA, WINE)

BISCUIT

FOOD	PORTION	CALORIES	IRON
FROZEN			
Egg, Canadian Bacon & Cheese (Great Starts)	5.2 oz	420	5
Sausage (Great Starts)	4.7 oz	410	2
HOME RECIPE			
buttermilk	1 (2 oz)	212	2
oatcakes	2 (4 oz)	115	1
plain	1 (2 oz)	212	2
MIX			
Bisquick	½ cup	240	1
Buttermilk Biscuit Mix, not prep (Health Valley)	1 oz	100	1
buttermilk	1 (2 oz)	191	1
plain	1 (2 oz)	191	1
REFRIGERATED			
1869 Brand Baking Powder	1	100	1
1869 Brand Butter Tastin'	1	100	1
1869 Brand Buttermilk	1	100	1
Ballard Ovenready	1	50	tr
Ballard Ovenready Buttermilk	1	50	tr
Big Country Southern Style	1	100	1

FOOD	PORTION	CALORIES	IRON
Hungry Jack Butter Tastin' Flaky	1	90	tr
Hungry Jack Buttermilk Flaky	1	90	tr
Hungry Jack Buttermilk Fluffy	1	90	tr
Hungry Jack Extra Rich Buttermilk	1	50	tr
Hungry Jack Flaky	1	80	tr
Hungry Jack Honey Tastin' Flaky	1	90	1
Pillsbury Big Country Butter Tastin'	1	100	1
Pillsbury Big Country Buttermilk	1	100	1
Pillsbury Butter	1	50	tr
Pillsbury Buttermilk	1	50	tr
Pillsbury Country	1	50	tr
Pillsbury Deluxe Heat 'n Eat Buttermilk	2	170	1
Pillsbury Good 'n Buttery Fluffy	1	90	1
Pillsbury Hearty Grains Multi-Grain	1	80	1
Pillsbury Heart Grains Oatmeal Raisin	1	90	1
Pillsbury Heat 'n Eat Big Premium	2	280	1
Pillsbury Tender Layer Buttermilk	1	50	tr
buttermilk	1 (1 oz)	98	1
plain	1 (1 oz)	98	1
TAKE-OUT			
buttermilk	1	127	1
plain	1	276	2
w/ egg	1	315	3
w/ egg & bacon	1	457	4
w/ egg & sausage	1	582	4
w/ egg & steak	1	474	5
w/ egg, cheese & bacon	1	477	3
w/ ham	1	387	3

FOOD	PORTION	CALORIES	IRON
w/ sausage	1	485	3
w/ steak	1	456	4

BISON

roasted	3 oz	122	3

BLACK BEANS

CANNED			
Health Valley Fast Menu Organic Black Beans w/ Tofu Wieners	7.5 oz	150	9
Health Valley Fast Menu Western Black Beans w/ Garden Vegetables	7.5 oz	160	14
DRIED			
cooked	1 cup	227	4

BLACKBERRIES

CANNED			
in heavy syrup	½ cup	118	1
FRESH			
blackberries	½ cup	37	tr
FROZEN			
unsweetened	1 cup	97	1

BLACKEYE PEAS

CANNED			
Trappey's	½ cup	90	1
Trappey's Jalapeno	½ cup	90	1
w/ pork	½ cup	199	3
DRIED			
cooked	1 cup	198	4

FOOD	PORTION	CALORIES	IRON

BLINTZE

TAKE-OUT

cheese	2	186	1

BLUEBERRIES

CANNED

In Heavy Syrup (S&W)	½ cup	111	tr
in heavy syrup	1 cup	225	1

FRESH

blueberries	1 cup	82	tr

FROZEN

Big Valley	4 oz	60	tr
unsweetened	1 cup	78	tr

BLUEFIN

fillet, baked	4.1 oz	186	1

BLUEFISH

fresh, baked	3 oz	135	1

BORAGE

cooked, chopped	3.5 oz	25	4
raw, chopped	½ cup	9	1

BOYSENBERRIES

CANNED

in heavy syrup	1 cup	226	1

FROZEN

Big Valley	3.5 oz	50	1
unsweetened	1 cup	66	1

FOOD	PORTION	CALORIES	IRON
JUICE			
Smucker's	8 oz	120	1
Smucker's Juice Sparkler	10 oz	130	tr

BRAINS

FOOD	PORTION	CALORIES	IRON
beef, pan-fried	3 oz	167	2
beef, simmered	3 oz	136	2
lamb, braised	3 oz	124	1
lamb, fried	3 oz	232	2
pork, braised	3 oz	117	2
veal, braised	3 oz	115	1
veal, fried	3 oz	181	1

BRAN

FOOD	PORTION	CALORIES	IRON
Fast Menu Oat Bran Pilaf w/ Garden Vegetables (Health Valley)	7.5 oz	210	2
Oat Bran (Mother's)	⅓ cup	92	2
Quaker Unprocessed Bran	2 tbsp	8	1
Super Bran (H-O)	⅓ cup	110	1
Toasted Wheat Bran (Kretschmer)	⅓ cup	57	4
corn	⅓ cup	56	tr
oat, cooked	½ cup	44	tr
oat, dry	½ cup	116	3
rice, dry	⅓ cup	88	5
wheat, dry	½ cup	65	3

BRAZIL NUTS

FOOD	PORTION	CALORIES	IRON
dried, unblanched	1 oz	186	1

BREAD

(*see also* BAGEL, BISCUIT, BREADSTICKS, CROISSANT, ENGLISH MUFFIN, MUFFIN, ROLL, SCONE)

FOOD	PORTION	CALORIES	IRON
CANNED			
Brown Bread New England Recipe (S&W)	2 slices	76	1
boston brown	1 slice (1.6 oz)	88	1
HOME RECIPE			
banana	1 slice (2 oz)	195	1
corn bread, as prep w/ 2% milk	1 piece (2.3 oz)	173	2
corn bread, as prep w/ whole milk	1 piece (2.3 oz)	176	2
date-nut	½" slice	92	1
hush puppies	5 (2.7 oz)	256	1
irish soda bread	1 slice (2 oz)	174	2
pumpkin	1 slice (1 oz)	94	tr
white, as prep w/ 2% milk	1 slice	81	1
white, as prep w/ nonfat dry milk	1 slice	78	1
white, as prep w/ whole milk	1 slice	82	1
whole wheat	1 slice	79	1
MIX			
Corn Bread (Ballard)	⅛ bread	140	tr
Corn Bread (Dromedary)	1 piece (2" × 2")	130	1
Corn Bread Easy Mix (Aunt Jemima)	⅙ cake	210	1
corn bread	1 piece (2 oz)	189	1
READY-TO-EAT			
7-Grain Hearty Slice (Pepperidge Farm)	2 slices	180	1
9-Grain & Nut (Matthew's)	1 slice	80	1
Apple Walnut (Arnold)	1 slice	64	1
Bran'nola			
Country Oat (Arnold)	1 slice	90	1
Country Oat (Brownberry)	1 slice	90	1
Dark Wheat (Arnold)	1 slice	83	1

FOOD	PORTION	CALORIES	IRON
Hearty Wheat (Arnold)	1 slice	88	2
Hearty Wheat (Brownberry)	1 slice	88	1
Nutty Grains (Arnold)	1 slice	85	1
Nutty Grains (Brownberry)	1 slice	85	1
Original (Arnold)	1 slice	85	2
Original (Brownberry)	1 slice	85	2
Cinnamon (Matthew's)	1 slice	70	1
Cinnamon (Pepperidge Farm)	1 slice	90	1
Cinnamon Raisin (Arnold)	1 slice	67	1
Cracked Wheat (Pepperidge Farm)	1 slice	70	1
Crunchy Oat 1½-lb Loaf (Pepperidge Farm)	2 slices	190	2
Date Walnut (Pepperidge Farm)	1 slice	90	1
Fiber Calcium (Thomas')	1 slice	52	tr
French Fully Baked (Pepperidge Farm)	2 oz	150	1
French Stick Extra Sour (Parisian)	2 oz	150	2
French Stick Sweet (Parisian)	2 oz	154	2
Frenchy Twin (Pepperidge Farm)	1 oz	80	1
Golden (Matthew's)	1 slice	70	1
Health Nut (Brownberry)	1 slice	71	1
Hi-Fibre (Monks' Bread)	1 slice	50	1
Honey Bran (Pepperidge Farm)	1 slice	90	1
Italian Bakery Light (Arnold)	1 slice	45	1
Brown & Serve (Pepperidge Farm)	1 oz	80	1
Francisco International Thick Sliced (Arnold)	1 slice	66	1
Francisco International Unsliced (Arnold)	1 slice (1 oz)	72	1
Light (Wonder)	1 slice	40	1

FOOD	PORTION	CALORIES	IRON
Italian *(cont.)*			
Sliced (Pepperidge Farm)	1 slice	70	tr
Malsovit	1 slice	66	1
Oat Bran (Matthew's)	1 slice	65	1
Oatmeal			
Pepperidge Farm	1 slice	70	1
1½-lb Loaf (Pepperidge Farm)	1 slice	90	1
Bakery (Arnold)	1 slice	59	1
Bakery Light (Arnold)	1 slice	44	1
Light (Pepperidge Farm)	1 slice	45	1
Natural (Brownberry)	1 slice	63	1
Raisin (Arnold)	1 slice	58	1
Soft (Brownberry)	1 slice	48	1
Very Thin Sliced (Pepperidge Farm)	1 slice	40	tr
Pita Oat Bran (Sahara)	½ pocket (1 oz)	66	1
Pita Wheat Mini (Sahara)	1 pocket (1 oz)	66	1
Pita White (Sahara)	½ pocket	78	tr
Pita White Mini (Sahara)	1 pocket	79	tr
Pita Whole Wheat (Matthew's)	1 pocket	210	3
Pumpernickel (Arnold)	1 slice	70	1
Pumpernickel Family (Pepperidge Farm)	1 slice	80	1
Pumpernickel Party (Pepperidge Farm)	4 slices	60	1
Raisin (Malsovit)	1 slice	77	1
Raisin (Monks' Bread)	1 slice	70	1
Raisin (Sunmaid)	1 slice	67	1
Raisin Bran (Brownberry)	1 slice	61	1
Raisin Cinnamon (Brownberry)	1 slice	66	1
Raisin Walnut (Brownberry)	1 slice	68	1

FOOD	PORTION	CALORIES	IRON
Raisin w/ Cinnamon (Pepperidge Farm)	1 slice	90	1
Rye			
Dijon (Pepperidge Farm)	1 slice	50	1
Dijon Thick Sliced (Pepperidge Farm)	1 slice	70	1
Dill (Arnold)	1 slice	71	1
Family (Pepperidge Farm)	3 oz	80	1
Jewish w/ Seeds (Arnold)	1 slice	69	1
Jewish w/o Seeds (Arnold)	1 slice	71	1
Melba Thin (Arnold)	1 slice	44	1
Party (Pepperidge Farm)	4 slices	60	1
Seedless Family (Pepperidge Farm)	1 slice	80	1
Soft (Pepperidge Farm)	1 slice	70	tr
Soft Bakery Light (Arnold)	1 slice	41	1
With Seeds (Levy's)	1 slice	76	1
Without Seeds (Levy's)	1 slice	75	1
Sesame Wheat (Pepperidge Farm)	2 slices	190	2
Sodium Free (Matthew's)	1 slice	70	1
Sourdough Light (Wonder)	1 slice	40	1
Sprouted Wheat (Pepperidge Farm)	1 slice	70	1
Sunflower & Bran (Monks' Bread)	1 slice	70	1
Vienna Light (Pepperidge Farm)	1 slice	45	1
Vienna Thick Sliced (Pepperidge Farm)	1 slice	70	1
Wheat			
1½-lb Loaf (Pepperidge Farm)	1 slice	90	1
Apple Honey (Brownberry)	1 slice	69	1
Berry Honey (Arnold)	1 slice	77	1
Brick Oven (Arnold)	1 slice	60	1

FOOD	PORTION	CALORIES	IRON
Wheat *(cont.)*			
Family (Pepperidge Farm)	1 slice	70	1
Family (Wonder)	1 slice	70	1
Golden Light (Arnold)	1 slice	44	1
Light (Pepperidge Farm)	1 slice	45	1
Light (Wonder)	1 slice	40	1
Lite (Thomas')	1 slice	41	1
Natural (Brownberry)	1 slice	80	1
Soft (Brownberry)	1 slice	74	1
Very Thin Sliced (Pepperidge Farm)	1 slice	35	tr
White			
(Monks' Bread)	1 slice	60	tr
(Wonder)	1 slice	70	1
Brick Oven (Arnold)	1 slice	61	1
Brick Oven Extra Fiber (Arnold)	1 slice	55	1
Country (Arnold)	1 slice	98	1
Country (Pepperidge Farm)	2 slices	190	2
Large Family Thin Sliced (Pepperidge Farm)	1 slice	70	1
Light (Wonder)	1 slice	40	1
Premium Light (Arnold)	1 slice	42	1
Sandwich (Pepperidge Farm)	2 slices	130	1
Thin Sliced (Pepperidge Farm)	1 slice	80	1
Toasting (Pepperidge Farm)	1 slice	90	1
Very Thin Sliced (Pepperidge Farm)	1 slice	40	tr
White Whole Special Recipe (Stroehmann)	1 slice	70	1
White Whole Special Recipe Kids (Stroehmann)	1 slice	60	1

FOOD	PORTION	CALORIES	IRON
Whole Wheat (Matthew's)	1 slice	70	1
100% Stoneground (Arnold)	1 slice	48	1
100% Stoneground (Monks' Bread)	1 slice	70	tr
100% Stoneground (Wonder)	1 slice	80	1
Thin Sliced (Pepperidge Farm)	1 slice	60	1
cracked wheat	1 slice	65	1
egg	1 slice (1.4 oz)	115	1
french	1 loaf (1 lb)	454	14
french	1 slice (1 oz)	78	1
gluten	1 slice	47	1
italian	1 loaf (1 lb)	454	13
italian	1 slice (1 oz)	81	1
navajo fry	1 (10.5" diam)	527	6
navajo fry	1 (5" diam)	296	3
oat bran	1 slice	71	1
oat bran reduced calorie	1 slice	46	1
oatmeal	1 slice	73	1
oatmeal reduced calorie	1 slice	48	1
pita	1 reg (2 oz)	165	2
pita	1 sm (1 oz)	78	1
protein	1 slice	47	1
pumpernickel	1 slice	80	1
raisin	1 slice	71	1
rice bran	1 slice	66	1
rye	1 slice	83	1
rye reduced calorie	1 slice	47	1
sourdough	1 slice (1 oz)	78	1
vienna	1 slice (1 oz)	78	1

FOOD	PORTION	CALORIES	IRON
wheat berry	1 slice	65	1
wheat bran	1 slice	89	1
wheat germ	1 slice	74	1
wheat reduced calorie	1 slice	46	1
white	1 slice	67	1
white cubed	1 cup	80	1
white reduced calorie	1 slice	48	1
white, toasted	1 slice	67	1
whole wheat	1 slice	70	1
REFRIGERATED			
Pillsbury			
Crusty French Loaf	1″ slice	60	1
Hearty Grains Country Oatmeal Twists	1	80	1
Hearty Grains Cracked Wheat Twists	1	80	1
Pipin'Hot Wheat Loaf	1″ slice	70	1
Pipin'Hot White Loaf	1″ slice	70	1
TAKE-OUT			
chapatis, as prep w/ fat	1 (2.5 oz)	230	2
chapatis, as prep w/o fat	1 (2.5 oz)	141	2
corn bread	2″ × 2″ piece (1.4 oz)	107	1
corn stick	1 (1.3 oz)	101	tr
naan	1 (6 oz)	571	2
papadums, fried	2 (1.5 oz)	81	2
paratha	1 (4.4 oz)	403	3

BREAD COATING

Golden Dipt Chicken Frying Mix	1 oz	90	tr
Golden Dipt Onion Ring Mix	1 oz	100	tr

FOOD	PORTION	CALORIES	IRON
Oven Fry Homestyle Flour Recipe for Chicken	¼ pkg	85	tr
Shake 'n Bake			
Extra Crispy Oven Fry for Pork	¼ pkg (1 oz)	120	tr
Italian Herb Recipe	¼ pkg (.5 oz)	77	1
Original Barbecue for Chicken	¼ pkg (.5 oz)	93	tr
Original Barbecue for Pork	¼ pkg (.5 oz)	38	tr
Original Country Mild	¼ pkg (.5 oz)	76	tr
Original for Chicken	¼ pkg (.5 oz)	75	tr
Original for Fish	¼ pkg (.5 oz)	73	tr
Original for Pork	¼ pkg (.5 oz)	41	tr

BREAD CRUMBS

FOOD	PORTION	CALORIES	IRON
4C Salt Free	1 tbsp (.5 oz)	50	tr
4C Seasoned	1 tbsp (.5 oz)	50	tr
4C Toasted	1 tbsp (.5 oz)	50	tr
4C Toasted Salt Free	1 tbsp (.5 oz)	50	tr
Devonsheer Italian Style	1 oz	104	1
Devonsheer Plain	1 oz	108	1
dry	1 cup	426	7
dry seasoned	1 cup	441	4
fresh	⅔ cup	76	1

BREADFRUIT

FOOD	PORTION	CALORIES	IRON
fresh	¼ small	99	1
seeds, cooked	1 oz	48	tr
seeds, raw	1 oz	54	1
seeds, roasted	1 oz	59	tr

BREADNUTTREE SEEDS

FOOD	PORTION	CALORIES	IRON
dried	1 oz	104	1

FOOD	PORTION	CALORIES	IRON
BREADSTICKS			
Garlic (Keebler)	2	30	tr
Onion (Keebler)	2	30	tr
Plain (Keebler)	2	30	tr
Sesame (Keebler)	2	30	tr
Soft Bread Sticks(Pillsbury)	1	100	1
plain	1	41	tr
plain	1 sm	25	tr
HOME RECIPE			
onion poppyseed	1	64	tr

BREAKFAST BARS
(*see also* BREAKFAST DRINKS, NUTRITIONAL SUPPLEMENTS)

Apple (Nutri-Grain)	1 (1.3 oz)	150	2
Blueberry (Nutri-Grain)	1 (1.3 oz)	150	2
Raspberry (Nutri-Grain)	1 (1.3 oz)	150	2
Strawberry (Nutri-Grain)	1 (1.3 oz)	150	2

BREAKFAST DRINKS
(*see also* BREAKFAST BARS, NUTRITIONAL SUPPLEMENTS)

Instant Breakfast (Pillsbury)			
Chocolate, as prep w/ whole milk	1 serving	290	5
Chocolate Malt, as prep w/ whole milk	1 serving	290	5
Strawberry, as prep w/ whole milk	1 serving	290	5
Vanilla, as prep w/ whole milk	1 serving	300	5
orange drink powder	3 rounded tsp	93	tr
orange drink powder, as prep w/ water	6 oz	86	tr

FOOD	PORTION	CALORIES	IRON
BROAD BEANS			
CANNED			
broad beans	1 cup	183	3
DRIED			
cooked	1 cup	186	3
FRESH			
cooked	3.5 oz	56	2
BROCCOLI			
FRESH			
chopped, cooked	½ cup	22	1
raw, chopped	½ cup	12	tr
FROZEN			
Baby Spears Deluxe (Birds Eye)	⅔ cup	30	1
Big Valley	3.5 oz	25	tr
Broccoli w/ Cheese in Pastry (Pepperidge Farm)	1	230	1
Chopped (Birds Eye)	⅔ cup	25	tr
Cuts (Green Giant)	½ cup	12	0
Farm Fresh Spears (Birds Eye)	¾ cup	30	1
Florets Deluxe (Birds Eye)	½ cup	25	1
Harvest Fresh Cuts (Green Giant)	½ cup	16	0
Harvest Fresh Spears (Green Giant)	½ cup	20	tr
In Butter Sauce (Green Giant)	½ cup	40	tr
In Cheese Sauce (Green Giant)	½ cup	60	tr
Mini Spears (Green Giant Select)	4–5 spears	18	1
One Serve Cuts in Butter Sauce (Green Giant)	1 pkg	45	1
One Serve Cuts in Cheese Sauce (Green Giant)	1 pkg	70	tr

FOOD	PORTION	CALORIES	IRON
Polybag Cuts (Birds Eye)	½ cup	25	1
Polybag Deluxe Florets (Birds Eye)	⅔ cup	25	1
Spears (Birds Eye)	⅔ cup	25	1
Valley Combinations Broccoli Fanfare (Green Giant)	½ cup	80	tr
With Cheese Sauce (Birds Eye)	½ pkg	110	tr
chopped, cooked	½ cup	25	1
spears, cooked	½ cup	25	1
spears, cooked	10-oz pkg	69	2

BROWNIE

FOOD	PORTION	CALORIES	IRON
FROZEN			
Monterey Hot Fudge Chocolate Chunk Brownie (Pepperidge Farm)	1	480	1
Newport Hot Fudge Brownie (Pepperidge Farm)	1	400	1
HOME RECIPE			
brownie w/ nuts	1 (.8 oz)	95	tr
MIX			
Brownie w/ Hot Fudge MicroRave Single (Betty Crocker)	1	350	2
Deluxe Family Size Fudge Brownie (Pillsbury)	2" sq	150	tr
Deluxe Fudge Brownie (Pillsbury)	2" sq	150	tr
Deluxe Fudge Brownie w/ Walnuts (Pillsbury)	2" sq	150	tr
Frosted MicroRave (Betty Crocker)	1	180	1
Fudge Family Size (Betty Crocker)	1	150	1
Fudge Light (Betty Crocker)	1	100	1
Fudge MicroRave (Betty Crocker)	1	150	1
Fudge Microwave (Pillsbury)	1	190	1

FOOD	PORTION	CALORIES	IRON
Fudge Regular Size (Betty Crocker)	1	150	1
Supreme Caramel (Betty Crocker)	1	120	tr
Supreme Frosted (Betty Crocker)	1	160	1
Supreme German Chocolate (Betty Crocker)	1	160	1
Supreme Original (Betty Crocker)	1	140	tr
Supreme Party (Betty Crocker)	1	160	1
Supreme Walnut (Betty Crocker)	1	140	1
The Ultimate Caramel Fudge Chunk Brownie (Pillsbury)	2" sq	170	1
The Ultimate Chunky Triple Fudge Brownie (Pillsbury)	2" sq	170	1
The Ultimate Double Fudge Brownie (Pillsbury)	2" sq	160	tr
The Ultimate Rocky Road Fudge Brownie (Pillsbury)	2" sq	170	tr
Walnut MicroRave (Betty Crocker)	1	160	1
READY-TO-EAT Charlotte Fudgey Brownie (Pepperidge Farm)	1	220	1
Little Debbie	1 pkg (2 oz)	230	2
Tahoe Milk Chocolate Pecan (Pepperidge Farm)	1	210	1
Westport Fudgey Brownies w/ Walnuts (Pepperidge Farm)	1	220	1
w/ nuts	1 (1 oz)	100	1
w/o nuts	1 (2 oz)	243	1

BRUSSELS SPROUTS

FRESH			
cooked	1 sprout	8	tr
cooked	½ cup	30	1

FOOD	PORTION	CALORIES	IRON
raw	1 sprout	8	tr
raw	½ cup	19	1
FROZEN			
Brussels Sprouts (Birds Eye)	½ cup	35	1
Green Giant	½ cup	7	tr
In Butter Sauce (Green Giant)	½ cup	40	tr
Whole (Big Valley)	3.5 oz	30	tr
cooked	½ cup	33	1

BUCKWHEAT

roasted groats, cooked	½ cup	91	tr
roasted groats, uncooked	½ cup	283	2

BUFFALO

water, roasted	3 oz	111	2

BULGUR

cooked	½ cup	76	tr
uncooked	½ cup	239	2

BURBOT (FISH)

fresh, baked	3 oz	98	1

BURDOCK ROOT

cooked	1 cup	110	1
raw	1 cup	85	1

BUTTER
(*see also* BUTTER BLENDS, MARGARINE)

REGULAR			
butter	1 pat	36	tr
butter	1 stick (4 oz)	813	tr

FOOD	PORTION	CALORIES	IRON
WHIPPED			
butter	1 tsp	27	tr
butter	4 oz	542	tr

BUTTER BEANS

CANNED			
S&W Tender Cooked	½ cup	100	2
Trappey's Large White	½ cup	80	1
Van Camp's	1 cup	162	4

BUTTER BLENDS

regular butter blend	1 stick	811	tr

BUTTERBUR

CANNED			
fuki, chopped	1 cup	3	1
FRESH			
fuki, raw	1 cup	13	tr

BUTTERFISH

baked	3 oz	159	1
fillet, baked	1 oz	47	tr

BUTTERNUTS

dried	1 oz	174	1

CABBAGE

FRESH			
chinese pak-choi, raw, shredded	½ cup	5	tr
chinese pak-choi, shredded, cooked	½ cup	10	1
chinese pe-tsai, raw, shredded	1 cup	12	tr

FOOD	PORTION	CALORIES	IRON
chinese pe-tsai, shredded, cooked	1 cup	16	tr
green, raw, shredded	1 head (2 lbs)	215	5
green, raw, shredded	½ cup	8	tr
green, shredded, cooked	½ cup	16	tr
red, raw, shredded	½ cup	10	tr
red, shredded, cooked	½ cup	16	tr
savoy, raw, shredded	½ cup	10	tr
savoy, shredded, cooked	½ cup	18	tr
HOME RECIPE			
coleslaw w/ dressing	¾ cup	147	tr
TAKE-OUT			
coleslaw w/ dressing	½ cup	42	tr
stuffed cabbage	1 (6 oz)	373	3
sweet & sour red cabbage	4 oz	61	1

CAKE

FROSTING/ICING			
Cake & Cookie Decorator, all flavors except chocolate (Pillsbury)	1 tbsp	70	0
Cake & Cookie Decorator Chocolate (Pillsbury)	1 tbsp	60	0
Chocolate Fudge (Pillsbury)	for ⅛ cake	110	0
Chocolate Fudge, as prep (Betty Crocker)	1/12 mix	180	tr
Coconut Almond Frosting Mix (Pillsbury)	for 1/12 cake	160	0
Coconut Pecan Frosting Mix (Pillsbury)	for 1/12 cake	150	0
Creamy Milk Chocolate, as prep (Betty Crocker)	1/12 mix	170	tr
Fluffy White Frosting Mix (Pillsbury)	for 1/12 cake	60	0

FOOD	PORTION	CALORIES	IRON
Frost It Hot Chocolate (Pillsbury)	for ⅛ cake	50	tr
Frost It Hot Fluffy White (Pillsbury)	for ⅛ cake	50	0
Frosting Supreme (Pillsbury)			
Caramel Pecan	for 1/12 cake	160	0
Chocolate Chip	for 1/12 cake	150	0
Chocolate Fudge	for 1/12 cake	150	0
Chocolate Mint	for 1/12 cake	150	0
Coconut Almond	for 1/12 cake	150	0
Coconut Pecan	for 1/12 cake	160	0
Cream Cheese	for 1/12 cake	160	0
Double Dutch	for 1/12 cake	140	0
Lemon	for 1/12 cake	160	0
Milk Chocolate	for 1/12 cake	150	0
Mocha	for 1/12 cake	150	0
Sour Cream Vanilla	for 1/12 cake	160	0
Strawberry	for 1/12 cake	160	0
Vanilla	for 1/12 cake	160	0
Funfetti Chocolate Fudge (Pillsbury)	1/12 can	140	0
Funfetti Vanilla Pink (Pillsbury)	1/12 can	150	0
Funfetti Vanilla White (Pillsbury)	1/12 can	150	0
Vanilla (Pillsbury)	for ⅛ cake	120	0
FROZEN			
Apple Crisp Light (Sara Lee)	1 (3 oz)	150	1
Apple Turnover (Pepperidge Farm)	1	300	1
Banana Single Layer Iced (Sara Lee)	1 slice (1.7 oz)	170	1
Berkshire Apple Crisp (Pepperidge Farm)	1	250	1
Black Forest Light (Sara Lee)	1 (3.6 oz)	170	1
Black Forest Two Layer (Sara Lee)	1 slice (2.5 oz)	190	1

FOOD	PORTION	CALORIES	IRON
Blueberry Turnover (Pepperidge Farm)	1	310	1
Boston Cream Supreme (Pepperidge Farm)	1 piece (2⅞ oz)	290	1
Carrot Classic (Pepperidge Farm)	1 cake	260	tr
Carrot Light (Sara Lee)	1 (2.5 oz)	170	1
Carrot Single Layer Iced (Sara Lee)	1 slice (2.4 oz)	250	1
Carrot w/ Cream Cheese Icing (Pepperidge Farm)	1 slice (1.5 oz)	150	tr
Charleston Peach Melba Shortcake (Pepperidge Farm)	1	220	1
Cheesecake Original Cherry (Sara Lee)	1 slice (3.2 oz)	243	1
Cheesecake Original Plain (Sara Lee)	1 slice (2.8 oz)	230	tr
Cheesecake Original Strawberry (Sara Lee)	1 slice (3.2 oz)	222	tr
Cherries Supreme Dessert Lights (Pepperidge Farm)	1 piece (3.25 oz)	170	1
Cherry Turnover (Pepperidge Farm)	1	310	1
Chocolate Free & Light (Sara Lee)	1 slice (1.7 oz)	110	1
Chocolate Fudge Large Layer (Pepperidge Farm)	1 slice (1⅝ oz)	180	1
Chocolate Fudge Strip Large Layer (Pepperidge Farm)	1 piece (1⅝ oz)	170	1
Chocolate Mousse Cake Dessert Lights (Pepperidge Farm)	1 piece (2.5 oz)	190	1
Chocolate Supreme (Pepperidge Farm)	1 piece (2⅞ oz)	300	1
Coconut Large Layer (Pepperidge Farm)	1 slice (1⅝ oz)	180	tr
Coffee Cake All Butter Cheese (Sara Lee)	1 slice (2 oz)	210	1
Coffee Cake All Butter Pecan (Sara Lee)	1 slice (1.4 oz)	160	1

FOOD	PORTION	CALORIES	IRON
Coffee Cake All Butter Streusel (Sara Lee)	1 slice (1.4 oz)	160	1
Devil's Food Large Layer (Pepperidge Farm)	1 slice (1⅝ oz)	180	tr
Double Chocolate Classic (Pepperidge Farm)	1 cake	250	1
Double Chocolate Light (Sara Lee)	1 (2.5 oz)	150	1
Double Chocolate Three Layer (Sara Lee)	1 slice (2.2 oz)	220	1
Elfin Loaves Apple Cinnamon	1	180	tr
Elfin Loaves Banana	1	190	1
Elfin Loaves Blueberry	1	170	1
Elfin Loaves Carrot	1	210	1
French Cheese (Sara Lee)	1 slice (2.9 oz)	250	1
French Cheesecake Light (Sara Lee)	1 (3.2 oz)	150	tr
Fruit Squares Apple (Pepperidge Farm)	1	220	1
Fruit Squares Cherry (Pepperidge Farm)	1	230	1
Fudge Golden Classic (Pepperidge Farm)	1 cake	260	tr
German Chocolate Large Layer (Pepperidge Farm)	1 slice (1⅝ oz)	180	tr
Golden Large Layer (Pepperidge Farm)	1 slice (1⅝ oz)	180	tr
Lemon Cake Supreme Dessert Lights (Pepperidge Farm)	1 piece (2.75 oz)	170	tr
Lemon Coconut Supreme (Pepperidge Farm)	1 piece (3 oz)	280	1
Lemon Cream Light (Sara Lee)	1 (3.2 oz)	180	1
Manhattan Strawberry Cheesecake (Pepperidge Farm)	1	300	1
Peach Melba Supreme (Pepperidge Farm)	1 (3⅛ oz)	270	1

FOOD	PORTION	CALORIES	IRON
Peach Turnover (Pepperidge Farm)	1	310	tr
Pineapple Cream Supreme (Pepperidge Farm)	1 piece (2 oz)	190	1
Pound All Butter Family Size (Sara Lee)	1 slice (1 oz)	130	1
Pound All Butter Original (Sara Lee)	1 slice (1 oz)	130	1
Pound Free & Light (Sara Lee)	1 slice (1 oz)	70	1
Raspberry Turnover (Pepperidge Farm)	1	310	1
Raspberry Vanilla Swirl Dessert Lights (Pepperidge Farm)	1 piece (3.25 oz)	160	tr
Strawberry Cream Supreme (Pepperidge Farm)	1 piece (2 oz)	190	1
Strawberry French Cheesecake Light (Sara Lee)	1 (3.5 oz)	150	1
Strawberry Shortcake Dessert Lights (Pepperidge Farm)	1 piece (3 oz)	170	1
Strawberry Shortcake Two Layer (Sara Lee)	1 slice (2.5 oz)	190	1
Strawberry Strip Large Layer (Pepperidge Farm)	1 piece (1.5 oz)	160	tr
Strawberry Yogurt Dessert Free & Light (Sara Lee)	1 slice (2.2 oz)	120	1
HOME RECIPE			
carrot w/ cream cheese icing	1 cake (10" diam)	6175	21
carrot w/ cream cheese icing	1/16 cake	385	1
eclair	1 (3 oz)	262	1
fruitcake dark	1 cake (7½" × 2¼")	5185	38
fruitcake dark	⅔" slice	165	1
pound	1 loaf (8½" × 3½")	1935	9

FOOD	PORTION	CALORIES	IRON
pound	1 slice (1 oz)	120	1
sheet cake w/ white frosting	1 cake (9" sq)	4020	11
sheet cake w/ white frosting	⅑ cake	445	1
sheet cake w/o frosting	1 cake (9" sq)	2830	12
sheet cake w/o frosting	⅑ cake	315	1
MIX			
Apple Cinnamon Coffee Cake (Pillsbury)	⅛ cake	240	1
Apple Streusel MicroRave (Betty Crocker)	⅙ cake	240	1
Apple Streusel MicroRave No Cholesterol Recipe (Betty Crocker)	⅙ cake	210	1
Banana Quick Bread (Pillsbury)	1/12 loaf	170	1
Blueberry Nut Quick Bread (Pillsbury)	1/12 loaf	150	1
Butter Chocolate (Betty Crocker)	1/12 cake	280	1
Butter Pecan No Cholesterol Recipe (Betty Crocker)	1/12 cake	220	1
Butter Pecan SuperMoist (Betty Crocker)	1/12 cake	250	1
Butter Recipe (Pillsbury Plus)	1/12 cake	260	1
Butter Yellow (Betty Crocker)	1/12 cake	260	1
Carrot (Betty Crocker)	1/12 cake	250	1
Carrot (Dromedary)	1/12 cake	232	1
Carrot No Cholesterol Recipe (Betty Crocker)	1/12 cake	210	1
Cheesecake (Jell-O)	⅛ cake	277	tr
Cheesecake Lite No-Bake (Royal)	⅛ pie	130	tr
Cheesecake New York Style (Jell-O)	⅛ cake	283	tr
Cherry Chip (Betty Crocker)	1/12 cake	190	1
Cherry Nut Quick Bread (Pillsbury)	1/12 loaf	180	1

FOOD	PORTION	CALORIES	IRON
Chocolate Chip (Betty Crocker)	1/12 cake	290	1
Chocolate Chip (Pillsbury Plus)	1/12 cake	270	1
Chocolate Chip No Cholesterol Recipe (Betty Crocker)	1/12 cake	220	1
Chocolate Chocolate Chip (Betty Crocker)	1/12 cake	260	1
Chocolate Fudge (Betty Crocker)	1/12 cake	260	1
Chocolate Microwave (Pillsbury)	1/8 cake	210	1
Chocolate Pudding Classic Dessert (Betty Crocker)	1/6 cake	230	1
Chocolate w/ Chocolate Frosting (Pillsbury)	1/8 cake	300	1
Chocolate w/ Vanilla Frosting (Pillsbury)	1/8 cake	300	1
Cinnamon Pecan Streusel MicroRave (Betty Crocker)	1/6 cake	280	1
Cinnamon Pecan Streusel MicroRave No Cholesterol (Betty Crocker)	1/6 cake	230	1
Cobbler Apple Crumb (Dromedary)	1/8 cake	237	1
Cobbler Cherry Crumb (Dromedary)	1/8 cake	231	1
Coffee Cake Easy Mix (Aunt Jemima)	1/8 cake	160	1
Cranberry Quick Bread (Pillsbury)	1/12 loaf	160	1
Date Quick Bread (Pillsbury)	1/12 loaf	160	1
Date Nut (Dromedary)	1/12 cake	183	1
Date Nut Roll (Dromedary)	1/2" slice	80	tr
Devil's Food (Betty Crocker)	1/12 cake	260	2
Devil's Food (Pillsbury Plus)	1/12 cake	270	1
Devil's Food No Cholesterol Recipe (Betty Crocker)	1/12 cake	220	2

FOOD	PORTION	CALORIES	IRON
Devil's Food SuperMoist Light (Betty Crocker)	1/12 cake	200	2
Devil's Food SuperMoist Light No Cholesterol Recipe (Betty Crocker)	1/12 cake	180	2
Devil's Food w/ Chocolate Frosting MicroRave (Betty Crocker)	1/6 cake	310	1
Devil's Food w/ Chocolate Frosting MicroRave Single (Betty Crocker)	1	440	2
Double Chocolate Supreme Microwave (Pillsbury)	1/8 cake	330	1
Double Lemon Supreme Microwave (Pillsbury)	1/8 cake	300	tr
Fudge Marble (Pillsbury Plus)	1/12 cake	270	1
German Chocolate (Betty Crocker)	1/12 cake	260	1
German Chocolate No Cholesterol Recipe (Betty Crocker)	1/12 cake	220	1
German Chocolate w/ Chocolate Frosting MicroRave (Betty Crocker)	1/6 cake	320	1
Gingerbread (Dromedary)	1 piece (2" sq)	100	1
Gingerbread (Pillsbury)	3" sq	190	tr
Gingerbread Classic Dessert (Betty Crocker)	1/9 cake	22	2
Gingerbread Classic Dessert No Cholesterol Recipe (Betty Crocker)	1/9 cake	21	2
Golden Pound Classic Dessert (Betty Crocker)	1/12 cake	200	1
Golden Vanilla (Betty Crocker)	1/12 cake	280	1
Golden Vanilla No Cholesterol Recipe (Betty Crocker)	1/12 cake	220	1
Golden Vanilla w/ Rainbow Chip Frosting MicroRave (Betty Crocker)	1/6 cake	320	1
Lemon (Betty Crocker)	1/12 cake	260	1
Lemon (Pillsbury Plus)	1/12 cake	250	1

FOOD	PORTION	CALORIES	IRON
Lemon Chiffon Classic Dessert (Betty Crocker)	¹⁄₁₂ cake	200	1
Lemon Microwave (Pillsbury)	⅛ cake	220	tr
Lemon No Cholesterol Recipe (Betty Crocker)	¹⁄₁₂ cake	220	1
Lemon Pudding Classic Dessert (Betty Crocker)	⅙ cake	230	tr
Lemon w/ Lemon Frosting (Pillsbury)	⅛ cake	300	tr
Marble (Betty Crocker)	¹⁄₁₂ cake	260	1
Marble No Cholesterol Recipe (Betty Crocker)	¹⁄₁₂ cake	220	1
Milk Chocolate (Betty Crocker)	¹⁄₁₂ cake	260	1
Milk Chocolate No Cholesterol Recipe (Betty Crocker)	¹⁄₁₂ cake	210	1
Nut Quick Bread (Pillsbury)	¹⁄₁₂ loaf	170	1
Pineapple Upsidedown Classic Dessert (Betty Crocker)	⅑ cake	250	1
Pound (Dromedary)	½" slice	150	tr
Rainbow Chip (Betty Crocker)	¹⁄₁₂ cake	250	1
Sour Cream Chocolate (Betty Crocker)	¹⁄₁₂ cake	260	1
Sour Cream Chocolate No Cholesterol Recipe (Betty Crocker)	¹⁄₁₂ cake	220	1
Sour Cream White (Betty Crocker)	¹⁄₁₂ cake	180	1
Spice (Betty Crocker)	¹⁄₁₂ cake	260	1
Spice No Cholesterol Recipe (Betty Crocker)	¹⁄₁₂ cake	220	1
Streusel Swirl Cinnamon (Pillsbury)	¹⁄₁₆ cake	260	1
Streusel Swirl Cinnamon Microwave (Pillsbury)	⅛ cake	240	tr
Streusel Swirl Lemon (Pillsbury)	¹⁄₁₆ cake	270	1

FOOD	PORTION	CALORIES	IRON
Tunnel of Fudge Bundt Microwave (Pillsbury)	1/8 cake	290	1
White (Betty Crocker)	1/12 cake	240	1
White (Pillsbury Plus)	1/12 cake	240	0
White No Cholesterol Recipe (Betty Crocker)	1/12 cake	220	1
White SuperMoist Light (Betty Crocker)	1/12 cake	180	1
Yellow (Betty Crocker)	1/12 cake	260	1
Yellow (Pillsbury Plus)	1/12 cake	260	1
Yellow Microwave (Pillsbury)	1/8 cake	220	tr
Yellow No Cholesterol Recipe (Betty Crocker)	1/12 cake	220	1
Yellow SuperMoist Light (Betty Crocker)	1/12 cake	200	1
Yellow SuperMoist Light No Cholesterol Recipe (Betty Crocker)	1/12 cake	190	1
Yellow w/ Chocolate Frosting (Pillsbury)	1/8 cake	300	1
Yellow w/ Chocolate Frosting MicroRave (Betty Crocker)	1/6 cake	300	tr
Yellow w/ Chocolate Frosting MicroRave Single (Betty Crocker)	1	440	1
angel food	1 (9.75″ diam)	1510	3
angel food	1/12 cake	125	tr
crumb coffee cake	1 (7¾″ × 5⅝″)	1385	7
crumb coffee cake	1/6 cake	230	1
devil's food w/ chocolate frosting	1 cake (9″ diam)	3755	22
devil's food w/ chocolate frosting	1/16 cake	235	1
gingerbread	1 cake (8″ sq)	1575	11
gingerbread	1/9 cake	175	1

FOOD	PORTION	CALORIES	IRON
yellow w/ chocolate frosting	1 cake (9″ diam)	3735	16
yellow w/ chocolate frosting	1/16 cake	235	1
READY-TO-USE Date Nut Loaf (Thomas')	1 oz	90	1
bakewell tart	1 slice (3 oz)	410	1
battenburg cake	1 slice (2 oz)	204	1
cheesecake	1 (9″ diam)	3350	5
cheesecake	1/12 cake	280	tr
crumpets, toasted	2 (4 oz)	119	1
eccles cake	1 slice (2 oz)	285	1
eclair	1 (1.4 oz)	149	tr
madeira cake	1 slice (1 oz)	98	tr
pound cake	1 cake (8½″ × 3½″ × 3″)	1935	8
pound cake	1 slice (1 oz)	110	1
strudel, apple	1 piece (2.5 oz)	195	tr
treacle tart	1 slice (2.5 oz)	258	1
vanilla slice	1 slice (2.5 oz)	248	1
white w/ white frosting	1 (9″ diam)	4170	16
white w/ white frosting	1/16 cake	260	1
yellow w/ chocolate frosting	1 (9″ diam)	3895	20
yellow w/ chocolate frosting	1/16 cake	245	1
REFRIGERATED Apple Turnover (Pillsbury)	1	170	1
Cheesecake (Baby Watson)	1 pkg (4 oz)	420	tr
Cherry Turnover (Pillsbury)	1	170	1
Coffee Cake Cinnamon Swirl (Pillsbury)	1/8 cake	180	1
Coffee Cake Pecan Streusel (Pillsbury)	1/8 cake	180	1

FOOD	PORTION	CALORIES	IRON
Pastry Pockets (Pillsbury)	1	240	1
SNACK			
All Butter Pound (Sara Lee)	1	200	tr
Apple Delights (Little Debbie)	1 pkg (1.25 oz)	160	1
Apple Spice (Little Debbie)	1 pkg (2.2 oz)	300	tr
Banana Twins (Little Debbie)	1 pkg (2.2 oz)	280	1
Be My Valentine (Little Debbie)	1 pkg (2.2 oz)	290	tr
Cherry Cordials (Little Debbie)	1 pkg (1.3 oz)	180	1
Choc-O-Jel (Little Debbie)	1 pkg (1.16 oz)	170	1
Chocolate Chip (Little Debbie)	1 pkg (2.4 oz)	310	1
Chocolate Fudge (Sara Lee)	1	190	1
Chocolate Twins (Little Debbie)	1 pkg (2.2 oz)	260	1
Christmas Tree (Little Debbie)	1 pkg (1.5 oz)	200	tr
Coconut (Little Debbie)	1 pkg (2.17 oz)	310	tr
Coconut Crunch (Little Debbie)	1 pkg (2 oz)	340	1
Coconut Rounds (Little Debbie)	1 pkg (1.13 oz)	160	tr
Coffee Cake			
(Drake's)	1 (1.1 oz)	140	tr
(Little Debbie)	1 pkg (2 oz)	220	1
Apple Cinnamon (Sara Lee)	1	290	1
Butter Streusel (Sara Lee)	1	230	1
Chocolate Crumb (Drake's)	1 (2.5 oz)	245	1
Cinnamon Crumb (Drake's)	1/12 cake (1.3 oz)	150	tr
Pecan (Sara Lee)	1	280	1
Small (Drake's)	1 (2 oz)	220	1
Deluxe Carrot (Sara Lee)	1	180	1
Devil Cremes (Little Debbie)	1 pkg (1.3 oz)	170	1
Devil Dog (Drake's)	1 (1.5 oz)	160	1
Devil Squares (Little Debbie)	1 pkg (2.2 oz)	300	1

FOOD	PORTION	CALORIES	IRON
Easter Bunny (Little Debbie)	1 pkg (2.5 oz)	320	2
Easter Puffs (Little Debbie)	1 pkg (1.25 oz)	150	1
Fancy (Little Debbie)	1 pkg (2.4 oz)	310	1
Figaroos (Little Debbie)	1 pkg (1.5 oz)	160	1
Fudge Crispy (Little Debbie)	1 pkg (2.08 oz)	330	1
Fudge Rounds (Little Debbie)	1 pkg (1.19 oz)	150	1
Funny Bones (Drake's)	1 (1.25 oz)	150	tr
Golden Cremes (Little Debbie)	1 pkg (1.47 oz)	160	1
Holiday Chocolate (Little Debbie)	1 pkg (2.4 oz)	330	1
Holiday Vanilla (Little Debbie)	1 pkg (2.5 oz)	350	tr
Jelly Rolls (Little Debbie)	1 pkg (2.17 oz)	240	tr
Lemon Stix (Little Debbie)	1 pkg (1.5 oz)	220	tr
Marshmallow Supremes (Little Debbie)	1 pkg (1.25 oz)	150	1
Mint Sprints (Little Debbie)	1 pkg (1.5 oz)	240	1
Nutty Bar (Little Debbie)	1 pkg (2 oz)	320	1
Pop-Tarts			
Apple Cinnamon	1	210	2
Blueberry	1	210	2
Brown Sugar Cinnamon	1	210	2
Cherry	1	210	2
Chocolate Graham	1	210	2
Frosted Brown Sugar Cinnamon	1	210	2
Frosted Cherry	1	210	2
Frosted Chocolate Fudge	1	200	2
Frosted Chocolate Vanilla Creme	1	200	2
Frosted Grape	1	200	2
Frosted Raspberry	1	200	2
Frosted Strawberry	1	200	2
Strawberry	1	210	2

FOOD	PORTION	CALORIES	IRON
Pound (Drake's)	1	110	tr
Pumpkin Delights (Little Debbie)	1 pkg (1.13 oz)	140	1
Ring Ding (Drake's)	1 (1.5 oz)	180	1
Ring Ding Mint (Drake's)	1 (1.5 oz)	190	1
Snack Cake Chocolate (Little Debbie)	1 pkg (2.5 oz)	340	1
Snack Cake Vanilla (Little Debbie)	1 pkg (2.6 oz)	360	tr
Star Crunch (Little Debbie)	1 pkg (1.08 oz)	150	tr
Sunny Doodle (Drake's)	1 (1 oz)	100	tr
Swiss Cake Roll (Little Debbie)	1 pkg (2.17 oz)	270	1
Toast-R-Cakes Blueberry	1	110	tr
Toast-R-Cakes Bran	1	103	1
Toast-R-Cakes Corn	1	120	tr
Toaster Tart Apple Cinnamon (Pepperidge Farm)	1	170	1
Toaster Tart Cheese (Pepperidge Farm)	1	190	1
Toaster Tart Strawberry (Pepperidge Farm)	1	190	1
Toastettes (Nabisco)			
Apple	1	190	2
Blueberry	1	190	2
Cherry	1	190	2
Frosted Apple	1	190	2
Frosted Blueberry	1	190	2
Frosted Brown Sugar Cinnamon	1	190	2
Frosted Cherry	1	190	2
Frosted Fruit Punch	1	190	2
Frosted Fudge	1	200	3
Frosted Strawberry	1	190	2
Strawberry	1	190	2

FOOD	PORTION	CALORIES	IRON
Vanilla Cremes (Little Debbie)	1 pkg (1.3 oz)	160	tr
Yankee Doodle (Drake's)	1 (1 oz)	100	tr
Yodels (Drake's)	1 (1 oz)	150	tr
devil's food cupcake w/ chocolate frosting	1	120	1
devil's food w/ creme filling	1 (1 oz)	105	1
sponge w/ creme filling	1 (1.5 oz)	155	1
toaster pastry apple	1 (1.75 oz)	204	2
toaster pastry blueberry	1 (1.75 oz)	204	2
toaster pastry brown sugar cinnamon	1 (1.75 oz)	206	2
toaster pastry cherry	1 (1.75 oz)	204	2
toaster pastry strawberry	1 (1.75 oz)	204	2
TAKE-OUT baklava	1 oz	126	1
strudel	1 piece (4.1 oz)	272	1
trifle w/ cream	6 oz	291	1

CANADIAN BACON

Oscar Mayer	1 slice	28	tr
unheated	2 slices (1.9 oz)	89	tr

CANDY

Almond Joy	1 (1.76 oz)	250	tr
Baby Ruth	2.2 oz	300	1
Bar None	1.5 oz	240	tr
Butterfinger	2.1 oz	280	1
Caramello	1 (1.6 oz)	220	tr
Chunky	1.4 oz	210	1

FOOD	PORTION	CALORIES	IRON
Golden Almond	½ bar	260	tr
Goobers	1.38 oz	220	tr
Hershey Bar w/ Almonds	1 (1.45 oz)	230	1
Hershey's Kisses	9 pieces	220	tr
Kit Kat Wafer	1 (1.63 oz)	250	tr
Milky Way II	1 bar (2 oz)	193	tr
Mounds	1 (1.9 oz)	260	1
Mr. GoodBar	1 (1.75 oz)	290	tr
Nestle Milk Chocolate w/ Almonds	1.45 oz	230	tr
Raisinets	1.38 oz	180	tr
Reese's Peanut Butter Cups	1.8 oz	280	tr
Reese's Pieces	1.85 oz	260	tr
Sno-Caps Nonpareils	1 oz	140	2
Solitaires w/ Almonds	½ bag	260	tr
Special Dark Sweet Chocolate Bar (Hershey)	1 (1.45 oz)	220	1
Symphony Almond Butterchips	1 (1.4 oz)	220	tr
York Peppermint Patty	1 (1.5 oz)	180	tr
boiled sweets	.25 lb	327	tr
candied cherries	1	12	tr
candied citron	1 oz	89	tr
candied pineapple slice	1 (2 oz)	179	tr
candy corn	1 oz	105	tr
caramels, chocolate	1 oz	115	tr
caramels, plain	1 oz	115	tr
chocolate	1 oz	145	tr
chocolate crisp	1 oz	140	tr
chocolate w/ almonds	1 oz	150	1
chocolate w/ peanuts	1 oz	155	tr
dark chocolate	1 oz	150	1

FOOD	PORTION	CALORIES	IRON
fruit pastilles	1 tube (1.4 oz)	101	1
fudge, chocolate	1 oz	115	tr
fudge, vanilla	1 oz	115	tr
gumdrops	1 oz	100	tr
hard candy	1 oz	110	tr
jelly beans	1 oz	105	tr
marzipan	3.5 oz	497	2
mint fondant	1 oz	105	tr
nougat nut cream	3.5 oz	342	4

CANTALOUPE

FRESH
cubed	1 cup	57	tr
half	½	94	1

CARAMBOLA

fresh	1	42	tr

CARAWAY

seeds	1 tsp	7	tr

CARDAMOM

seeds, ground	1 tsp	6	tr

CARDOON

fresh, cooked	3.5 oz	22	1
raw, shredded	½ cup	36	1

CARIBOU

roasted	3 oz	142	5

FOOD	PORTION	CALORIES	IRON

CARISSA PLUM

fresh	1	12	tr

CAROB

flour	1 cup	185	3
flour	1 tbsp	14	tr
mix	3 tsp	45	1
mix, as prep w/ whole milk	9 oz	195	1

CARP

FRESH
cooked	3 oz	138	1
fillet, cooked	6 oz	276	3
raw	3 oz	108	1

CARROTS

CANNED
Diced Fancy (S&W)	½ cup	30	tr
Julienne French Style Fancy (S&W)	½ cup	30	tr
Sliced Fancy (S&W)	½ cup	30	tr
Sliced Water Pack (S&W)	½ cup	30	1
Whole Tiny Fancy (S&W)	½ cup	30	tr
slices	½ cup	17	tr
slices low sodium	½ cup	17	tr

FRESH
raw	1 (2.5 oz)	31	tr
raw, shredded	½ cup	24	tr
slices, cooked	½ cup	35	tr

FROZEN
Baby Whole Deluxe (Birds Eye)	½ cup	40	1
Crinkle Cut (Big Valley)	3.5 oz	40	tr

FOOD	PORTION	CALORIES	IRON
Harvest Fresh Baby (Green Giant)	½ cup	18	0
Polybag Slices (Birds Eye)	¾ cup	35	1
Whole (Big Valley)	3.5 oz	40	tr
slices, cooked	½ cup	26	tr
JUICE			
canned	6 oz	73	1

CASABA

cubed	1 cup	45	1
fresh	⅒ melon	43	1

CASHEWS

Fancy (Planters)	1 oz	170	1
Honey Roasted (Eagle)	1 oz	170	1
Honey Roasted (Planters)	1 oz	170	1
Low Salt (Eagle)	1 oz	170	2
Unsalted Halves (Planters)	1 oz	170	1
cashew butter w/o salt	1 tbsp	94	1
dry roasted	1 oz	163	2
dry roasted, salted	1 oz	163	2
oil roasted	1 oz	163	1
oil roasted, salted	1 oz	163	1

CASSAVA

raw	3.5 oz	120	4

CATFISH

FRESH			
channel, breaded & fried	3 oz	194	1
channel, raw	3 oz	99	1

FOOD	PORTION	CALORIES	IRON
CATSUP			
Hunt's	1 tbsp	15	tr
Hunt's No Salt Added	1 tbsp	20	tr
catsup	1 pkg (.2 oz)	6	tr
catsup	1 tbsp	16	tr
low sodium	1 tbsp	16	tr
CAULIFLOWER			
FRESH			
cooked	½ cup	15	tr
raw	½ cup	12	tr
FROZEN			
Big Valley	3.3 oz	25	tr
Birds Eye	⅔ cup	25	tr
Cuts (Green Giant)	½ cup	12	0
In Cheese Sauce (Green Giant)	½ cup	60	tr
One Serve in Cheese Sauce (Green Giant)	1 pkg	80	tr
Polybag (Birds Eye)	½ cup	20	tr
With Cheddar Cheese Sauce (Budget Gourmet)	1 pkg	130	tr
With Cheese Sauce (Birds Eye)	½ pkg	90	tr
cooked	½ cup	17	tr
JARRED			
Hot & Spicy (Vlasic)	1 oz	4	tr
CELERIAC			
fresh, cooked	3.5 oz	25	tr
raw	½ cup	31	1

FOOD	PORTION	CALORIES	IRON
CELERY			
DRIED			
seed	1 tsp	8	1
FRESH			
diced, cooked	½ cup	13	tr
raw	1 stalk (1.3 oz)	6	tr
raw, diced	½ cup	10	tr
CELTUCE			
raw	3.5 oz	22	1
CEREAL			
COOKED			
5-Bran Kashi (Kashi)	2.5 oz	281	3
Barley Plus (Erewhon)	1 oz	110	tr
Brown Rice Cream (Erewhon)	1 oz	110	1
Coco Wheat (Little Crow)	3 tbsp	130	2
Cream of Rice (Nabisco)	1 oz	100	1
Cream of Wheat Instant (Nabisco)	1 oz	100	9
Cream of Wheat Quick (Nabisco)	1 oz	100	8
Cream of Wheat Regular (Nabisco)	1 oz	100	8
Enriched White Hominy Grits Quick (Quaker)	3 tbsp	101	1
Enriched White Hominy Grits Regular (Aunt Jemima)	3 tbsp	101	1
Enriched Yellow Hominy Grits Quick (Quaker)	3 tbsp	101	1
Farina (H-O)	3 tbsp	120	tr
Farina Instant (H-O)	1 pkg	110	tr
Farina, as prep (Pillsbury)	⅔ cup	80	1

FOOD	PORTION	CALORIES	IRON
High Fiber Hot Cereal, as prep (Ralston)	⅔ cup	90	1
Instant Grits White Hominy (Quaker)	1 pkg	79	8
Instant Grits w/ Imitation Bacon Bits (Quaker)	1 pkg	101	8
Instant Grits w/ Imitation Ham Bits (Quaker)	1 pkg	99	8
Instant Grits w/ Real Cheddar Cheese (Quaker)	1 pkg	104	8
Kashi (Kashi)	2 oz	177	2
Mix 'n Eat Cream of Wheat (Nabisco)			
Brown Sugar Cinnamon	1 pkg (1.25 oz)	130	8
Apple & Cinnamon	1 pkg (1.25 oz)	130	8
Maple Brown Sugar	1 pkg (1.25 oz)	130	8
Original	1 pkg (1.25 oz)	100	8
Oat Bran (Quaker)	⅓ cup	92	1
Oat Bran Natural Apples & Cinnamon (Health Valley)	¼ cup	100	1
Oat Bran Natural Raisins & Spice (Health Valley)	¼ cup	100	1
Oat Bran w/ Toasted Wheat Germ (Erewhon)	1 oz	115	1
Oatmeal, Instant			
(H-O)	1 pkg	110	1
(H-O)	½ cup	130	1
Apple Cinnamon (Erewhon)	1.25 oz	145	tr
Apple Cinnamon (H-O)	1 pkg	130	1
Apple Raisin (Erewhon)	1.3 oz	150	tr
Apples & Cinnamon (Quaker)	1 pkg	118	6
Cinnamon & Spice (Quaker)	1 pkg	164	8
Dates & Walnuts (Erewhon)	1.2 oz	130	1

FOOD	PORTION	CALORIES	IRON
Oatmeal, Instant *(cont.)*			
Extra Fortified Apples & Spice (Quaker)	1 pkg	133	18
Extra Fortified Raisins & Cinnamon (Quaker)	1 pkg	129	18
Extra Fortified Regular (Quaker)	1 pkg	95	18
Maple & Brown Sugar (Quaker)	1 pkg	152	8
Maple Brown Sugar (H-O)	1 pkg	160	1
Maple Spice (Erewhon)	1.2 oz	140	tr
Peaches & Cream (Quaker)	1 pkg	129	6
Raisin & Spice (H-O)	1 pkg	150	1
Raisin & Spice (Quaker)	1 pkg	149	6
Raisin, Dates & Walnuts (Quaker)	1 pkg	141	5
Regular (Quaker)	1 pkg	94	8
Strawberries & Cream (Quaker)	1 pkg	129	5
Sweet 'n Mellow (H-O)	1 pkg	150	1
With Added Oat Bran (Erewhon)	1.25 oz	125	1
Oats 'n Fiber (H-O)	1 pkg	110	1
Oats 'n Fiber (H-O)	⅓ cup	100	1
Oats 'n Fiber Apple & Bran (H-O)	1 pkg	130	1
Oats 'n Fiber Raisin & Bran (H-O)	1 pkg	150	1
Oats Gourmet (H-O)	⅓ cup	100	1
Oats Old Fashioned (Quaker)	⅔ cup	99	1
Oats Quick (H-O)	½ cup	130	1
Oats Quick (Quaker)	⅔ cup	99	1
Whole Wheat Hot Natural (Quaker)	⅔ cup	92	tr
corn grits instant, as prep	1 pkg (.8 oz)	82	1
corn grits quick	1 tbsp	36	tr
corn grits quick	1 cup	146	2

FOOD	PORTION	CALORIES	IRON
corn grits regular	1 cup	579	6
corn grits regular	1 cup	146	2
farina, cooked	¾ cup	87	tr
farina, dry	1 tbsp	40	tr
oatmeal, cooked	1 cup	145	2
oatmeal, dry	1 cup	311	3
oatmeal instant, cooked w/o salt	1 cup	145	2
oatmeal quick, cooked w/o salt	1 cup	145	2
oatmeal regular, cooked w/o salt	1 cup	145	2
READY-TO-EAT			
100% Bran (Nabisco)	⅓ cup	70	3
100% Natural Bran w/ Apples & Cinnamon (Health Valley)	¼ cup	100	tr
All-Bran (Kellogg's)	⅓ cup (1 oz)	70	5
All-Bran w/ Extra Fiber (Kellogg's)	½ cup (1 oz)	50	5
Almond Delight (Ralston)	¾ cup	110	2
Alpha-Bits (Post)	1 cup	111	3
Alpha-Bits Marshmallow Sweetened (Post)	1 cup	110	3
Apple Cinnamon Squares (Kellogg's)	½ cup (1 oz)	90	8
Apple Jacks (Kellogg's)	1 cup (1 oz)	110	5
Apple Raisin Crisp (Kellogg's)	⅔ cup (1 oz)	130	2
Aztec (Erewhon)	1 oz	100	1
Basic 4 (General Mills)	¾ cup	130	5
Batman (Ralston)	1 cup	110	5
Blue Corn Flakes 100% Organic (Health Valley)	½ cup	90	4
Blueberry Squares (Kellogg's)	½ cup (1 oz)	90	8
Body Buddies Natural Fruit (General Mills)	1 cup (1 oz)	110	8

FOOD	PORTION	CALORIES	IRON
Booberry (General Mills)	1 cup (1 oz)	110	5
Bran Buds (Kellogg's)	⅓ cup (1 oz)	70	5
Bran Cereal w/ ¼ cup Dates 100% Organic (Health Valley)	¼ cup	100	1
Bran Cereal w/ Raisins 100% Organic (Health Valley)	¼ cup	100	1
Bran Flakes (Kellogg's)	⅔ cup (1 oz)	90	18
Bran News (Ralston)	¾ cup	100	5
Breakfast With Barbie (Ralston)	1 cup	110	5
Cap'n Crunch (Quaker)	¾ cup	113	5
Cap'n Crunch's Crunchberries (Quaker)	¾ cup	113	5
Cap'n Crunch's Peanut Butter Crunch (Quaker)	¾ cup	119	5
Cheerios (General Mills)	1¼ cup (1 oz)	110	8
Cheerios Apple Cinnamon (General Mills)	¾ cup (1 oz)	110	5
Cheerios Honey Nut (General Mills)	¾ cup (1 oz)	110	5
Cheerios-to-Go (General Mills)	¾-oz pkg	80	6
Cheerios-to-Go Apple Cinnamon (General Mills)	1-oz pkg	110	5
Cheerios-to-Go Honey Nut (General Mills)	1-oz pkg	110	5
Chex Corn (Ralston)	1 cup	110	8
Chex Double (Ralston)	⅔ cup	100	8
Chex Honey Graham (Ralston)	⅔ cup	110	2
Chex Honey Nut Oat (Ralston)	½ cup	100	8
Chex Multi-Bran (Ralston)	⅔ cup	90	8
Chex Rice (Ralston)	1⅛ cup	110	8
Chex Wheat (Ralston)	⅔ cup	100	8

FOOD	PORTION	CALORIES	IRON
Cinnamon Mini Buns (Kellogg's)	¾ cup (1 oz)	110	5
Cinnamon Toast Crunch (General Mills)	¾ cup (1 oz)	120	5
Clusters (General Mills)	½ cup (1 oz)	110	5
Cocoa Krispies (Kellogg's)	¾ cup (1 oz)	110	2
Cocoa Pebbles (Post)	⅞ cup	113	2
Cocoa Puffs (General Mills)	1 cup (1 oz)	110	5
Common Sense Oat Bran (Kellogg's)	¾ cup (1 oz)	100	8
Common Sense Oat Bran w/ Raisins (Kellogg's)	¾ cup (1 oz)	130	8
Cookie-Crisp Chocolate Chip (Ralston)	1 cup	110	5
Cookie-Crisp Vanilla Wafer (Ralston)	1 cup	110	5
Corn Flakes (Kellogg's)	1 cup (1 oz)	100	2
Corn Pops (Kellogg's)	1 cup (1 oz)	110	2
Count Chocula (General Mills)	1 cup (1 oz)	110	5
Country Corn Flakes (General Mills)	1 cup (1 oz)	110	8
Cracklin' Oat Bran (Kellogg's)	½ cup (1 oz)	110	2
Crispix (Kellogg's)	1 cup (1 oz)	110	2
Crispy Brown Rice (Erewhon)	1 oz	110	1
Crispy Critters (Post)	1 cup	110	8
Crispy Wheats 'n Raisins (General Mills)	¾ cup (1 oz)	100	5
Crunchy Bran (Quaker)	⅔ cup	89	9
Crunchy Not Oh!s (Quaker)	1 cup	127	6
Dinersaurs (Ralston)	1 cup	110	5
Double Dip Crunch (Kellogg's)	⅔ cup (1 oz)	120	2
Fiber 7 Flakes 100% Organic (Health Valley)	½ cup	90	1

FOOD	PORTION	CALORIES	IRON
Fiber 7 Flakes w/ Raisins 100% Organic (Health Valley)	½ cup	90	1
Fiber One (General Mills)	½ cup (1 oz)	60	5
Fiberwise (Kellogg's)	⅔ cup (1 oz)	90	5
Frankenberry (General Mills)	1 cup (1 oz)	110	5
Froot Loops (Kellogg's)	1 cup (1 oz)	110	5
Frosted Mini-Wheats (Kellogg's)	4 biscuits (1 oz)	100	2
Frosted Mini-Wheats Bite Size (Kellogg's)	½ cup	100	2
Frosted Bran (Kellogg's)	1.5 oz	150	6
Frosted Flakes (Kellogg's)	¾ cup (1 oz)	110	2
Frosted Krispies (Kellogg's)	¾ cup (1 oz)	110	2
Fruit & Fiber Dates, Raisins, Walnuts w/ Oat Clusters (Post)	⅔ cup	120	6
Fruit & Fiber Tropical Fruit w/ Oat Clusters (Post)	⅔ cup	125	5
Fruit & Fitness (Health Valley)	1 cup	220	2
Fruit 'n Wheat (Erewhon)	1 oz	100	i.
Fruit Lites Corn (Health Valley)	½ cup	45	3
Fruit Lites Rice (Health Valley)	½ cup	45	5
Fruit Lites Wheat (Health Valley)	½ cup	45	1
Fruit Muesli Raisins, Apples & Almonds (Ralston)	½ cup	150	4
Fruit Muesli Raisins, Dates & Almonds (Ralston)	½ cup	140	4
Fruit Muesli Raisins, Peaches & Pecans (Ralston)	½ cup	150	4
Fruit Muesli Raisins, Walnuts & Cranberries (Ralston)	½ cup	150	4
Fruit Wheats Apple (Nabisco)	1 oz	90	2
Fruitful Bran (Kellogg's)	⅔ cup (1.4 oz)	120	5

FOOD	PORTION	CALORIES	IRON
Fruity Marshmallow Krispies (Kellogg's)	1¼ cups (1.3 oz)	140	2
Fruity Pebbles (Post)	⅞ cup	113	2
Fruity Yummy Mummy (General Mills)	1 cup (1 oz)	110	5
Golden Grahams (General Mills)	¾ cup (1 oz)	110	5
Grape-Nuts (Post)	¼ cup	105	8
Grape-Nuts Raisin (Post)	¼ cup	102	2
Healthy Crunch Almond Date (Health Valley)	½ cup	110	tr
Healthy Crunch Apple Cinnamon (Health Valley)	¼ cup	110	tr
Healthy O's 100% Organic (Health Valley)	¾ cup	90	1
Honey Bunches of Oats Honey Roasted (Post)	⅔ cup	111	3
Honey Bunches of Oats w/ Almonds (Post)	⅔ cup	115	3
Honey Graham Oh!s (Quaker)	1 cup	122	6
Honeycomb (Post)	1⅓ cup	110	3
Hot Wheels (Ralston)	1 cup	110	5
Just Right w/ Fiber Nuggets (Kellogg's)	⅔ cup (1 oz)	100	18
Just Right w/ Raisins, Dates & Nuts (Kellogg's)	¾ cup (1.3 oz)	140	18
Kaboom (General Mills)	1 cup (1 oz)	110	8
Kashi Brittles Sesame/Maple (Kashi)	3.5 oz	473	2
Kashi Puffed (Kashi)	.75 oz	74	1
Kenmei (Kellogg's)	¾ cup (1 oz)	110	1
King Vitaman (Quaker)	1½ cup	110	8
Kix (General Mills)	1½ cup (1 oz)	110	8

FOOD	PORTION	CALORIES	IRON
Life (Quaker)	⅔ cup	101	8
Life Cinnamon (Quaker)	⅔ cup	101	8
Lites Puffed Corn (Health Valley)	½ cup	50	tr
Lites Puffed Rice (Health Valley)	½ cup	50	tr
Lites Puffed Wheat (Health Valley)	½ cup	50	1
Lucky Charms (General Mills)	1 cup (1 oz)	110	5
Morning Funnies (Ralston)	1 cup	110	5
Mueslix Crispy Blend (Kellogg's)	⅔ cup (1.5 oz)	150	5
Mueslix Golden Crunch (Kellogg's)	½ cup (1.2 oz)	120	5
Natural Bran Flakes (Post)	⅔ cup	88	8
Nintendo Cereal System (Ralston)	1 cup	110	5
Nut & Honey Crunch (Kellogg's)	⅔ cup (1 oz)	110	2
Nut & Honey Crunch O's (Kellogg's)	⅔ cup (1 oz)	110	2
Nutri-Grain Almond Raisin (Kellogg's)	⅔ cup (1.4 oz)	140	1
Nutri-Grain Raisin Bran (Kellogg's)	1 cup (1.4 oz)	130	2
Nutri-Grain Wheat (Kellogg's)	⅔ cup (1 oz)	90	1
Oat Bran Flakes 100% Organic (Health Valley)	½ cup	100	1
Oat Bran Flakes w/ Almonds & Dates 100% Organic (Health Valley)	½ cup	100	1
Oat Bran Flakes w/ Raisins 100% Organic (Health Valley)	½ cup	100	1
Oat Bran Options (Ralston)	¾ cup	130	8
Oat Bran O's 100% Organic (Health Valley)	½ cup	110	2
Oat Bran O's Fruit & Nuts (Health Valley)	½ cup	110	2
Oat Flakes (Post)	⅔ cup	107	8
Oat Squares (Quaker)	½ cup	105	7

FOOD	PORTION	CALORIES	IRON
Oatbake Honey Bran (Kellogg's)	⅓ cup (1 oz)	110	5
Oatbake Raisin Nut (Kellogg's)	⅓ cup (1 oz)	110	5
Oatmeal Crisp (General Mills)	½ cup (1 oz)	110	5
Oatmeal Raisin Crisp (General Mills)	½ cup (1.2 oz)	130	5
Orangeola Almonds & Dates (Health Valley)	¼ cup	110	1
Orangeola Bananas & Hawaiian Fruit (Health Valley)	¼ cup	120	tr
Popeye Sweet Crunch (Quaker)	1 cup	113	6
Poppets (US Mills)	1 oz	110	1
Post Toasties Corn Flakes	1¼ cup	111	tr
Product 19 (Kellogg's)	1 cup (1 oz)	100	18
Puffed Rice (Quaker)	1 cup	54	tr
Puffed Wheat (Quaker)	1 cup	50	1
Quaker 100% Natural	¼ cup	127	1
Quaker 100% Natural Apples & Cinnamon	¼ cup	126	1
Quaker 100% Natural Raisins & Date	¼ cup	123	1
Raisin Bran (Erewhon)	1 oz	100	tr
Raisin Bran (Kellogg's)	¾ cup (1.4 oz)	120	18
Raisin Bran (Post)	⅔ cup	122	6
Raisin Bran Flakes 100% Organic (Health Valley)	½ cup	100	1
Raisin Nut Bran (General Mills)	½ cup (1 oz)	110	5
Raisin Squares (Kellogg's)	½ cup (1 oz)	90	8
Real Oat Bran Almond Crunch (Health Valley)	¼ cup	110	1
Real Oat Bran Hawaiian Fruit (Health Valley)	¼ cup	130	1

FOOD	PORTION	CALORIES	IRON
Real Oat Bran Raisin Nut (Health Valley)	¼ cup	130	1
Rice Bran Options (Ralston)	⅔ cup	120	8
Rice Bran O's (Health Valley)	½ cup	110	1
Rice Bran w/ Almonds & Dates (Health Valley)	½ cup	110	1
Rice Krispies (Kellogg's)	1 cup (1 oz)	110	2
S'Mores Grahams (General Mills)	¾ cup (1 oz)	120	5
Shredded Wheat 'n Bran (Nabisco)	⅔ cup	90	1
Shredded Wheat (Quaker)	2 biscuits	132	1
Shredded Wheat (Sunshine)	1 biscuit	90	1
Shredded Wheat Bite Size (Sunshine)	⅔ cup	110	1
Shredded Wheat Spoon Size (Nabisco)	⅔ cup	90	1
Shredded Wheat w/ Oat Bran (Nabisco)	⅔ cup	100	1
Slimer! And the Real Ghostbusters (Ralston)	1 cup	110	5
Special K (Kellogg's)	1 cup (1 oz)	100	5
Sprouts 7 Bananas & Hawaiian Fruit (Health Valley)	¼ cup	90	1
Sprouts 7 Raisin (Health Valley)	¼ cup	90	1
Strawberry Squares (Kellogg's)	½ cup (1 oz)	90	8
Sunflakes Multi-Grain (Ralston)	1 cup	100	2
Super Golden Crisp (Post)	⅞ cup	104	3
Super-O's (Erewhon)	1 oz	110	2
Swiss Breakfast Raisin Nut (Health Valley)	¼ cup	100	1
Swiss Breakfast Tropical Fruit (Health Valley)	¼ cup	100	1
Team (Nabisco)	1 cup	110	8

FOOD	PORTION	CALORIES	IRON
Teenage Mutant Ninja Turtles (Ralston)	1 cup	110	2
Total (General Mills)	1 cup (1 oz)	100	18
Total Corn Flakes (General Mills)	1 cup (1 oz)	110	18
Total Raisin Bran (General Mills)	1 cup (1.5 oz)	140	18
Triples (General Mills)	¾ cup (1 oz)	110	5
Trix (General Mills)	1 cup (1 oz)	110	5
Uncle Sam Cereal (US Mills)	1 oz	110	1
Weetabix	2 (1.3 oz)	142	2
Wheat Flakes (Erewhon)	1 oz	100	tr
Wheaties (General Mills)	1 cup (1 oz)	100	8
Whole Grain Shredded Wheat (Kellogg's)	½ cup (1 oz)	90	2
all bran	½ cup (1 oz)	76	3
bran flakes	¾ cup (1 oz)	90	8
corn flakes	1¼ cup (1 oz)	110	2
corn flakes low sodium	1 cup	100	1
crispy rice	1 cup	111	1
fortified oat flakes	1 cup	177	14
granola	¼ cup	138	1
puffed rice	1 cup	57	tr
puffed wheat	1 cup	44	1
shredded wheat	1 biscuit	83	1
sugar-coated corn flakes	¾ cup (1 oz)	110	2

CHAYOTE

FOOD	PORTION	CALORIES	IRON
fresh, cooked	1 cup	38	tr
raw	1 (7 oz)	49	1
raw, cut up	1 cup	32	1

FOOD	PORTION	CALORIES	IRON

CHEESE

NATURAL

FOOD	PORTION	CALORIES	IRON
Blue (Sargento)	1 oz	100	tr
Breakfast (Marin French Cheese)	1 oz	86	tr
Brie (Marin French Cheese)	1 oz	86	tr
Brie (Sargento)	1 oz	95	tr
Burger Cheese (Sargento)	1 oz	106	tr
Cajun (Sargento)	1 oz	110	tr
Camembert (Marin French Cheese)	1 oz	86	tr
Camembert (Sargento)	1 oz	85	tr
Cheddar (Sargento)	1 oz	114	tr
Cheddar New York (Sargento) ·	1 oz	114	tr
Cheddar Sharp Nut Log (Sargento)	1 oz	97	1
Colby (Sargento)	1 oz	112	tr
Colby Jack (Sargento)	1 oz	109	tr
Edam (Sargento)	1 oz	101	tr
Feta (Sargento)	1 oz	75	tr
Finland Swiss (Sargento)	1 oz	107	tr
Fontina (Sargento)	1 oz	110	tr
Fruit Moos Apricot (Dannon)	3.5 oz	150	0
Fruit Moos Banana (Dannon)	3.5 oz	150	0
Fruit Moos Raspberry (Dannon)	3.5 oz	150	0
Fruit Moos Strawberry (Dannon)	3.5 oz	150	0
Gouda (Sargento)	1 oz	101	tr
Havarti (Sargento)	1 oz	118	tr
Italian Style Grated Cheeses (Sargento)	1 oz	108	tr
Limburger (Sargento)	1 oz	93	tr
Monterey Jack (Sargento)	1 oz	106	tr

FOOD	PORTION	CALORIES	IRON
Mozzarella Low Moisture Part Skim (Sargento)	1 oz	79	tr
Mozzarella Whole Milk (Sargento)	1 oz	90	tr
Muenster Red Rind (Sargento)	1 oz	104	tr
Parmazest (Frigo)	1 oz	120	tr
Parmesan & Romano Grated (Sargento)	1 oz	111	tr
Parmesan Fresh (Sargento)	1 oz	111	tr
Parmesan Grated (Sargento)	1 oz	129	tr
Port Wine Nut Log (Sargento)	1 oz	97	1
Provolone (Sargento)	1 oz	100	tr
Queso Blanco (Sargento)	1 oz	104	tr
Queso de Papa (Sargento)	1 oz	114	tr
Ricotta Part Skim (Sargento)	1 oz	32	tr
Ricotta Lite (Sargento)	1 oz	24	tr
Schloss (Marin French Cheese)	1 oz	86	tr
Smokestick (Sargento)	1 oz	103	tr
String (Sargento)	1 oz	79	tr
String Smoked (Sargento)	1 oz	79	tr
Swiss (Sargento)	1 oz	107	tr
Swiss Almond Nut Log (Sargento)	1 oz	94	tr
Taco (Sargento)	1 oz	109	tr
Tilsit (Sargento)	1 oz	96	tr
Tybo Red Wax (Sargento)	1 oz	98	tr
blue	1 oz	100	tr
blue, crumbled	1 cup	477	tr
brick	1 oz	105	tr
brie	1 oz	95	tr
caerphilly	1.4 oz	150	tr
camembert	1 oz	85	tr

FOOD	PORTION	CALORIES	IRON
camembert	1 wedge (1.33 oz)	114	tr
cheddar	1 oz	114	tr
cheddar reduced fat	1.4 oz	104	tr
cheddar, shredded	1 cup	455	1
cheshire	1 oz	110	tr
cheshire reduced fat	1.4 oz	108	tr
colby	1 oz	112	tr
derby	1.4 oz	161	tr
double gloucester	1.4 oz	162	tr
edam	1 oz	101	tr
emmenthaler	3.5 oz	403	tr
feta	1 oz	75	tr
fontina	1 oz	110	tr
fromage frais	1.6 oz	51	0
goat, hard	1 oz	128	1
goat, semi-soft	1 oz	103	tr
goat, soft	1 oz	76	1
gorgonzola	3.5 oz	376	tr
gouda	1 oz	101	tr
lancashire	1.4 oz	149	tr
leicester	1.4 oz	160	tr
limburger	1 oz	93	tr
lymeswold	1.4 oz	170	tr
monterey	1 oz	106	tr
mozzarella	1 lb	1276	1
mozzarella	1 oz	80	tr
mozzarella low moisture	1 oz	90	tr
mozzarella low moisture part skim	1 oz	79	tr
mozzarella part skim	1 oz	72	tr

FOOD	PORTION	CALORIES	IRON
muenster	1 oz	104	tr
parmesan, grated	1 oz	129	tr
parmesan, grated	1 tbsp	23	tr
parmesan, hard	1 oz	111	tr
provolone	1 oz	100	tr
quark 20% fat	3.5 oz	116	tr
quark 40% fat	3.5 oz	167	tr
quark made w/ skim milk	3.5 oz	78	tr
ricotta	1 cup	428	1
ricotta	½ cup	216	tr
ricotta part skim	1 cup	340	1
ricotta part skim	½ cup	171	1
roquefort	1 oz	105	tr
stilton blue	1.4 oz	164	tr
stilton white	1.4 oz	145	tr
swiss	1 oz	107	tr
tilsit	1 oz	96	tr
wensleydale	1.4 oz	151	tr
PROCESSED			
Lactaid American	3.5 oz	328	1
Sargento American Hot Pepper	1 oz	106	tr
Sargento American Sharp Spread	1 oz	106	tr
Sargento American w/ Pimento	1 oz	106	tr
Sargento Imitation Cheddar	1 oz	85	tr
Sargento Imitation Mozzarella	1 oz	80	tr
Sargento Brick	1 oz	95	tr
Sargento Swiss	1 oz	95	tr
american	1 oz	106	tr
american	1 oz	93	tr

FOOD	PORTION	CALORIES	IRON
american cheese food	1 pkg (8 oz)	745	2
american cheese spread	1 jar (5 oz)	412	tr
american cheese spread	1 oz	82	tr
american cold pack	1 pkg (8 oz)	752	2
pimento	1 oz	106	tr
swiss	1 oz	95	tr
swiss	1 oz	92	tr
swiss cheese food	1 pkg (8 oz)	734	1

CHEESE DISHES

HOME RECIPE			
welsh rarebit, as prep w/ 1 white toast	1 slice	228	1
TAKE-OUT			
cheese omelet, as prep w/ 2 eggs	1 (6.8 oz)	519	2
fondue	½ cup	303	tr
macaroni & cheese	6.3 oz	320	1

CHERIMOYA

fresh	1	515	3

CHERRIES

CANNED			
sour in heavy syrup	½ cup	232	3
sour in light syrup	½ cup	189	3
sour water pack	1 cup	87	3
sweet in heavy syrup	½ cup	107	tr
sweet in light syrup	½ cup	85	tr
sweet juice pack	½ cup	68	1
sweet water pack	½ cup	57	tr

FOOD	PORTION	CALORIES	IRON
DRIED			
Bing (Chukar)	2 oz	160	1
Rainer (Chukar)	2 oz	160	1
FRESH			
sour	1 cup	51	tr
sweet	10	49	tr
FROZEN			
Dark Sweet (Big Valley)	4 oz	60	tr
sour, unsweetened	1 cup	72	1
sweet, sweetened	1 cup	232	1
JUICE			
Dole Pure & Light	6 oz	90	tr
Kool-Aid Koolers	1 (8.45 oz)	142	tr
Smucker's Black Cherry	8 oz	130	1
Smucker's Black Cherry Sparkler	10 oz	120	1
Tang Fruit Box	8.45 oz	121	tr
Wylers Drink Mix Wild Cherry	8 oz	81	0

CHERVIL

seed	1 tsp	1	tr

CHESTNUTS

chinese, cooked	1 oz	44	tr
chinese, dried	1 oz	103	1
chinese, raw	1 oz	64	tr
chinese, roasted	1 oz	68	tr
cooked	1 oz	37	tr
dried, peeled	1 oz	105	1
japanese, cooked	1 oz	16	tr
japanese, dried	1 oz	102	1

FOOD	PORTION	CALORIES	IRON
japanese, raw	1 oz	44	tr
japanese, roasted	1 oz	57	1
raw, peeled	1 oz	56	tr
roasted	1 cup	350	1
roasted	1 oz	70	tr

CHIA SEEDS

dried	1 oz	134	3

CHICKEN
(see also CHICKEN DISHES, DINNERS)

FOOD	PORTION	CALORIES	IRON
CANNED			
Chunk Style Mixin' Chicken (Swanson)	2.5 oz	130	1
White (Swanson)	2.5 oz	100	tr
White & Dark (Swanson)	2.5 oz	100	1
chicken spread	1 oz	55	1
chicken spread	1 tbsp	25	tr
chicken spread barbeque flavor	1 oz	55	1
w/ broth	1 can (5 oz)	234	2
w/ broth	½ can (2.5 oz)	117	1
FRESH			
broiler/fryer			
back w/ skin, batter dipped & fried	½ back (2.5 oz)	238	1
back w/ skin, floured & fried	1.5 oz	146	1
back w/ skin, roasted	1 oz	96	tr
back w/ skin, stewed	½ back (2.1 oz)	158	1
back w/o skin, fried	½ back (2 oz)	167	1
breast w/ skin, batter dipped & fried	½ breast (4.9 oz)	364	1

FOOD	PORTION	CALORIES	IRON
breast w/ skin, batter dipped & fried	2.9 oz	218	1
breast w/ skin, roasted	½ breast (3.4 oz)	193	1
breast w/ skin, roasted	2 oz	115	1
breast w/ skin, stewed	½ breast (3.9 oz)	202	1
breast w/o skin, fried	½ breast (3 oz)	161	1
breast w/o skin, roasted	½ breast (3 oz)	142	1
breast w/o skin, stewed	2 oz	86	1
dark meat w/ skin, batter dipped & fried	5.9 oz	497	2
dark meat w/ skin, floured & fried	3.9 oz	313	2
dark meat w/ skin, roasted	3.5 oz	256	1
dark meat w/ skin, stewed	3.9 oz	256	1
dark meat w/o skin, fried	1 cup (5 oz)	334	2
dark meat w/o skin, roasted	1 cup (5 oz)	286	2
dark meat w/o skin, stewed	1 cup (5 oz)	269	2
dark meat w/o skin, stewed	3 oz	165	1
drumstick w/ skin, batter dipped & fried	1 (2.6 oz)	193	1
drumstick w/ skin, floured & fried	1 (1.7 oz)	120	1
drumstick w/ skin, roasted	1 (1.8 oz)	112	1
drumstick w/ skin, stewed	1 (2 oz)	116	1
drumstick w/o skin, fried	1 (1.5 oz)	82	1
drumstick w/o skin, roasted	1 (1.5 oz)	76	1
drumstick w/o skin, stewed	1 (1.6 oz)	78	1
leg w/ skin, batter dipped & fried	1 (5.5 oz)	431	2
leg w/ skin, floured & fried	1 (3.9 oz)	285	2

FOOD	PORTION	CALORIES	IRON
Fresh Broiler/Fryer *(cont.)*			
leg w/ skin, roasted	1 (4 oz)	265	2
leg w/ skin, stewed	1 (4.4 oz)	275	2
leg w/o skin, fried	1 (3.3 oz)	195	1
leg w/o skin, roasted	1 (3.3 oz)	182	1
leg w/o skin, stewed	1 (3.5 oz)	187	1
light meat w/ skin, batter dipped & fried	4 oz	312	1
light meat w/ skin, floured & fried	2.7 oz	192	1
light meat w/ skin, roasted	2.8 oz	175	1
light meat w/ skin, stewed	3.2 oz	181	1
light meat w/o skin, fried	1 cup (5 oz)	268	2
light meat w/o skin, roasted	1 cup (5 oz)	242	1
light meat w/o skin, stewed	1 cup (5 oz)	223	1
neck w/ skin, stewed	1 (1.3 oz)	94	1
neck w/o skin, stewed	1 (.6 oz)	32	tr
skin, batter dipped & fried	4 oz	449	2
skin, batter dipped & fried	½ chicken (6.7 oz)	748	3
skin, floured & fried	1 oz	166	1
skin, floured & fried	½ chicken (2 oz)	281	1
skin, roasted	½ chicken (2 oz)	254	1
skin, stewed	½ chicken (2.5 oz)	261	1
thigh w/ skin, batter dipped & fried	1 (3 oz)	238	1
thigh w/ skin, floured & fried	1 (2.2 oz)	162	1
thigh w/ skin, roasted	1 (2.2 oz)	153	1
thigh w/ skin, stewed	1 (2.4 oz)	158	1

FOOD	PORTION	CALORIES	IRON
thigh w/o skin, fried	1 (1.8 oz)	113	1
thigh w/o skin, roasted	1 (1.8 oz)	109	1
thigh w/o skin, stewed	1 (1.9 oz)	107	1
wing w/ skin, batter dipped & fried	1 (1.7 oz)	159	1
wing w/ skin, floured & fried	1 (1.1 oz)	103	tr
wing w/ skin, roasted	1 (1.2 oz)	99	tr
wing w/ skin, stewed	1 (1.4 oz)	100	tr
skin, floured & fried	½ chicken (11 oz)	844	4
w/ skin, fried	½ chicken (16.4 oz)	1347	6
w/ skin, neck & giblets, batter dipped & fried	1 chicken (2.3 lbs)	2987	18
w/ skin, neck & giblets, roasted	1 chicken (1.5 lbs)	1598	11
w/ skin, neck & giblets, stewed	1 chicken (1.6 lbs)	1625	12
w/ skin, roasted	½ chicken (10.5 oz)	715	4
w/ skin, stewed	½ chicken (11.7 oz)	730	4
capon w/ skin, neck & giblets, roasted	1 chicken (3.1 lbs)	3211	25
roaster dark meat w/o skin, roasted	1 cup (5 oz)	250	2
roaster light meat w/o skin, roasted	1 cup (5 oz)	214	2
roaster w/ skin, neck & giblets, roasted	1 chicken (2.4 lbs)	2363	17
roaster w/ skin, roasted	½ chicken (1.1 lbs)	1071	6
roaster w/o skin, roasted	1 cup (5 oz)	469	2

FOOD	PORTION	CALORIES	IRON
stewing dark meat w/o skin, stewed	1 cup (5 oz)	361	2
stewing w/ skin neck & giblets, stewed	1 chicken (1.3 lbs)	1636	11
stewing w/ skin, stewed	½ chicken (9.2 oz)	744	4
stewing w/ skin, stewed	6.2 oz	507	2
FROZEN PREPARED Banquet			
Boneless Breast Tenders	2.25 oz	150	tr
Boneless Chicken Nuggets	2.5 oz	200	1
Boneless Chicken Nuggets w/ Cheddar	2.5 oz	240	tr
Boneless Chicken Patties	2.5 oz	190	tr
Boneless Chicken Sticks	2.5 oz	210	tr
Boneless Drum Snackers	2.5 oz	210	tr
Boneless Fried Breast Tenders	2.25 oz	160	tr
Boneless Southern Fried Chicken Nuggets	2.5 oz	210	tr
Boneless Southern Fried Chicken Patties	2.5 oz	200	tr
Hot 'n Spicy Chicken Nuggets	2.5 oz	240	tr
Country Skillet			
Chicken Chunks	3 oz	260	1
Chicken Nuggets	3 oz	250	1
Chicken Patties	3 oz	230	1
Southern Fried Chicken Chunks	3 oz	270	1
Southern Fried Chicken Patties	3 oz	240	1
Swanson			
Chicken Nibbles	3.25 oz	300	1
Chicken Nuggets	3 oz	230	1
Fried Chicken Breast Portion	4.5 oz	360	1

FOOD	PORTION	CALORIES	IRON
Pre-fried Chicken Parts	3.25 oz	270	1
Thighs & Drumsticks	3.25 oz	290	1
READY-TO-USE			
Carl Buddig	1 oz	60	tr
Louis Rich Deluxe Oven Roasted Breast	1 slice (1 oz)	30	tr
Louis Rich Hickory Smoked Breast	1 slice (1 oz)	30	tr
Louis Rich Oven Roasted Thin Sliced Breast	1 slice	12	tr
Louis Rich Oven Roasted White	1 slice (1 oz)	35	tr
Oscar Mayer Breast Roast Thin Sliced	1 slice (.4 oz)	13	tr
Oscar Mayer Smoked Breast	1 slice (1 oz)	25	tr
chicken roll light meat	1 pkg (6 oz)	271	2
chicken roll light meat	2 oz	90	1
poultry salad sandwich spread	1 oz	238	tr
poultry salad sandwich spread	1 tbsp	109	tr
TAKE-OUT			
boneless, breaded & fried w/ barbecue sauce	6 pieces (4.6 oz)	330	1
boneless, breaded & fried w/ honey	6 pieces (4 oz)	339	1
boneless, breaded & fried w/ mustard sauce	6 pieces (4.6 oz)	323	1
boneless, breaded & fried w/ sweet & sour sauce	6 pieces (4.6 oz)	346	1
breast & wing, breaded & fried	2 pieces (5.7 oz)	494	1
drumstick, breaded & fried	2 pieces (5.2 oz)	430	2
thigh, breaded & fried	2 pieces (5.2 oz)	430	2

FOOD	PORTION	CALORIES	IRON

CHICKEN DISHES

CANNED

Chicken & Dumplings (Swanson)	7.5 oz	220	1
Chicken a la King (Swanson)	5.25 oz	190	tr
Chicken Stew (Swanson)	7.62 oz	160	1

FROZEN

MicroMagic Chicken Sandwich	1 pkg (4.5 oz)	390	1

HOME RECIPE

chicken & noodles	1 cup	365	2
chicken a la king	1 cup	470	3

MIX

Lipton Microeasy Barbeque Chicken	¼ pkg	108	1
Lipton Microeasy Country Chicken	¼ pkg	78	1
Skillet Chicken Helper Cheesy Broccoli, as prep	⅕ pkg (7.5 oz)	270	1
Skillet Chicken Helper Creamy Chicken, as prep	⅕ pkg (8.25 oz)	290	1
Skillet Chicken Helper Creamy Mushroom, as prep	⅕ pkg (8 oz)	280	1
Skillet Chicken Helper Fettucine Alfredo, as prep	⅕ pkg (7.5 oz)	270	1
Skillet Chicken Helper Stir-Fried Chicken, as prep	⅕ pkg (7 oz)	330	2

TAKE-OUT

chicken & dumplings	¾ cup	256	2
chicken cacciatore	¾ cup	394	4
chicken pie w/ top crust	1 slice (5.6 oz)	472	1
fillet sandwich plain	1	515	5
fillet sandwich w/ cheese, lettuce, mayonnaise & tomato	1	632	4

FOOD	PORTION	CALORIES	IRON

CHICKPEAS

CANNED
Goya Spanish Style	7.5 oz	150	3
Green Giant Garbanzos	½ cup	90	1
S&W Garbanzos Lite 50% Less Salt	½ cup	110	2
S&W Garbanzos Premium Large	½ cup	110	tr
S&W Garbanzos Water Pack	½ cup	105	1
chickpeas	1 cup	285	3

DRIED
cooked	1 cup	269	5

CHICORY

FRESH
greens, raw, chopped	½ cup	21	1
roots, raw, cut up	½ cup	33	tr
witloof, raw	½ cup	7	tr

CHILI

CANNED
Gebhardt Hot w/ Beans	1 cup	470	6
Gebhardt Plain	1 cup	530	5
Gebhardt w/ Beans	1 cup	495	7
Health Valley Mild Vegetarian w/ Beans	5 oz	160	2
Health Valley Mild Vegetarian w/ Beans No Salt Added	5 oz	160	3
Health Valley Mild Vegetarian w/ Lentils	5 oz	140	1
Health Valley Mild Vegetarian w/ Lentils No Salt Added	5 oz	140	1

FOOD	PORTION	CALORIES	IRON
Health Valley Spicy Vegetarian w/ Beans	5 oz	160	3
Healthy Choice Spicy w/ Beans & Ground Turkey	½ can (7.5 oz)	210	3
Healthy Choice Turkey w/ Beans	½ can (7.5 oz)	200	3
Hunt's Chili Beans	4 oz	100	2
Just Rite Hot w/ Beans	4 oz	195	2
Just Rite w/ Beans	4 oz	200	2
Just Rite w/o Beans	4 oz	180	2
Manwich Chili Fixin's, as prep	8 oz	290	5
S&W Chili Beans	½ cup	130	2
S&W Chili Makin's Original	½ cup	100	2
Van Camp's Chili Weenee	1 cup	309	5
Van Camp's Chili w/ Beans	1 cup	352	5
Van Camp's Chili w/o Beans	1 cup	412	3
Wolf Brand Chili-Mac	7.5 oz	317	2
Wolf Brand Extra Spicy w/ Beans	7.5 oz	324	3
Wolf Brand Extra Spicy w/o Beans	7.5 oz	363	4
Wolf Brand Plain	7.5 oz	330	5
Wolf Brand w/ Beans	7.5 oz	345	3
Wolf Brand w/o Beans	1 cup	387	4
chili w/ beans	1 cup	286	9
DRIED			
Gebhardt Chili Quik Seasoning	1 tsp	10	tr
powder	1 tsp	8	tr
FROZEN			
Swanson Homestyle Chili Con Carne	8.25 oz	270	4
TAKE-OUT			
con carne w/ beans	8.9 oz	254	5

FOOD	PORTION	CALORIES	IRON
cooked	½ cup	11	tr

CHIPS

FOOD	PORTION	CALORIES	IRON
CORN			
Health Valley	1 oz	160	tr
Health Valley No Salt Added	1 oz	160	tr
Health Valley w/ Cheddar Cheese	1 oz	160	tr
Snyder's	1 oz	160	tr
Snyder's BBQ	1 oz	160	tr
Snyder's Chili 'n Cheese	1 oz	160	tr
POTATO			
Eagle BBQ Thins	1 oz	150	tr
Eagle Ranch Ridged	1 oz	160	tr
Eagle Ridged	1 oz	150	tr
Eagle Thins	1 oz	150	tr
Eagle Kettle Fry			
BBQ Crunchy	1 oz	150	tr
Cape Cod	1 oz	150	tr
Cape Code No Salt	1 oz	150	tr
Cape Cod Waves	1 oz	150	tr
Cape Cod Waves No Salt	1 oz	150	tr
Dill & Sour Cream	1 oz	150	tr
Dill & Sour Cream No Salt	1 oz	150	tr
Extra Crunchy	1 oz	150	tr
Idaho Russet	1 oz	150	tr
Louisiana BBQ	1 oz	150	tr
Health Valley Country Ripple	1 oz	160	1
Health Valley Country Ripple No Salt Added	1 oz	160	1
Health Valley Dip Chips	1 oz	160	1

FOOD	PORTION	CALORIES	IRON
Health Valley Dip Chips No Salt Added	1 oz	160	1
Health Valley Natural	1 oz	160	1
Health Valley Natural No Salt Added	1 oz	160	1
Kelly's	1 oz	150	tr
Kelly's Bar-B-Q	1 oz	150	tr
Kelly's Crunchy	1 oz	150	tr
Kelly's Rippled	1 oz	150	tr
Kelly's Sour Cream 'n Onion	1 oz	150	tr
Kelly's Unsalted	1 oz	150	tr
Old Dutch Foods	1 oz	150	tr
Old Dutch Foods Au Gratin	1 oz	150	tr
Old Dutch Foods BBQ	1 oz	140	tr
Old Dutch Foods Dill Flavored	1 oz	150	tr
Old Dutch Foods Onion & Garlic	1 oz	150	tr
Old Dutch Foods Ripple	1 oz	150	tr
Old Dutch Foods Sour Cream & Onion	1 oz	150	tr
Snyder's	1 oz	150	tr
Snyder's Au Gratin	1 oz	150	tr
Snyder's BBQ	1 oz	150	tr
Snyder's Cajun	1 oz	150	tr
Snyder's Coney Island	1 oz	150	tr
Snyder's Grilled Steak & Onion	1 oz	150	tr
Snyder's Hot Chili	1 oz	150	tr
Snyder's Kosher Dill	1 oz	150	tr
Snyder's No Salt	1 oz	150	tr
Snyder's Salt & Vinegar	1 oz	150	tr
Snyder's Smokey Bacon	1 oz	150	tr
Snyder's Sour Cream & Onion	1 oz	150	tr

FOOD	PORTION	CALORIES	IRON
Snyder's Sour Cream & Onion Unsalted	1 oz	150	tr
Snyder's Zesty Italian	1 oz	150	tr
potato	1 oz	148	tr
potato	10 chips	105	tr
sticks	1-oz pkg	148	1
sticks	½ cup	94	tr
TORTILLA			
Eagle	1 oz	150	tr
Eagle Nacho	1 oz	150	tr
Eagle Ranch	1 oz	150	tr
Eagle Restaurant Style	1 oz	150	tr
Eagle Strips	1 oz	150	tr
Snyder's	1 oz	140	tr
Snyder's Enchilada	1 oz	140	tr
Snyder's Nacho Cheese	1 oz	140	tr
Snyder's No Salt	1 oz	140	tr
Snyder's Ranch	1 oz	140	tr

CHITTERLINGS

FOOD	PORTION	CALORIES	IRON
pork, simmered	3 oz	258	3
freeze dried	1 tbsp	1	tr
fresh, chopped	1 tbsp	1	tr
fresh, chopped	1 tsp	0	tr

CHOCOLATE

FOOD	PORTION	CALORIES	IRON
BAKING			
Baker's German Sweet	1 oz	143	1
Baker's German Sweet	¼ cup	200	1

FOOD	PORTION	CALORIES	IRON
Baker's Semi-Sweet	1 oz	135	1
Baker's Unsweetened	1 oz	141	2
Hershey Premium Unsweetened	1 oz	190	2
Nestle Pre-Melted Unsweetened	1 oz	190	2
Nestle Semi-Sweet	1 oz	160	1
Nestle Unsweetened	1 oz	180	1
baking	1 oz	145	2
CHIPS Baker's	1 oz	143	tr
Baker's Big Milk Chocolate	¼ cup	239	tr
Baker's Big Semi-Sweet	¼ cup	220	1
Baker's Real Semi-Sweet	¼ cup	198	1
Baker's Semi-Sweet	¼ cup	197	1
Hershey Milk Chocolate	1 oz	150	tr
Hershey Miniature Semi-Sweet	¼ cup	220	1
Hershey Mint Chocolate	¼ cup	230	1
Hershey Semi-Sweet	¼ cup	220	1
Nestle Morsels Mint Chocolate	1 oz	140	tr
Nestle Morsels Semi-Sweet	1 oz	140	tr
Toll House Merry Morsels	1 oz	140	tr
Toll House Morsels Semi-Sweet	1 oz	140	tr
Toll House Treasures Semi-Sweet	1 oz	150	1
MIX powder	2–3 heaping tsp	75	1
powder, as prep w/ whole milk	9 oz	226	1
SYRUP Hershey	2 tbsp	80	tr
chocolate	1 cup	653	6
chocolate	2 tbsp	82	1
chocolate, as prep w/ whole milk	9 oz	232	1

FOOD	PORTION	CALORIES	IRON
CHUTNEY			
apple	1.2 oz	68	tr
apple cranberry	1 tbsp	16	tr
tomato	1.2 oz	54	tr
CILANTRO			
fresh	¼ cup	1	tr
CINNAMON			
ground	1 tsp	6	1
CISCO			
smoked	1 oz	50	tr
smoked	3 oz	151	tr
CLAMS			
CANNED			
Empress Whole Baby	4 oz	60	16
Gorton's Minced & Chopped	½ can	70	3
S&W Fancy Chopped	2 oz	28	1
S&W Whole Baby Chowder Clams	2 oz	33	3
meat only	1 cup	236	45
meat only	3 oz	126	24
FRESH			
cooked	20 sm	133	25
cooked	3 oz	126	24
raw	20 sm	133	25
raw	3 oz	63	12
raw	9 lg	133	25

FOOD	PORTION	CALORIES	IRON
FROZEN			
Fried (Mrs. Paul's)	2.5 oz	200	1
Microwave Crunchy Clam Strips (Gorton's)	3.5 oz	330	1
Microwave Fried Clams (Mrs. Paul's)	2.5 oz	260	1
HOME RECIPE			
breaded & fried	20 sm	379	26
breaded & fried	3 oz	171	12
TAKE-OUT			
breaded & fried	¾ cup	451	3

CLOVES

ground	1 tsp	7	tr

COCOA

Hershey	⅓ cup	120	5
Hershey European Cocoa	1 oz	90	9
Nestle	⅓ cup (1 oz)	80	5
Nestle Hot Cocoa Mix	1 oz	110	tr
Nestle Hot Cocoa Mix, as prep w/ 2% milk	6 oz	210	1
Nestle Hot Cocoa Mix, as prep w/ skim milk	6 oz	180	1
Nestle Hot Cocoa Mix, as prep w/ whole milk	6 oz	230	1
Nestle Hot Cocoa Mix w/ Marshmallows	1 oz	120	1
Nestle Hot Cocoa Mix w/ Marshmallows, as prep w/ 2% milk	6 oz	220	1
Nestle Hot Cocoa Mix w/ Marshmallows, as prep w/ skim milk	6 oz	190	1

FOOD	PORTION	CALORIES	IRON
Nestle Hot Cocoa Mix w/ Marshmallows, as prep w/ whole milk	6 oz	240	1
Swiss Miss Cocoa Diet	4 oz	20	tr
Swiss Miss Cocoa Sugar Free w/ Sugar Free Marshmallows, as prep	6 oz	50	tr
Swiss Miss Cocoa Sugar Free, as prep	6 oz	60	tr
Swiss Miss Hot Cocoa Bavarian Chocolate	6 oz	110	1
Swiss Miss Hot Cocoa Double Rich	4 oz	110	1
Swiss Miss Hot Cocoa Milk Chocolate	6 oz	110	tr
Swiss Miss Hot Cocoa w/ Mini Marshmallows	4 oz	110	tr
Ultra Slim-Fast Hot Cocoa, as prep w/ water	8 oz	190	6
hot cocoa	1 cup	218	1
mix, as prep w/ water	7 oz	103	tr
mix w/ Nutrasweet, as prep w/ water	7 oz	48	1
powder	1 oz	102	tr

COCONUT

FOOD	PORTION	CALORIES	IRON
Angel Flake Toasted (Baker's)	⅓ cup	212	1
Premium Shred (Baker's)	⅓ cup	135	1
coconut water	1 cup	46	1
coconut water	1 tbsp	3	tr
cream, canned	1 cup	568	2
cream, canned	1 tbsp	36	tr
dried, sweetened, flaked	1 cup	351	1
dried, sweetened, flaked	7-oz. pkg	944	4
dried, sweetened, flaked, canned	1 cup	341	1

FOOD	PORTION	CALORIES	IRON
dried, sweetened, shredded	1 cup	466	2
dried, sweetened, shredded	7-oz pkg	997	4
dried, toasted	1 oz	168	1
dried, unsweetened	1 oz	187	1
fresh	1 piece (1.5 oz)	159	1
fresh, shredded	1 cup	283	2
milk, canned	1 cup	445	7
milk, canned	1 tbsp	30	1
milk, frozen	1 cup	486	2
milk, frozen	1 tbsp	30	tr

COD

FOOD	PORTION	CALORIES	IRON
CANNED			
atlantic	1 can (11 oz)	327	2
atlantic	3 oz	89	tr
DRIED			
atlantic	3 oz	246	2
FRESH			
atlantic, cooked	3 oz	89	tr
atlantic fillet, cooked	6.3 oz	189	1
atlantic, raw	3 oz	70	tr
pacific, baked	3 oz	95	tr
FROZEN			
Light Fillets (Mrs. Paul's)	1 fillet	240	1

COFFEE
(*see also* COFFEE SUBSTITUTES)

FOOD	PORTION	CALORIES	IRON
INSTANT			
cappuccino mix, as prep	7 oz	62	tr
decaffeinated	1 rounded tsp	4	tr

FOOD	PORTION	CALORIES	IRON
decaffeinated, as prep	6 oz	4	tr
french mix, as prep	7 oz	57	tr
mocha mix, as prep	7 oz	51	tr
regular	1 rounded tsp	4	tr
regular w/ chicory	1 rounded tsp	6	tr
regular w/ chicory, as prep	6 oz	6	tr
regular, as prep	6 oz	4	tr
REGULAR			
brewed	6 oz	4	tr

COFFEE SUBSTITUTES

Postum Instant	6 oz	11	tr
Postum Instant Coffee Flavored	6 oz	11	tr
powder	1 tsp	9	tr
powder, as prep	6 oz	9	tr
powder, as prep w/ milk	6 oz	121	tr

COFFEE WHITENERS

LIQUID			
nondairy, frzn	1 tbsp	20	tr
POWDER			
nondairy	1 tsp	11	tr

COLLARDS

FRESH			
cooked	½ cup	17	tr
raw, chopped	½ cup	6	tr
FROZEN			
chopped, cooked	½ cup	31	1

FOOD	PORTION	CALORIES	IRON

COOKIES

HOME RECIPE

FOOD	PORTION	CALORIES	IRON
chocolate chip	4 (1.5 oz)	185	1
peanut butter	4 (1.7 oz)	245	1
shortbread	2 (1 oz)	145	1

MIX

FOOD	PORTION	CALORIES	IRON
Chocolate Chip Big Batch (Betty Crocker)	2	120	tr

READY-TO-EAT

FOOD	PORTION	CALORIES	IRON
Almond Crescents (Sunshine)	2	70	tr
Almost Home Oatmeal Raisin (Nabisco)	1	70	tr
Amaranth Cookies (Health Valley)	1	70	tr
Animal Crackers (Sunshine)	7	70	tr
Animal Crackers Barnum's	5	60	tr
Baked Apple Bar (Sunbelt)	1 pkg (1.31 oz)	130	1
Bakers Bonus Oatmeal (Nabisco)	1	80	tr
Bavarian Fingers (Sunshine)	1	70	tr
Beacon Hill Chocolate Chocolate Walnut (Pepperidge Farm)	1	120	1
Brown Edge Wafers (Nabisco)	2½	70	tr
Brownie Chocolate Nut (Pepperidge Farm)	2	110	1
Brownie Nut Large Cookie (Pepperidge Farm)	1	140	tr
Bugs Bunny Graham Cookies (Nabisco)	5	60	tr
Butter Flavored Cookies (Sunshine)	2	60	tr
Buttercup (Keebler)	3	70	tr
Cheyenne Peanut Butter Milk Chocolate Chunk (Pepperidge Farm)	1	110	tr

FOOD	PORTION	CALORIES	IRON
Chip-a-Roos (Sunshine)	1	60	tr
Chips Ahoy! Chocolate Chocolate Chunk	1	90	tr
Chips Ahoy! Chocolate Chocolate Walnut	1	100	tr
Chips Ahoy! Chocolate Chunk Pecan	1	100	tr
Chips Ahoy! Chunky Chocolate Chip	1	90	tr
Chips Ahoy! Mini	6	70	tr
Chips Ahoy! Oatmeal Chocolate Chip	1	90	tr
Chips Ahoy! Striped	1	90	tr
Chocolate Chip (Drake's)	2 (1 oz)	140	tr
Chocolate Chip Snaps (Nabisco)	3	70	tr
Chocolate Chocolate Chip (Drake's)	2 (1 oz)	130	1
Chocolate Cookiesaurus (Sunshine)	7	120	1
Chocolate Fudge Sandwich (Keebler)	1	80	tr
Chocolate Snaps (Nabisco)	4	70	tr
Coconut (Drake's)	2 (1 oz)	130	tr
Coconut Macaroon (Drake's)	1 (1 oz)	135	tr
Commodore (Keebler)	1	60	tr
Cookie Caramel Bars (Little Debbie)	1 pkg (1.17 oz)	170	tr
Cookies Mates (Keebler)	2	50	tr
Cookies 'n Fudge Striped Shortbread	1	60	tr
Cookies 'n Fudge Striped Wafers (Nabisco)	1	70	tr
Devil's Food Cakes (Nabisco)	1	70	tr

FOOD	PORTION	CALORIES	IRON
Dinosaur Grrrahams (Mother's)	1	70	tr
Dixi Vanilla (Sunshine)	2	130	tr
Famous Chocolate Wafers (Nabisco)	2½	70	tr
Fancy Fruit Chunks (Health Valley)			
Apricot Almond	2	90	1
Date Pecan	2	90	1
Raisin Oat Bran	2	70	1
Tropical Fruit	2	90	1
Fancy Peanut Chunks (Health Valley)	2	90	1
Fat Free (Health Valley)			
Apple Spice	3	75	1
Apricot Delight	3	75	1
Date Delight	3	75	1
Hawaiian Fruit	3	75	1
Jumbos Apple Raisin	1	70	1
Jumbos Raisin	1	70	7
Jumbos Raspberry	1	70	1
Raisin Oatmeal	3	75	1
Fiber Jumbos Blueberry Nut (Health Valley)	1	100	1
Fiber Jumbos Chunky Pecan (Health Valley)	1	100	1
Fiber Jumbos Raisin Nut (Health Valley)	1	100	1
Fig Bar (Mother's)	1 oz	100	tr
Fig Newtons (Nabisco)	1	60	tr
Fortune (La Choy)	1	15	tr
French Vanilla Creme (Keebler)	1	80	tr
Fruit & Fitness (Health Valley)	5	200	2

FOOD	PORTION	CALORIES	IRON
Fruit Jumbos Almond Date (Health Valley)	1	70	tr
Fruit Jumbos Oat Bran (Health Valley)	1	70	1
Fruit Jumbos Raisin Nut (Health Valley)	1	70	tr
Fruit Jumbos Tropical Fruit (Health Valley)	1	70	tr
Fudge Family Bears Chocolate w/ Vanilla Filling (Sunshine)	1	70	1
Fudge Family Bears Peanut Butter (Sunshine)	1	70	1
Fudge Family Bears Vanilla w/ Fudge Filling (Sunshine)	1	60	tr
Fudge Striped Shortbread (Sunshine)	3	160	tr
Geneva (Pepperidge Farm)	2	130	tr
Ginger Snaps (Bakery Wagon)	4–5 (1 oz)	140	1
Ginger Snaps (Sunshine)	3	60	tr
Ginger Snaps Old Fashioned (Nabisco)	2	60	1
Golden Fruit (Sunshine)	1	70	tr
Graham (Nabisco)	2	60	tr
Graham Amaranth (Health Valley)	7	110	2
Graham Chocolate (Nabisco)	1	50	tr
Graham Honey (Health Valley)	7	100	1
Graham Honey (Honey Maid)	2	60	tr
Graham Honey Fiber Enriched (Keebler)	2	90	tr
Graham Kitchen Rich (Keebler)	2	60	tr
Graham Oat Bran (Health Valley)	7	120	2
Grahamy Bears (Sunshine)	4	60	tr
Hermit (Drake's)	1 (2 oz)	230	1

FOOD	PORTION	CALORIES	IRON
Heyday Caramel & Peanut (Nabisco)	1	110	tr
Heyday Fudge (Nabisco)	1	110	tr
Honey Jumbos Crisp Cinnamon (Health Valley)	1	70	1
Honey Jumbos Crisp Peanut Butter (Health Valley)	1	70	1
Honey Jumbos Fancy Oat Bran (Health Valley)	2	130	1
Hydrox	1	50	tr
Hydrox Doubles Peanut Butter	1	60	tr
Iced Gingerbread Cookies (Sunshine)	3	70	1
Ideal Bars (Nabisco)	1	90	tr
Jingles (Sunshine)	3	70	tr
Keebies (Keebler)	1	80	tr
Lemon Nut Crunch (Pepperidge Farm)	2	110	tr
Linzer (Pepperidge Farm)	1	120	tr
Lorna Doone	2	70	tr
Mallomars	1	60	tr
Marshmallow Puffs (Nabisco)	1	90	1
Marshmallow Twirls (Nabisco)	1	130	1
Mini Chocolate Chip Cookies (Sunshine)	2	70	tr
Mint Milano (Pepperidge Farm)	2	150	tr
Molasses Iced (Bakery Wagon)	1	100	tr
My Goodness Banana Nut (Nabisco)	1	90	1
My Goodness Chocolate Chip & Raisin (Nabisco)	1	90	tr
My Goodness Oatmeal Raisin (Nabisco)	1	90	1

FOOD	PORTION	CALORIES	IRON
Mystic Mint	1	90	1
Newtons Apple (Nabisco)	1	70	tr
Newtons Raspberry (Nabisco)	1	70	tr
Newtons Strawberry (Nabisco)	1	70	tr
Nilla Wafers (Nabisco)	3½	60	tr
Nutter Butter Peanut Butter (Nabisco)	1	70	tr
Nutter Butter Peanut Creme (Nabisco)	2	80	tr
Oat Bran Animal Cookies (Health Valley)	7	110	1
Oat Bran Fruit & Nut (Health Valley)	2	110	1
Oat Bran w/ Nuts & Raisins (Sunshine)	1	60	tr
Oatmeal (Drake's)	2 (1 oz)	120	tr
Oatmeal Large Cookie (Pepperidge Farm)	1	120	tr
Oatmeal Creme (Drake's)	1 (2 oz)	240	tr
Oatmeal Date Filled (Bakery Wagon)	1	90	tr
Oatmeal Raisin (Pepperidge Farm)	2	110	tr
Oatmeal Soft (Bakery Wagon)	1	100	tr
Old Fashion Double Fudge (Keebler)	1	80	tr
Old Fashion Oatmeal (Keebler)	1	80	tr
Old Fashion Peanut Butter (Keebler)	1	80	tr
Old Fashion Sugar (Keebler)	1	80	tr
Orange Milano (Pepperidge Farm)	2	150	tr
Oreo	1	50	tr
Oreo Big Stuf	1	200	1

FOOD	PORTION	CALORIES	IRON
Oreo Double Stuf	1	70	tr
Oreo Fudge Covered	1	110	1
Oreo Mini	5	70	tr
Orleans (Pepperidge Farm)	3	90	tr
Pantry Molasses (Nabisco)	1	80	1
Peanut Butter Bars (Little Debbie)	1 pkg (1.83 oz)	290	1
Peanut Butter Naturals (Sunbelt)	1 pkg (1.2 oz)	170	1
Peanut Butter Wafers (Drake's)	1 (2.25 oz)	324	tr
Peanut Butter & Jelly Sandwiches (Little Debbie)	1 pkg (1.13 oz)	150	1
Peanut Clusters (Little Debbie)	1 pkg (1.44 oz)	210	1
Pecan Shortbread (Nabisco)	1	80	tr
Pinwheels (Nabisco)	1	130	1
Pitter Patter (Keebler)	1	90	tr
Pure Chocolate Middles (Nabisco)	1	80	tr
School House Cookies (Sunshine)	15	120	1
Sea Flappers (Sunshine)	7	140	tr
Social Tea (Nabisco)	3	70	tr
Suddenly S'Mores (Nabisco)	1	100	tr
Sugar Wafers Chocolate (Sunshine)	2	90	tr
Taffy Creme Sandwich (Mother's)	1–2 (1 oz)	140	tr
Teddy Grahams (Nabisco)			
Bearwich Chocolate w/ Vanilla Creme	4	70	tr
Bearwich Cinnamon w/ Vanilla Creme	4	70	tr
Bearwich Vanilla w/ Chocolate Creme	4	70	tr
Chocolate Graham	11	60	tr
Cinnamon Graham	11	60	tr
Honey Graham	11	60	tr

FOOD	PORTION	CALORIES	IRON
Vanilla Graham	11	60	tr
The Great Tofu (Health Valley)	2	90	2
The Great Wheat Free (Health Valley)	2	80	4
Tru Blu Chocolate (Sunshine)	2	160	1
Tru Blu Lemon (Sunshine)	1	70	tr
Tru Blu Vanilla (Sunshine)	1	8	tr
Vanilla Wafers (Keebler)	4	80	tr
Vienna Fingers (Sunshine)	12	70	tr
animal crackers	1 box (2.4 oz)	299	1
chocolate chip	1 box (1.9 oz)	233	1
chocolate chip	4 (1.5 oz)	180	1
chocolate sandwich	4 (1.4 oz)	195	1
digestive biscuits plain	2	141	1
fig bars	4 (2 oz)	210	1
graham	2 squares	60	tr
oatmeal raisin	4 (1.8 oz)	245	1
shortbread	4 (1 oz)	155	1
vanilla sandwich	4 (1.4 oz)	195	1
vanilla wafers	10 (1.25 oz)	185	1
REFRIGERATED			
Chocolate Chip (Pillsbury)	1	70	0
Oatmeal Raisin (Pillsbury)	1	60	tr
Peanut Butter (Pillsbury)	1	70	0
Sugar (Pillsbury)	1	70	0
chocolate chip	4 (1.7 oz)	225	1
sugar	4 (1.7 oz)	235	1

CORIANDER

leaf, dried	1 tsp	2	tr

FOOD	PORTION	CALORIES	IRON
leaf, fresh	¼ cup	1	tr
seed	1 tsp	5	tr

CORN

FOOD	PORTION	CALORIES	IRON
CANNED			
50% Less Salt No Sugar Added (Green Giant)	½ cup	50	0
Corn (Green Giant)	½ cup	70	tr
Cream Style (Green Giant)	½ cup	100	0
Cream Style Diet (S&W)	½ cup	100	1
Cream Style Premium Homestyle (S&W)	½ cup	105	tr
Deli Corn (Green Giant)	½ cup	80	tr
Golden Kernel 50% Less Salt (Green Giant)	½ cup	70	0
Golden Vacuum Packed (Green Giant)	½ cup	80	tr
Mexi Corn (Green Giant)	½ cup	80	0
No Salt No Sugar (Green Giant)	½ cup	80	tr
Sweet 'n Natural (S&W)	½ cup	90	tr
Sweet Select (Green Giant)	½ cup	60	tr
White Vacuum Packed (Green Giant)	½ cup	80	tr
Whole Kernel Tender Young (S&W)	½ cup	90	tr
cream style	½ cup	93	tr
white	½ cup	66	1
w/ red & green peppers	½ cup	86	1
yellow	½ cup	66	1
FRESH			
on-the-cob, cooked, w/ butter	1 ear	155	tr
white, cooked	½ cup	89	1

FOOD	PORTION	CALORIES	IRON
white, raw	½ cup	66	tr
yellow, cooked	1 ear (2.7 oz)	83	tr
yellow, cooked	½ cup	89	1
yellow, raw	1 ear (3 oz)	77	tr
yellow, raw	½ cup	66	tr
FROZEN			
Big Ears (Birds Eye)	1 ear	160	1
Cob Corn (Ore Ida)	1 ear (5.3 oz)	190	1
Cream Style (Green Giant)	½ cup	110	0
Cut (Big Valley)	3.5 oz	80	tr
Fritters (Mrs. Paul's)	2	240	1
Harvest Fresh Niblets (Green Giant)	½ cup	80	0
Harvest Fresh White Shoepeg (Green Giant)	½ cup	90	0
In Butter Sauce (Birds Eye)	½ cup	90	tr
In Butter Sauce (Green Giant)	½ cup	100	tr
Little Ears (Birds Eye)	2 ears	130	1
Nibblers Corn on the Cob (Green Giant)	2 ears	120	1
Niblet Ears (Green Giant)	1 ear	120	1
Niblets (Green Giant)	½ cup	90	0
On the Cob (Birds Eye)	1 ear	120	1
One Serve Niblets in Butter Sauce (Green Giant)	1 pkg	120	0
One Serve on the Cob (Green Giant)	1 pkg	120	1
Polybag Cut (Birds Eye)	½ cup	80	tr
Polybag Deluxe Tender Sweet (Birds Eye)	½ cup	80	tr
Super Sweet Nibblers Corn on the Cob (Green Giant)	2 ears	90	tr

FOOD	PORTION	CALORIES	IRON
Super Sweet Niblet (Green Giant Select)	½ cup	60	tr
Super Sweet Niblet Ears (Green Giant)	1 ear	90	tr
Sweet (Birds Eye)	½ cup	80	tr
White (Green Giant Select)	½ cup	90	0
White in Butter Sauce (Green Giant)	½ cup	100	2
cooked	½ cup	67	tr
on-the-cob, cooked	1 ear (2.2 oz)	59	tr
TAKE-OUT fritters	1 (1 oz)	62	tr
scalloped	½ cup	258	1

CORNMEAL

FOOD	PORTION	CALORIES	IRON
Aunt Jemima White	3 tbsp	102	1
Aunt Jemima Yellow	3 tbsp	102	1
Quaker White	3 tbsp	102	1
Quaker Yellow	3 tbsp	102	1
corn grits, cooked	1 cup	146	2
corn grits, uncooked	1 cup	579	6
degermed	1 cup	506	6
self-rising degermed	1 cup	489	7
whole grain	1 cup	442	4
HOME RECIPE hush puppies	1 (.75 oz)	74	1
MIX Aunt Jemima Bolted White Mix	3 tbsp	99	1
Aunt Jemima Buttermilk Self-Rising White Mix	3 tbsp	101	1

FOOD	PORTION	CALORIES	IRON
Aunt Jemima Self-Rising White Mix	3 tbsp	98	1
Aunt Jemima Self-Rising Yellow Mix	3 tbsp	100	1
Golden Dipt Corny Dog Batter Mix	1 oz	100	1
Golden Dipt Hush Puppy Jalapeno Mix	1.25 oz	120	1
Golden Dipt Hush Puppy w/ Onion	1.25 oz	120	tr

CORNSTARCH

cornstarch	⅓ cup	164	tr

COTTAGE CHEESE

Lactaid 1%	4 oz	72	tr
Sargento Pot Cheese	1 oz	26	tr
creamed	1 cup	217	tr
creamed	4 oz	117	tr
creamed, w/ fruit	4 oz	140	tr
dry curd	1 cup	123	tr
dry curd	4 oz	96	tr
lowfat 1%	1 cup	164	tr
lowfat 1%	4 oz	82	tr
lowfat 2%	1 cup	203	tr
lowfat 2%	4 oz	101	tr

COTTONSEED

kernels, roasted	1 tbsp	51	1

COUSCOUS

cooked	½ cup	101	tr
dry	½ cup	346	1

FOOD	PORTION	CALORIES	IRON

COWPEAS

CANNED

common	1 cup	184	2

FRESH

leafy tips, chopped, cooked	1 cup	12	1
leafy tips, raw, chopped	1 cup	10	1

FROZEN

cooked	½ cup	112	2

CRAB

CANNED

Dungeness Crab (S&W)	3.25 oz	81	1
blue	1 cup	133	1
blue	3 oz	84	1

FRESH

alaska king, cooked	1 leg (4.7 oz)	129	1
alaska king, cooked	3 oz	82	1
alaska king, raw	1 leg (6 oz)	144	1
alaska king, raw	3 oz	71	1
blue, cooked	1 cup	138	1
blue, cooked	3 oz	87	1
blue, raw	1 crab (.7 oz)	18	tr
blue, raw	3 oz	74	1
dungeness, raw	1 crab (5.7 oz)	140	1
dungeness, raw	3 oz	73	tr

FROZEN

Deviled Crab (Mrs. Paul's)	1 cake	180	1
Deviled Crab Miniatures (Mrs. Paul's)	3.5 oz	240	1

FOOD	PORTION	CALORIES	IRON
READY-TO-USE			
crab cakes	1 cake (2.1 oz)	93	1
TAKE-OUT			
baked	1 (3.8 oz)	160	1
cake	1 (2 oz)	160	1
soft-shell, fried	1 (4.4 oz)	334	2

CRACKER CRUMBS

FOOD	PORTION	CALORIES	IRON
Corn Flake Crumbs (Kellogg's)	¼ cup (1 oz)	100	2
Cracker Meal (Golden Dipt)	1 oz	100	tr
Cracker Meal (Keebler)	1 cup	100	tr
Graham Crumbs (Keebler)	1 cup	520	4
Zesty Meal (Keebler)	1 cup	85	4

CRACKERS

FOOD	PORTION	CALORIES	IRON
American Classic (Nabisco)			
Cracked Wheat	4	70	tr
Dairy Butter	4	70	tr
Golden Sesame	4	70	1
Minced Onion	4	70	tr
Toasted Poppy	4	70	1
Armenian Cracker Bread (Venus)	5	60	tr
Bacon Cheese (Eagle)	1 oz	140	1
Bacon Flavored Thins (Nabisco)	7	70	tr
Better Cheddars (Nabisco)	10	70	tr
Better Cheddars Low Salt (Nabisco)	10	70	tr
Bran Wafers Salt Free (Venus)	5 (.5 oz)	60	tr
Breadflats (J.J. Flats)			
Caraway	1	52	tr
Caraway & Salt	1	51	tr

FOOD	PORTION	CALORIES	IRON
Breadflats *(cont.)*			
Cinnamon	1	53	tr
Flavorall	1	52	tr
Garlic	1	52	tr
Oat Bran	1	49	tr
Onion	1	53	tr
Plain	1	53	tr
Poppy	1	53	tr
Sesame	1	55	tr
Butter Crackers (Goya)	1	40	tr
Cheddar Wedges (Nabisco)	31	70	1
Cheese (Eagle)	1 oz	130	1
Cheese Crackers w/ Peanut Butter (Little Debbie)	1 pkg (.93 oz)	140	1
Cheez 'n Crackers (Handi-Snacks)	1 pkg	120	tr
Cheez 'n Crackers Bacon (Handi-Snacks)	1 pkg	130	tr
Cheez-It	12	70	tr
Cheez-It Low Salt	12	70	tr
Chicken in a Biskit (Nabisco)	7	80	tr
Corn Crackers Salt Free (Venus)	5 (.5 oz)	60	tr
Cracker Wheat Wafers Salt Free (Venus)	5 (.5 oz)	60	tr
Crown Pilot (Nabisco)	1	70	1
Escort (Nabisco)	3	70	tr
Garden Vegetable (Pepperidge Farm)	5	60	tr
Goldfish Cheddar Cheese (Pepperidge Farm)	1 oz	120	tr
Goldfish Cheddar Cheese (Pepperidge Farm)	1 pkg (1.5 oz)	190	tr

FOOD	PORTION	CALORIES	IRON
Goldfish Pizza Flavored (Pepperidge Farm)	1 oz	130	1
Goldfish Pretzel (Pepperidge Farm)	1 oz	110	tr
Goya Crackers	1	30	tr
Harvest Crisps 5 Grain (Nabisco)	6	60	1
Harvest Crisps Oat (Nabisco)	6	60	tr
Harvest Crisps Rice (Nabisco)	6	60	1
Hearty Wheat (Pepperidge Farm)	4	100	tr
Herb Stoned Wheat (Health Valley)	13	55	tr
Herb Stoned Wheat No Salt (Health Valley)	13	55	tr
Krispy Saltine (Sunshine)	5	60	tr
Krispy Unsalted Tops (Sunshine)	5	60	tr
Lavash Wafer Bread (Venus)	2 (.5 oz)	60	tr
Lavash Wafer Bread Sesame (Venus)	2 (.5 oz)	60	tr
Meal Mates Sesame Bread Wafers (Nabisco)	3	70	tr
Melba Rounds (Devonsheer)			
Garlic	.5 oz	56	1
Honey Bran	.5 oz	52	1
Onion	.5 oz	51	tr
Plain	.5 oz	53	1
Plain Unsalted	.5 oz	52	tr
Rye	.5 oz	53	tr
Sesame	.5 oz	57	1
Melba Toast			
Garlic (Keebler)	2	25	tr
Onion (Keebler)	2	25	tr
Plain (Keebler)	2	25	tr
Pumpernickel (Old London)	.5 oz	54	1

FOOD	PORTION	CALORIES	IRON
Melba Toast *(cont.)*			
Rye (Old London)	.5 oz	52	1
Sesame (Keebler)	2	25	tr
Sesame (Old London)	.5 oz	55	1
Sesame Unsalted (Old London)	.5 oz	55	1
Wheat (Old London)	.5 oz	51	1
White (Old London)	.5 oz	51	1
White Unsalted (Old London)	.5 oz	51	1
Whole Grain (Old London)	.5 oz	52	1
Whole Grain Unsalted (Old London)	.5 oz	53	1
Nips Cheese (Nabisco)	13	70	tr
Oat Bran Wafers (Venus)	5 (.5 oz)	60	tr
Oat Bran Wafers Salt Free (Venus)	5 (.5 oz)	60	tr
Oat Bran Krisp (Ralston)	2	60	tr
Oat Thins (Nabisco)	8	70	tr
Oyster Crackers Large (Keebler)	26	80	tr
Oyster Crackers Small (Keebler)	50	80	tr
Oysterettes (Nabisco)	18	60	1
Peanut Butter & Cheese (Eagle)	1 oz	280	1
Peanut Butter 'n Cheez Crackers (Handi-Snacks)	1 pkg	190	1
Premium Plus Saltines Whole Wheat (Nabisco)	5	60	1
Premium Saltine (Nabisco)	5	60	1
Premium Saltine Fat Free (Nabisco)	5	50	1
Premium Saltine Low Salt (Nabisco)	5	60	1
Premium Saltine Unsalted Tops (Nabisco)	5	60	1
Premium Soup & Oyster (Nabisco)	20	60	1

FOOD	PORTION	CALORIES	IRON
Rice Bran (Health Valley)	7	130	2
Ritz (Nabisco)	4	70	tr
Ritz Bits (Nabisco)	22	70	tr
Ritz Bits Cheese (Nabisco)	22	70	tr
Ritz Bits Cheese Sandwiches (Nabisco)	6	80	tr
Ritz Bits Low Salt (Nabisco)	22	70	tr
Ritz Bits Peanut Butter Sandwiches (Nabisco)	6	80	tr
Ritz Low Salt (Nabisco)	4	70	tr
Ritz Whole Wheat (Nabisco)	5	70	tr
Rounds Bacon (Old London)	.5 oz	53	1
Rounds Garlic (Old London)	.5 oz	56	1
Rounds Onion (Old London)	.5 oz	52	1
Rounds Rye (Old London)	.5 oz	52	1
Rounds Sesame (Old London)	.5 oz	56	1
Rounds White (Old London)	.5 oz	48	1
Rounds Whole Grain (Old London)	.5 oz	54	1
Royal Lunch (Nabisco)	1	60	tr
Rye Wafers Salt Free (Venus)	5 (.5 oz)	60	tr
Rykrisp Natural	2	40	tr
Rykrisp Seasoned	2	45	tr
Rykrisp Seasoned Twindividuals	2	45	tr
Rykrisp Sesame	2	50	tr
Sesame (Pepperidge Farm)	4	80	tr
Sesame Stoned Wheat (Health Valley)	13	55	tr
Sesame Stoned Wheat No Salt Added (Health Valley)	13	55	tr
Seven Grain Vegetable Stoned Wheat (Health Valley)	13	55	tr

FOOD	PORTION	CALORIES	IRON
Seven Grain Vegetable Stoned Wheat No Salt Added (Health Valley)	13	55	tr
Snack Mix Classic (Pepperidge Farm)	1 oz	140	1
Snack Mix Lightly Smoked (Pepperidge Farm)	1 oz	150	tr
Snack Sticks Pumpernickel (Pepperidge Farm)	8	140	1
Snack Sticks Sesame (Pepperidge Farm)	8	140	1
Sociables (Nabisco)	6	70	tr
Stoned Wheat (Health Valley)	13	55	tr
Stoned Wheat No Salt Added (Health Valley)	13	55	tr
Swiss Cheese (Nabisco)	7	70	tr
Tam Tams (Manischewitz)	10	147	1
Tam Tams No Salt (Manischewitz)	10	138	1
Tams Garlic (Manischewitz)	10	153	1
Tams Onion (Manischewitz)	10	150	1
Tams Wheat (Manischewitz)	10	150	1
Tid Bits Cheese (Nabisco)	15	70	tr
Toast Peanut Butter Sandwich (Planters)	6 (1.4 oz)	200	1
Toasty Crackers w/ Peanut Butter (Little Debbie)	1 pkg (.93 oz)	140	1
Triscuit (Nabisco)	3	60	tr
Triscuit Bits (Nabisco)	15	60	tr
Triscuit Deli-Style Rye (Nabisco)	3	60	tr
Triscuit Low Salt (Nabisco)	3	60	tr
Triscuit Wheat 'n Bran (Nabisco)	3	60	tr
Twigs Sesame & Cheese Sticks (Nabisco)	5	70	tr

FOOD	PORTION	CALORIES	IRON
Uneeda Biscuit Unsalted Tops (Nabisco)	2	60	1
Vegetable Thins (Nabisco)	7	70	tr
Water Crackers Fat Free (Venus)	5 (.5 oz)	55	1
Waverly (Nabisco)	4	70	tr
Waverly Low Salt (Nabisco)	4	70	tr
Wheat Thins (Nabisco)	8	70	tr
Wheat Thins Low Salt (Nabisco)	8	70	tr
Wheat Thins Nutty (Nabisco)	7	70	tr
Wheat Wafers (Venus)	5 (.5 oz)	60	tr
Wheat Wafers Salt Free (Venus)	5 (.5 oz)	60	tr
Wheatsworth Stone Ground (Nabisco)	4	70	1
Zings! (Nabisco)	15	70	tr
Zwieback (Nabisco)	2	60	tr
cheese	10 (.33 oz)	50	tr
crispbread	3	61	tr
crispbread rye	3	77	1
melba toast plain	1	20	tr
peanut butter sandwich	1 (.33 oz)	40	tr
saltines	4	50	1
water biscuits	3	92	tr
zwieback	3.5 oz	374	2

CRANBERRIES

CANNED			
sauce sweetened	½ cup	209	tr
FRESH			
chopped	1 cup	54	tr

FOOD	PORTION	CALORIES	IRON
JUICE			
Smucker's Juice Sparkler	10 oz	140	tr
Veryfine	8 oz	160	1
cranberry juice cocktail	1 cup	147	tr
cranberry juice cocktail	6 oz	108	tr
cranberry juice cocktail low calorie	6 oz	33	tr
cranberry juice cocktail, frzn	12-oz can	821	1
cranberry juice cocktail, frzn, as prep	6 oz	102	tr

CRANBERRY BEANS

FOOD	PORTION	CALORIES	IRON
CANNED			
cranberry beans	1 cup	216	4
DRIED			
cooked	1 cup	240	4

CRAYFISH

FOOD	PORTION	CALORIES	IRON
cooked	3 oz	97	3
raw	3 oz	76	2

CREAM

FOOD	PORTION	CALORIES	IRON
LIQUID			
half & half	1 cup	315	tr
half & half	1 tbsp	20	tr
heavy whipping	1 tbsp	52	tr
light coffee	1 cup	496	tr
light coffee	1 tbsp	29	tr
light whipping	1 tbsp	44	tr
WHIPPED			
heavy whipping	1 cup	411	tr
light whipping	1 cup	345	tr

FOOD	PORTION	CALORIES	IRON

CREAM CHEESE

neufchatel	1 oz	74	tr
neufchatel	1 pkg (3 oz)	221	tr

REGULAR
cream cheese	1 oz	99	tr
cream cheese	1 pkg (3 oz)	297	1

CREAM OF TARTAR

cream of tartar	1 tsp	8	tr

CRESS

garden, cooked	½ cup	16	1
garden, raw	½ cup	8	tr

CROAKER

FRESH
atlantic, breaded & fried	3 oz	188	1
atlantic, raw	3 oz	89	tr

CROISSANT

All Butter (Sara Lee)	1	170	1
All Butter Petite Size (Sara Lee)	1	120	1
Croissant Sandwich Quartet (Pepperidge Farm)	1	170	1
Petite All Butter (Pepperidge Farm)	1	120	1
croissant	1 (2 oz)	235	2

TAKE-OUT
w/ egg & cheese	1	369	2
w/ egg, cheese & bacon	1	413	2
w/ egg, cheese & ham	1	475	2
w/ egg, cheese & sausage	1	524	3

FOOD	PORTION	CALORIES	IRON

CROUTONS

FOOD	PORTION	CALORIES	IRON
Arnold Crispy Cheddar Romano	.5 oz	64	tr
Arnold Crispy Cheese Garlic	.5 oz	60	1
Arnold Crispy Fine Herbs	.5 oz	53	1
Brownberry Caesar Salad	.5 oz	62	tr
Brownberry Cheddar Cheese	.5 oz	63	tr
Brownberry Onion & Garlic	.5 oz	60	1
Brownberry Seasoned	.5 oz	59	1
Brownberry Toasted	.5 oz	56	1
Kellogg's Croutettes	1 cup (1 oz)	100	2
Pepperidge Farm Cheddar & Romano Cheese	.5 oz	60	1
Pepperidge Farm Cheese & Garlic	.5 oz	70	tr
Pepperidge Farm Onion & Garlic	.5 oz	70	tr
Pepperidge Farm Seasoned	.5 oz	70	tr
Pepperidge Farm Sour Cream & Chives	.5 oz	70	tr

CUCUMBER

FOOD	PORTION	CALORIES	IRON
FRESH			
raw	1 (11 oz)	39	1
raw, sliced	½ cup	7	tr

CUMIN

FOOD	PORTION	CALORIES	IRON
seed	1 tsp	8	1

CURRANTS

FOOD	PORTION	CALORIES	IRON
DRIED			
zante	½ cup	204	2
FRESH			
black	½ cup	36	1

FOOD	PORTION	CALORIES	IRON
JUICE			
black currant nectar	3.5 oz	55	tr
red currant nectar	3.5 oz	54	tr
CUSK			
fresh fillet, baked	3 oz	106	1
CUSTARD			
Flan (Jell-O)	½ cup	151	tr
Golden Egg Americana (Jell-O)	½ cup	160	tr
baked	1 cup	305	1
CUTTLEFISH			
steamed	3 oz	134	9
DANDELION GREENS			
fresh, cooked	½ cup	17	1
raw, chopped	½ cup	13	1
DANISH PASTRY			
FROZEN			
Apple (Pepperidge Farm)	1	220	1
Apple (Sara Lee)	1	120	1
Apple Danish Twist (Sara Lee)	1 slice (1.9 oz)	190	1
Apple Free & Light (Sara Lee)	1 slice (2 oz)	130	1
Cheese (Pepperidge Farm)	1	240	1
Cheese (Sara Lee)	1	130	tr
Cheese Danish Twist (Sara Lee)	1 slice (1.9 oz)	200	1
Cinnamon Raisin (Pepperidge Farm)	1	250	1
Cinnamon Raisin (Sara Lee)	1	150	1

FOOD	PORTION	CALORIES	IRON
Raspberry (Pepperidge Farm)	1	220	1
Raspberry Danish Twist (Sara Lee)	1 slice (1.9 oz)	200	1
READY-TO-EAT			
cheese	1 (3 oz)	353	2
cinnamon	1 (3 oz)	349	2
fruit	1 (2.3 oz)	235	1
fruit	1 (3.3 oz)	335	1
plain	1 (2 oz)	220	1
plain ring	1 (12 oz)	1305	7
REFRIGERATED			
Caramel Danish w/ Nuts (Pillsbury)	1	160	1
Cinnamon Raisin Danish w/ Icing (Pillsbury)	1	150	tr
Orange Danish w/ Icing (Pillsbury)	1	150	1

DATES

DRIED			
Bordo Diced	2 oz	203	5
Dole Chopped	½ cup	280	1
Dole Pitted	½ cup	280	1
Dromedary Chopped	¼ cup	130	1
Dromedary Pitted	5	100	1
chopped	1 cup	489	2
whole	10	228	1

DILL

seed	1 tsp	6	tr
weed, dry	1 tsp	3	tr

FOOD	PORTION	CALORIES	IRON

DINNERS

FROZEN

Armour Classics

FOOD	PORTION	CALORIES	IRON
Chicken & Noodles	11 oz	230	2
Chicken Fettucini	11 oz	260	2
Chicken Mesquite	9.5 oz	370	2
Chicken Parmigiana	11.5 oz	370	3
Chicken w/ Wine & Mushroom Sauce	10.75 oz	280	1
Glazed Chicken	10.75 oz	300	2
Meat Loaf	11.25 oz	360	4
Salisbury Parmigiana	11.5 oz	410	5
Salisbury Steak	11.25 oz	350	5
Swedish Meatballs	11.25 oz	330	3
Turkey w/ Dressing & Gravy	11.5 oz	320	3
Veal Parmigiana	11.25 oz	400	4

Armour Lite

FOOD	PORTION	CALORIES	IRON
Beef Pepper Steak	11.25 oz	220	2
Beef Stroganoff	11.25 oz	250	3
Chicken a la King	11.25 oz	290	2
Chicken Burgundy	10 oz	210	2
Chicken Marsala	10.5 oz	250	3
Chicken Oriental	10 oz	180	2
Salisbury Steak	11.5 oz	300	5
Shrimp Creole	11.25 oz	260	3
Sweet & Sour Chicken	11 oz	240	1

Banquet

FOOD	PORTION	CALORIES	IRON
Boneless Chicken Drum Snacker Platter	7 oz	290	1
Southern Fried Chicken Platter	8.75 oz	400	5
White Meat Fried Chicken Platter	8.75 oz	390	2

FOOD	PORTION	CALORIES	IRON
Banquet *(cont.)*			
White Meat Hot 'n Spicy Fried Chicken Platter	9 oz	440	3
Banquet Extra Helping			
Beef Dinner	15.5 oz	430	5
Chicken Nuggets w/ Barbecue Sauce	10 oz	540	3
Chicken Nuggets w/ Sweet & Sour Sauce	10 oz	540	3
Fried Chicken All White Meat	14.25 oz	760	3
Fried Chicken Dinner	14.25 oz	790	4
Meat Loaf	16.25 oz	640	5
Mexican Style Dinner	19 oz	680	8
Salisbury Steak Dinner	16.25 oz	590	4
Southern Fried Chicken Dinner	13.25 oz	790	5
Turkey Dinner	17 oz	460	4
Birds Eye Easy Recipe Beef Burgundy, not prep	½ pkg	120	2
Birds Eye Easy Recipe Beef Fajitas, not prep	½ pkg	80	1
Budget Gourmet			
Beef Cantonese	1 pkg	260	1
Beef Stroganoff	1 pkg	290	1
Breast of Chicken in Wine Sauce	1 pkg	250	1
Chicken Cacciatore	1 pkg	470	2
Chicken & Egg Noodle w/ Broccoli	1 pkg	440	2
Chicken au Gratin	1 pkg	250	1
Chicken Marsala	1 pkg	270	2
Chicken w/ Fettucini	1 pkg	400	1
French Recipe Chicken	1 pkg	240	tr
Glazed Turkey	1 pkg	270	tr

FOOD	PORTION	CALORIES	IRON
Ham & Asparagus au Gratin	1 pkg	290	1
Mandarin Chicken	1 pkg	300	tr
Orange Glazed Chicken	1 pkg	250	1
Oriental Beef	1 pkg	290	1
Pepper Steak w/ Rice	1 pkg	330	1
Roast Chicken w/ Herb Gravy	1 pkg	270	1
Roast Sirloin Supreme	1 pkg	320	2
Scallops & Shrimp Marinara	1 pkg	330	tr
Seafood Newburg	1 pkg	350	1
Sirloin Beef in Herb Sauce	1 pkg	270	1
Sirloin Cheddar Melt	1 pkg	390	2
Sirloin Salisbury Steak	1 pkg	260	6
Sirloin Salisbury Steak Dinner	1 pkg	450	2
Sirloin Tips in Burgundy Sauce	1 pkg	340	1
Sirloin Tips w/ Country Vegetables	1 pkg	300	2
Sliced Turkey Breast w/ Herb Gravy	1 pkg	290	1
Swedish Meatballs w/ Noodles	1 pkg	580	2
Sweet & Sour Chicken	1 pkg	340	1
Swiss Steak w/ Zesty Tomato Sauce	1 pkg	410	2
Turkey a la King w/ Rice	1 pkg	390	1
Veal Parmigiana	1 pkg	490	2
Yankee Pot Roast	1 pkg	360	2
Budget Gourmet Light & Healthy Chicken Breast Parmigiana	1 pkg	260	1
Herbed Chicken Breast w/ Fettucini	1 pkg	240	2
Italian Style Meatloaf	1 pkg	270	3
Pot Roast	1 pkg	210	2
Sirloin Beef in Wine Sauce	1 pkg	230	2

FOOD	PORTION	CALORIES	IRON
Budget Gourmet Light & Healthy *(cont.)*			
Sirloin Salisbury Steak	1 pkg	260	2
Special Recipe Sirloin of Beef	1 pkg	250	2
Stuffed Turkey Breast	1 pkg	230	1
Teriyaki Chicken Breast	1 pkg	310	1
Dining Light			
Chicken a la King	9 oz	240	1
Chicken w/ Noodles	9 oz	240	2
Salisbury Steak	9 oz	200	4
Sauce & Swedish Meatballs	9 oz	280	2
Healthy Choice			
Barbecue Beef Ribs	11 oz	330	2
Beef Pepper Steak	11 oz	290	2
Breast of Turkey	10.5 oz	290	2
Cacciatore Chicken	12.5 oz	310	3
Chicken a l'Orange	9 oz	240	1
Chicken & Pasta Divan	11.5 oz	310	2
Chicken & Vegetables	11.5 oz	210	3
Chicken Dijon	11 oz	260	1
Chicken Oriental	11.25 oz	230	2
Chicken Parmigiana	11.5 oz	270	3
Glazed Chicken	8.5 oz	220	1
Herb Roasted Chicken	12.3 oz	290	2
Lemon Pepper Fish	10.7 oz	300	1
Mandarin Chicken	11 oz	260	2
Mesquite Chicken	10.5 oz	340	2
Roasted Turkey & Mushroom Gravy	8.5 oz	200	1
Salisbury Steak	11.5 oz	300	3
Salisbury Steak w/ Mushroom Gravy	11 oz	280	3

FOOD	PORTION	CALORIES	IRON
Salsa Chicken	11.25 oz	240	1
Seafood Newburg	8 oz	200	1
Shrimp Creole	11.25 oz	230	2
Shrimp Marinara	10.25 oz	260	3
Sirloin Beef w/ Barbecue Sauce	11 oz	300	2
Sirloin Tips	11.75 oz	280	3
Sliced Turkey w/ Gravy & Dressing	10 oz	270	2
Sole au Gratin	11 oz	270	1
Sole w/ Lemon Butter	8.25 oz	230	1
Sweet & Sour Chicken	11.5 oz	280	1
Turkey Tetrazzini	12.6 oz	340	2
Yankee Pot Roast	11 oz	250	2
Kid Cuisine			
Chicken Nuggets	6.8 oz	360	2
Chicken Sandwich	8.2 oz	470	3
Fried Chicken	7.5 oz	430	1
Hot Dogs w/ Buns	6.7 oz	450	5
Mexican Style	5.7 oz	290	2
Le Menu			
Beef Sirloin Tips	11.5 oz	400	4
Beef Stroganoff	10 oz	430	3
Chicken a la King	10.25 oz	330	1
Chicken Cordon Bleu	11 oz	460	1
Chicken in Wine Sauce	10 oz	280	2
Chicken Parmigiana	11.75 oz	410	3
Chopped Sirloin Beef	12.25 oz	430	4
Ham Steak	10 oz	300	2
Pepper Steak	11.5 oz	370	4
Salisbury Steak	10.5 oz	370	3

FOOD	PORTION	CALORIES	IRON
Le Menu *(cont.)*			
Sliced Breast of Turkey w/ Mushroom Gravy	10.5 oz	300	1
Sweet & Sour Chicken	11.25 oz	400	2
Veal Parmigiana	11.5 oz	390	3
Yankee Pot Roast	10 oz	330	4
Le Menu Entree LightStyle			
Chicken a la King	8.25 oz	240	1
Chicken Dijon	8 oz	240	1
Empress Chicken	8.25 oz	210	1
Glazed Turkey	8.25 oz	260	1
Herb Roast Chicken	7.75 oz	260	1
Swedish Meatballs	8 oz	260	3
Traditional Turkey	8 oz	200	3
Le Menu LightStyle			
Glazed Chicken Breast	10 oz	230	1
Herb Roasted Chicken	10 oz	240	1
Salisbury Steak	10 oz	280	3
Sliced Turkey	10 oz	210	1
Sweet & Sour Chicken	10 oz	250	1
Turkey Divan	10 oz	260	1
Veal Marsala	10 oz	230	1
Lean Cuisine			
Beefsteak Ranchero	9.25 oz	260	1
Breaded Breast of Chicken Parmesan	10.88 oz	270	2
Breast of Chicken Marsala w/ Vegetables	8.13 oz	190	1
Chicken a l'Orange w/ Almond Rice	8 oz	280	1
Chicken & Vegetables w/ Vermicelli	11.75 oz	250	2

FOOD	PORTION	CALORIES	IRON
Chicken Cacciatore w/ Vermicelli	10.88 oz	280	1
Chicken in Barbecue Sauce	8.75 oz	260	1
Chicken Italiano	9 oz	290	1
Chicken Oriental w/ Vegetables & Vermicelli	9 oz	280	2
Chicken Tenderloins in Herb Cream Sauce	9.5 oz	240	1
Chicken Tenderloins in Peanut Sauce	9 oz	290	2
Fiesta Chicken	8.5 oz	240	tr
Fillet of Fish Divan	10.38 oz	210	1
Fillet of Fish Florentine	9.63 oz	220	1
Glaxed Chicken w/ Vegetable Rice	8.5 oz	260	tr
Homestyle Turkey w/ Vegetables & Pasta	9.38 oz	230	1
Oriental Beef w/ Vegetables & Rice	8.63 oz	290	2
Salisbury Steak w/ Gravy & Scalloped Potatoes	9.5 oz	240	3
Sliced Turkey Breast in Mushroom Sauce	8 oz	220	1
Sliced Turkey Breast w/ Dressing	7.88 oz	200	1
Stuffed Cabbage w/ Meat in Tomato Sauce	10.75 oz	210	3
Swedish Meatballs in Gravy w/ Pasta	9.13 oz	290	4
Turkey Dijon	9.5 oz	230	1
Morton			
Beans & Franks w/ Sauce	8.5 oz	300	3
Fish w/ Mashed Potatoes & Carrots	9.25 oz	350	2
Glazed Ham	8 oz	230	1
Gravy & Charbroiled Beef Patty	9 oz	270	2

FOOD	PORTION	CALORIES	IRON
Morton *(cont.)*			
Gravy & Salisbury Steak	9 oz	270	2
Tomato Sauce & Meatloaf	9 oz	280	2
Veal Parmagian	8.75 oz	230	2
Swanson			
Beans & Franks	10.5 oz	440	4
Beef	11.25 oz	310	5
Beef in Barbecue Sauce	11 oz	460	5
Chopped Sirloin Beef	10.75 oz	340	3
Fish 'n' Chips	10 oz	500	2
Fried Chicken Dark Meat	9.75 oz	560	3
Fried Chicken White Meat	10.25 oz	550	3
Loin of Pork	10.75 oz	280	1
Macaroni & Beef	12 oz	370	2
Meatloaf	10.75 oz	360	4
Noodles & Chicken	10.5 oz	280	1
Salisbury Steak	10.75 oz	400	3
Swedish Meatballs	8.5 oz	360	3
Swiss Steak	10 oz	350	4
Turkey	11.5 oz	350	2
Veal Parmigiana	12.25 oz	430	3
Western Style	11.5 oz	430	4
Swanson Homestyle			
Chicken Cacciatore	10.95 oz	260	3
Chicken Nibbles	4.25 oz	340	1
Fish & Fries	6.5 oz	340	2
Fried Chicken	7 oz	390	2
Salisbury Steak	10 oz	320	3
Scalloped Potatoes & Ham	9 oz	300	2
Seafood Creole w/ Rice	9 oz	240	1

FOOD	PORTION	CALORIES	IRON
Sirloin Tips in Burgundy Sauce	7 oz	160	2
Turkey w/ Dressing & Potatoes	9 oz	290	2
Veal Parmigiana	10 oz	330	2
Swanson Hungry-Man			
Boneless Chicken	17.75 oz	700	5
Chopped Beef Steak	16.75 oz	640	5
Fried Chicken Dark Meat	14.25 oz	860	4
Fried Chicken White Meat	14.25 oz	870	4
Salisbury Steak	16.5 oz	680	6
Sliced Beef	15.25 oz	450	5
Turkey	17 oz	550	5
Veal Parmigiana	10.25 oz	590	5
Ultra Slim-Fast			
Beef Pepper Steak	12 oz	270	1
Chicken & Vegetable	12 oz	290	4
Chicken Fettucini	12 oz	380	3
Country Style Vegetable & Beef Tips	12 oz	230	2
Mesquite Chicken	12 oz	360	2
Roasted Chicken in Mushroom Sauce	12 oz	280	1
Shrimp Creole	12 oz	240	1
Shrimp Marinara	12 oz	290	4
Sweet & Sour Chicken	12 oz	330	1
Turkey Medallions in Herb Sauce	12 oz	280	1

DIP

Bean (Eagle)	1 oz	35	tr

DOCK

fresh, cooked	3.5 oz	20	2
raw, chopped	½ cup	15	2

FOOD	PORTION	CALORIES	IRON
DOGFISH			
raw	3.5 oz	193	1
DOLPHINFISH			
fresh, baked	3 oz	93	1
fresh fillet, baked	5.6 oz	174	2
DOUGHNUTS			
Donut Sticks (Little Debbie)	1 pkg (1.67 oz)	200	1
Old Fashion Donuts (Drake's)	1 (1.7 oz)	182	1
Powdered Sugar Donut Delites (Drake's)	7 (2.5 oz)	300	1
cake type	1 (1.8 oz)	210	1
glazed	1 (2 oz)	235	1
jelly	1	235	1
DRINK MIXERS			
Bloody Mary Mix (Libby's)	6 oz	40	2
Bloody Mary Mix (Tabasco)	6 oz	56	1
whiskey sour mix	2 oz	55	tr
DRUM			
FRESH			
freshwater, baked	3 oz	130	1
freshwater fillet, baked	5.4 oz	236	2
DUCK			
w/ skin, roasted	½ duck (13.4 oz)	1287	10
w/ skin, roasted	6 oz	583	5
w/o skin, roasted	½ duck (7.8 oz)	445	6

FOOD	PORTION	CALORIES	IRON
w/o skin, roasted	3.5 oz	201	3
wild breast w/o skin, raw	½ breast (2.9 oz)	102	4
wild w/ skin, raw	½ duck (9.5 oz)	571	11

DUMPLING

FROZEN
Apple Dumpling (Pepperidge Farm)	1 (3 oz)	260	tr

DURIAN

fresh	3.5 oz	141	1

EEL

FRESH
cooked	3 oz	200	1
fillet, cooked	5.6 oz	375	1
raw	3 oz	156	tr

EGG

(see also EGG DISHES, EGG SUBSTITUTES)

CHICKEN
Simply Eggs Reduced Cholesterol	1.75 oz	70	1
fried w/ margarine	1	91	1
frozen	1	75	1
frozen	1 cup	363	4
hard cooked	1	77	1
hard cooked, chopped	1 cup	210	2
poached	1	74	1
raw	1	75	1
scrambled plain	2	200	2

FOOD	PORTION	CALORIES	IRON
scrambled w/ whole milk & margarine	1	101	1
scrambled w/ whole milk & margarine	1 cup	365	3
white only	1	17	tr
white only	1 cup	121	tr
OTHER POULTRY duck, raw	1	130	3
quail, raw	1	14	tr
turkey, raw	1	135	3

EGG DISHES

FROZEN

Great Starts

FOOD	PORTION	CALORIES	IRON
Egg, Sausage & Cheese	5.5 oz	460	2
Omelet w/ Cheese & Ham	7 oz	390	2
Reduced Cholesterol Eggs w/ Mini Oatbran Muffins	4.75 oz	250	1
Scrambled Eggs w/ Bacon & Home Fries	5.6 oz	340	2
Scrambled Eggs w/ Cheese & Cinnamon Pancakes	3.4 oz	290	2
Scrambled Eggs w/ Home Fries	4.6 oz	260	1
Scrambled Eggs w/ Sausage & Hash Browns	6.5 oz	430	2
Quaker Scrambled Eggs & Cheddar Cheese w/ Fried Potatoes	1 pkg (5.9 oz)	250	1
Quaker Scrambled Eggs & Sausage w/ Hash Browns	1 pkg (5.7 oz)	290	1
Quaker Scrambled Eggs & Sausage w/ Pancakes	1 pkg (5.2 oz)	270	3

FOOD	PORTION	CALORIES	IRON
HOME RECIPE			
deviled	2 halves	145	1
TAKE-OUT			
salad	½ cup	307	2
sandwich w/ cheese	1	340	3
sandwich w/ cheese & ham	1	348	3
scotch egg	1 (4.2 oz)	301	2

EGG SUBSTITUTES

Egg Beaters	¼ cup	25	1
Egg Beaters Cheese Omelet	½ cup	110	2
Egg Beaters Vegetable Omelet	½ cup	50	1
Egg Watchers	2 oz	50	1
Healthy Choice Cholesterol Free	¼ cup	30	1
frozen	1 cup	384	5
frozen	¼ cup	96	1
liquid	1.5 oz	40	1
liquid	1 cup	211	5
powder	.35 oz	44	tr
powder	.7 oz	88	1

EGGNOG

eggnog	1 cup	342	1
eggnog	1 qt	1368	2
eggnog flavor mix, as prep w/ milk	9 oz	260	tr

EGGPLANT

FRESH			
cubed, cooked	½ cup	13	tr
raw, cut up	½ cup	11	tr

FOOD	PORTION	CALORIES	IRON
FROZEN			
Parmigiana (Mrs. Paul's)	5 oz	240	1

ELDERBERRIES

fresh	1 cup	105	2

ELK

roasted	3 oz	124	3

ENDIVE

fresh	3.5 oz	9	1
raw, chopped	½ cup	4	tr

ENGLISH MUFFIN

FROZEN			
Great Starts Egg, Beefsteak & Cheese	5.9 oz	360	3
Great Starts Egg, Canadian Bacon & Cheese	4.1 oz	290	3
Healthy Choice English Muffin Sandwich	1 (4.5 oz)	200	4
Healthy Choice Turkey Sausage Omelet on English Muffin	1 (4.75 oz)	210	4
Healthy Choice Western Style Omelet on English Muffin	1 (4.75 oz)	200	4
HOME RECIPE			
cinnamon raisin	1	186	2
english muffin	1	158	2
honey bran	1	153	2
whole wheat	1	167	1
READY-TO-USE			
Matthew's 9 Grain & Nut	1	140	2

FOOD	PORTION	CALORIES	IRON
Matthew's Cinnamon Raisin	1	160	3
Matthew's Golden White	1	140	1
Matthew's Whole Wheat	1	150	2
Pepperidge Farm Cinnamon Apple	1	140	1
Pepperidge Farm Cinnamon Chip	1	160	1
Pepperidge Farm Cinnamon Raisin	1	150	1
Pepperidge Farm Plain	1	140	1
Pepperidge Farm Sourdough	1	135	2
Thomas'	1	130	1
Thomas' Honey Wheat	1	128	1
Thomas' Oat Bran	1	116	1
Thomas' Raisin Cinnamon	1	151	1
Thomas' Sourdough	1	131	1
apple cinnamon	1	138	1
granola	1	155	2
mixed grain	1	155	2
plain	1	134	1
plain, toasted	1	133	1
raisin cinnamon	1	138	1
sourdough	1	134	1
wheat	1	127	2
whole wheat	1	134	2
TAKE-OUT			
w/ butter	1	189	2
w/ cheese & sausage	1	394	2
w/ egg, cheese & bacon	1	487	3
w/ egg, cheese & canadian bacon	1	383	3

EPPAW

FOOD	PORTION	CALORIES	IRON
raw	½ cup	75	1

FOOD	PORTION	CALORIES	IRON

FALAFEL

FOOD	PORTION	CALORIES	IRON
falafel	1 (1.2 oz)	57	1
falafel	3 (1.8 oz)	170	2

FAT

FOOD	PORTION	CALORIES	IRON
Wesson Shortening	1 tbsp	100	0
beef, cooked	1 oz	193	tr
new zealand lamb, raw	1 oz	182	tr
pork, cooked	1 oz	200	tr
salt pork	1 oz	212	tr

FEIJOA

FOOD	PORTION	CALORIES	IRON
fresh	1 (1.75 oz)	25	tr
puree	1 cup	119	tr

FENNEL

FOOD	PORTION	CALORIES	IRON
seed	1 tsp	7	tr

FENUGREEK

FOOD	PORTION	CALORIES	IRON
seed	1 tsp	12	1

FIBER

FOOD	PORTION	CALORIES	IRON
Natural Delta Fiber	½ cup (1 oz)	20	5

FIGS

CANNED

FOOD	PORTION	CALORIES	IRON
Kadota Figs Whole Fancy (S&W)	½ cup	100	tr
in heavy syrup	3	75	tr
in light syrup	3	58	tr
water pack	3	42	tr

FOOD	PORTION	CALORIES	IRON
DRIED			
cooked	½ cup	140	1
whole	10	477	4
FRESH			
fig	1 med	50	tr

FILBERTS

dried, blanched	1 oz	191	1
dried, unblanched	1 oz	179	1
dry roasted, unblanched	1 oz	188	1
oil roasted, unblanched	1 oz	187	1

FISH
(*see also individual fish names*)

FROZEN			
Gorton's			
Crispy Batter Dipped Fillets	2	290	tr
Cripsy Batter Sticks	4	260	tr
Crunch Fillets	2	230	tr
Crunchy Sticks	4	210	tr
Light Recipe Lightly Breaded Fish Fillets	1	180	tr
Light Recipe Tempura Fillets	1	200	tr
Microwave Fillets	2	340	tr
Microwave Larger Cut Fillets	1	320	1
Microwave Larger Cut Ranch Fillets	1	330	tr
Microwave Sticks	6	340	1
Potato Crisp Fillets	2	300	1
Potato Crisp Sticks	4	260	tr
Value Pack Portions	1 portion	180	tr

FOOD	PORTION	CALORIES	IRON
Mrs. Paul's			
40 Crunchy Fish Sticks	4 (2.75 oz)	200	tr
Batter Dipped Fish Fillets	2	330	tr
Battered Fish Portions	2 portions	300	1
Battered Fish Sticks	4	210	1
Combination Seafood Platter	9 oz	600	tr
Crispy Crunchy Breaded Fish Portions	2 portions	230	1
Crispy Crunchy Breaded Fish Sticks	4	140	1
Crispy Crunchy Fish Fillets	2	220	1
Crispy Crunchy Fish Sticks	4	190	1
Crunchy Batter Fish Fillets	2	280	tr
Fish Cakes	2	190	tr
Light Seafood Entrees Fish Dijon	8.75 oz	200	1
Light Seafood Entrees Fish Florentine	8 oz	220	1
Light Seafood Entrees Fish Mornay	9 oz	230	1
Microwave Buttered Fillet	1	80	tr
Microwave Fillet Sandwich	1	280	1
Microwave Fillets	1	280	tr
Microwave Fish Sticks	5	290	tr
breaded fillet	1 (2 oz)	155	tr
sticks	1 (1 oz)	76	tr
MIX			
Cajun Style Fish Fry (Golden Dipt)	.66 oz	60	1
Fish & Chips Batter Mix (Golden Dipt)	1.25 oz	120	tr
Fish Fry (Golden Dipt)	.66 oz	60	tr
TAKE-OUT			
kedgeree	5.6 oz	242	1

FOOD	PORTION	CALORIES	IRON
sandwich w/ tartar sauce	1	431	3
sandwich w/ tartar sauce & cheese	1	524	4
taramasalata	3.5 oz	446	tr

FISH PASTE

fish paste	2 tsp	15	1

FLATFISH

FRESH			
cooked	3 oz	99	tr
fillet, cooked	4.5 oz	148	tr
TAKE-OUT			
battered & fried	3.2 oz	211	2
breaded & fried	3.2 oz	211	2

FLOUNDER

FROZEN			
Crunchy Batter Fillets (Mrs. Paul's)	2	220	tr
Light Fillets (Mrs. Paul's)	1	240	1
Microwave Entree Stuffed (Gorton's)	1 pkg	350	2

FLOUR

All Purpose (Ballard)	1 cup	400	5
All Purpose (Ceresota)	1 cup	390	5
All Purpose (Gold Medal)	1 cup	400	5
All Purpose (Heckers)	1 cup	390	5
All Purpose (Pillsbury Best)	1 cup	400	5
All Purpose (Robin Hood)	1 cup	400	5
All Purpose Unbleached (Pillsbury Best)	1 cup	400	5

FOOD	PORTION	CALORIES	IRON
Better for Bread (Gold Medal)	1 cup	400	5
Bohemian Style, Rye and Wheat (Pillsbury Best)	1 cup	400	4
Bread (Pillsbury Best)	1 cup	400	5
Medium Rye (Pillsbury Best)	1 cup	400	3
Oat Blend (Gold Medal)	1 cup	390	4
Rye Stone Ground (Robin Hood)	1 cup	360	4
Self-Rising (Aunt Jemima)	¼ cup	109	2
Self-Rising (Ballard)	1 cup	380	5
Self-Rising (Gold Medal)	1 cup	380	5
Self-Rising (Pillsbury Best)	1 cup	380	5
Self-Rising (Robin Hood)	1 cup	380	5
Shake & Blend (Pillsbury Best)	2 tbsp	50	tr
Unbleached (Gold Medal)	1 cup	400	5
Unbleached (Robin Hood)	1 cup	400	5
Whole Wheat (Ceresota)	1 cup	400	4
Whole Wheat (Gold Medal)	1 cup	350	5
Whole Wheat (Heckers)	1 cup	400	4
Whole Wheat (Pillsbury Best)	1 cup	400	4
Whole Wheat Blend (Gold Medal)	1 cup	380	5
corn masa	1 cup	416	8
corn whole grain	1 cup	422	3
cottonseed lowfat	1 oz	94	4
peanut defatted	1 cup	196	1
peanut defatted	1 oz	92	1
peanut lowfat	1 cup	257	3
potato	1 cup	628	31
rice, brown	1 cup	574	3
rice, white	1 cup	578	tr
rye, dark	1 cup	415	8

FOOD	PORTION	CALORIES	IRON
rye, light	1 cup	374	2
rye, medium	1 cup	361	2
sesame lowfat	1 oz	95	4
triticale whole grain	1 cup	440	3
white, all purpose	1 cup	455	6
white, bread	1 cup	495	6
white, cake	1 cup	395	8
white self-rising	1 cup	442	6
whole wheat	1 cup	407	5

FRENCH BEANS

FOOD	PORTION	CALORIES	IRON
dried, cooked	1 cup	228	2

FRENCH TOAST

FOOD	PORTION	CALORIES	IRON
FROZEN			
Aunt Jemima	3 oz	166	2
Aunt Jemima Cinnamon Swirl	3 oz	171	2
Great Starts Cinnamon Swirl w/ Sausage	5.5 oz	390	3
Great Starts French Toast w/ Sausage	5.5 oz	380	3
Great Starts Mini French Toast w/ Sausage	2.5 oz	190	1
Great Starts Oatmeal French Toast w/ Lite Links	4.65 oz	310	2
Quaker French Toast Sticks & Syrup	1 pkg (5.2 oz)	400	2
Quaker French Toast Wedges & Sausage	1 pkg (5.3 oz)	360	4
french toast	1 slice (2 oz)	126	1
HOME RECIPE			
as prep w/ 2% milk	1 slice	149	1

FOOD	PORTION	CALORIES	IRON
as prep w/ whole milk	1 slice	151	1
TAKE-OUT w/ butter	2 slices	356	2

FROG'S LEGS

FOOD	PORTION	CALORIES	IRON
frog leg, as prep w/ seasoned flour & fried	1 (.8 oz)	70	tr

FRUIT DRINKS

FROZEN

FOOD	PORTION	CALORIES	IRON
Tree Top Apple Citrus, as prep	6 oz	90	1
Tree Top Apple Cranberry, as prep	6 oz	100	1
Tree Top Apple Grape, as prep	6 oz	100	1
Tree Top Apple Pear, as prep	6 oz	90	1
Tree Top Apple Raspberry, as prep	6 oz	80	1
citrus juice drink	12-oz can	684	17
citrus juice drink, as prep	1 cup	114	3
fruit punch	12-oz can	678	1
fruit punch, as prep w/ water	1 cup	113	tr
lemonade	6-oz can	397	2
lemonade, as prep w/ water	1 cup	100	tr
limeade	6-oz can	408	tr
limeade, as prep w/ water	1 cup	102	tr

MIX

FOOD	PORTION	CALORIES	IRON
fruit punch, as prep w/ water	9 oz	97	tr
lemonade powder, as prep w/ water	9 oz	113	tr
lemonade powder w/ Nutrasweet	1 pitcher (67 oz)	40	1

READY-TO-USE

FOOD	PORTION	CALORIES	IRON
Dole New Breakfast Juice Pineapple Orange Banana	6 oz	90	tr

FOOD	PORTION	CALORIES	IRON
Dole New Breakfast Juice Pineapple Orange Guava	6 oz	100	tr
Dole New Breakfast Juice Pineapple Passion Banana	6 oz	100	tr
Dole Pinneapple Grapefruit	6 oz	90	tr
Dole Pineapple Orange	6 oz	90	tr
Dole Pineapple Orange Banana	6 oz	90	tr
Dole Pineapple Pink Grapefruit	6 oz	100	tr
Juice & More Apple Cherry	8 oz	120	tr
Juice & More Apple Grape	8 oz	120	tr
Juice & More Apple Raspberry	8 oz	120	tr
Juicy Juice Berry	8.45 oz	130	tr
Juicy Juice Punch	6 oz	100	tr
Juicy Juice Punch	8.45 oz	140	tr
Kern's Apricot Orange Nectar	6 oz	112	tr
Kern's Apricot Pineapple Nectar	6 oz	110	1
Kern's Strawberry Banana Nectar	6 oz	100	tr
Kool-Aid Koolers Lemonade	8.45 oz	120	tr
Kool-Aid Koolers Mountainberry Punch	8.45 oz	142	tr
Kool-Aid Koolers Rainbow Punch	8.45 oz	135	tr
Kool-Aid Koolers Sharkleberry Fin	8.45 oz	140	tr
Kool-Aid Koolers Tropical Punch	8.45 oz	132	tr
Libby's Passion Fruit Orange Nectar	8 oz	150	tr
Libby's Strawberry Banana Nectar	8 oz	150	tr
S&W Apricot Pineapple Nectar	6 oz	120	1
S&W Apricot Pineapple Nectar Diet	6 oz	80	tr
Smucker's Apple Cranberry Juice	8 oz	120	tr
Smucker's Orange Banana Juice	8 oz	120	tr
Tang Mixed Fruit	8.45 oz	137	tr

FOOD	PORTION	CALORIES	IRON
Tang Strawberry	8.45 oz	121	tr
Tang Tropical Orange	8.45 oz	146	tr
Tree Top Apple Citrus	6 oz	90	1
Tree Top Apple Cranberry	6 oz	100	1
Tree Top Apple Grape	6 oz	100	1
Tree Top Apple Pear	6 oz	90	1
Tree Top Apple Raspberry	6 oz	80	1
Veryfine Apple Raspberry	8 oz	110	1
Veryfine Lemonade	8 oz	120	1
Veryfine Papaya Punch	8 oz	120	3
Veryfine Passion Fruit Orange	8 oz	110	tr
Veryfine Pineapple Orange	8 oz	130	1
Wylers Lemonade	6-oz can	64	0
Wylers Tropical Punch	6-oz can	82	0
cranberry apple drink	6 oz	123	tr
cranberry apricot drink	6 oz	118	tr
fruit punch	6 oz	87	tr
orange & apricot	1 cup	128	tr
orange grapefruit juice	1 cup	107	1
pineapple & grapefruit	1 cup	117	1
pineapple & orange drink	1 cup	125	1

FRUIT, MIXED

CANNED

Chunky Mixed Natural Style (S&W)	½ cup	90	1
Fruit Cocktail (Hunt's)	4 oz	90	tr
Fruit Cocktail Natural Lite (S&W)	½ cup	60	tr
Fruit Cocktail Natural Style (S&W)	½ cup	90	1
fruit cocktail in heavy syrup	½ cup	93	tr
fruit cocktail juice pack	½ cup	56	tr

FOOD	PORTION	CALORIES	IRON
fruit cocktail water pack	½ cup	40	tr
fruit salad in heavy syrup	½ cup	94	tr
fruit salad in light syrup	½ cup	73	tr
fruit salad juice pack	½ cup	62	tr
fruit salad water pack	½ cup	37	tr
mixed fruit in heavy syrup	½ cup	92	tr
tropical fruit salad in heavy syrup	½ cup	110	1
DRIED			
Fruit 'n Nut Mix (Planters)	1 oz	150	1
mixed	11-oz pkg	712	8
FROZEN			
Mixed Fruit (Birds Eye)	½ cup	120	tr
mixed fruit, sweetened	1 cup	245	1

FRUIT SNACKS

FOOD	PORTION	CALORIES	IRON
Health Valley Bakes Apple	1 bar	100	2
Health Valley Bakes Date	1 bar	100	1
Health Valley Bakes Raisin	1 bar	100	3
Health Valley Fat Free Fruit Bars 100% Organic Apple	1 bar	140	2
Health Valley Fat Free Fruit Bars 100% Organic Apricot	1 bar	140	2
Health Valley Fat Free Fruit Bars 100% Organic Date	1 bar	140	2
Health Valley Fat Free Fruit Bars 100% Organic Raisin	1 bar	140	2
Health Valley Fruit & Fitness Bars	2 bars	200	1
Health Valley Oat Bran Bakes Apricot	1 bar	100	1
Health Valley Oat Bran Bakes Fig & Nut	1 bar	110	1
Health Valley Oat Bran Jumbo Fruit Bar Almond & Date	1 bar	170	3

FOOD	PORTION	CALORIES	IRON
Health Valley Oat Bran Jumbo Fruit Bar Raisin & Cinnamon	1 bar	160	4
Sunkist Fruit Flippits Cherry	.8 oz	107	0
Sunkist Fruit Flippits Strawberry	.8 oz	107	0
Sunkist Fruit Roll Apricot	1	76	tr
Sunkist Fruit Roll Cherry	1	75	tr
Sunkist Fruit Roll Grape	1	76	tr
Sunkist Fruit Roll Raspberry	1	75	tr
Sunkist Fruit Roll Strawberry	1	74	tr
Sunkist Fun Fruit Animals	.9 oz	100	0
Sunkist Fun Fruit Dinosaurs Strawberry	.9 oz	100	0
Sunkist Fun Fruit Spooky Fruit	1 pkg	100	0
Sunkist Fun Fruit Strawberry	.9 oz	100	0

GARLIC

clove	1	4	tr
powder	1 tsp	9	tr

GEFILTE FISH

READY-TO-USE			
sweet	1 piece (1.5 oz)	35	1

GELATIN

MIX			
fruit flavored	½ cup	70	tr
low calorie	½ cup	8	tr

GIBLETS

capon, simmered	1 cup (5 oz)	238	10
chicken, floured & fried	1 cup (5 oz)	402	15

FOOD	PORTION	CALORIES	IRON
chicken, simmered	1 cup (5 oz)	228	9
turkey, simmered	1 cup (5 oz)	243	10

GINGER

ground	1 tsp	6	tr
root, fresh	¼ cup	17	tr
root, fresh	5 slices	8	tr
root, fresh, sliced	¼ cup	17	tr
root, fresh, sliced	5 slices	8	tr

GINKGO NUTS

canned	1 oz	32	tr
dried	1 oz	99	tr
raw	1 oz	52	tr

GIZZARDS

chicken, simmered	1 cup (5 oz)	222	6
turkey, simmered	1 cup (5 oz)	236	8

GOAT

roasted	3 oz	122	3

GOOSE

FRESH

w/ skin, roasted	½ goose (1.7 lbs)	2362	22
w/ skin, roasted	6.6 oz	574	5
w/o skin, roasted	½ goose (1.3 lbs)	1406	17
w/o skin, roasted	5 oz	340	4

FOOD	PORTION	CALORIES	IRON

GOOSEBERRIES

FOOD	PORTION	CALORIES	IRON
fresh	1 cup	67	tr
CANNED in light syrup	½ cup	93	tr

GRANOLA

FOOD	PORTION	CALORIES	IRON
BARS Hershey Chocolate Covered Chocolate Chip	1 (1.2 oz)	170	tr
Hershey Chocolate Covered Cocoa Creme	1 (1.2 oz)	180	tr
Hershey Chocolate Covered Cookies & Creme	1 (1.2 oz)	170	tr
Hershey Chocolate Covered Peanut Butter	1 (1.2 oz)	180	tr
Nature Valley Cinnamon	1	120	1
Nature Valley Oat Bran Honey Graham	1	110	1
Nature Valley Oats 'n Honey	1	120	1
Nature Valley Peanut Butter	1	120	1
Nature Valley Rice Bran Cinnamon Graham	1	90	1
New Trail Chocolate Covered Cookies & Creme	1	200	tr
Quaker Chewy Chocolate Chip	1	128	1
Quaker Chewy Chunky Nut & Raisin	1	131	1
Quaker Chewy Cinnamon Raisin	1	128	1
Quaker Chewy Honey & Oats	1	125	1
Quaker Chewy Peanut Butter	1	128	1
Quaker Chewy Peanut Butter Chocolate Chip	1	131	1

FOOD	PORTION	CALORIES	IRON
Quaker Dipps Caramel Nut	1	148	1
Quaker Dipps Chocolate Chip	1	139	1
Quaker Dipps Chocolate Fudge	1	160	tr
Quaker Dipps Peanut Butter	1	170	1
Quaker Dipps Peanut Butter Chocolate Chip	1	174	tr
Sunbelt Chewy Chocolate Chip	1 (1.25 oz)	150	1
Sunbelt Chewy Oats & Honey	1 (1 oz)	130	1
Sunbelt Chewy w/ Almonds	1 (oz)	120	tr
Sunbelt Chewy w/ Raisins	1 (1.25 oz)	150	1
Sunbelt Fudge Dipped Chewy Chocolate Chip	1 (1.5 oz)	210	1
Sunbelt Fudge Dipped Chewy Macaroo	1 (1.4 oz)	200	1
Sunbelt Fudge Dipped Chewy w/ Peanuts	1 (1.5 oz)	200	1

CEREAL

FOOD	PORTION	CALORIES	IRON
Erewhon Date Nut	1 oz	130	1
Erewhon Honey Almond	1 oz	130	1
Erewhon Maple	1 oz	130	1
Erewhon Spiced Apple	1 oz	130	1
Erewhon Sunflower Crunch	1 oz	130	1
Erewhon w/ Bran	1 oz	130	1
Kellogg's Low Fat	⅓ cup (1 oz)	120	2
Nature Valley Cinnamon & Raisin	⅓ cup (1 oz)	120	1
Nature Valley Fruit & Nut	⅓ cup (1 oz)	130	1
Nature Valley Toasted Oat	⅓ cup (1 oz)	130	1
Post Hearty	¼ cup	128	7
Quaker Sun Country 100% Natural w/ Almonds	¼ cup	130	1

FOOD	PORTION	CALORIES	IRON
Quaker Sun Country 100% Natural w/ Raisins & Dates	¼ cup	123	1
Quaker Sun Country w/ Raisins	¼ cup	125	1
Sunbelt Banana Almond	1 oz	130	1
Sunbelt Fruit & Nut	1 oz	120	1

GRAPEFRUIT

FOOD	PORTION	CALORIES	IRON
CANNED			
juice pack	½ cup	46	tr
unsweetened	1 cup	93	1
water pack	½ cup	44	1
FRESH			
pink	½	37	tr
pink sections	1 cup	69	tr
red	½	37	tr
red sections	1 cup	69	tr
white	½	39	tr
white sections	1 cup	76	tr
JUICE			
S&W Unsweetened	6 oz	80	1
Tree Top	6 oz	80	tr
Veryfine 100%	8 oz	101	tr
Veryfine Pink Grapefruit	8 oz	120	2
fresh	1 cup	96	tr
frzn, as prep	1 cup	102	tr
frzn, not prep	6 oz	302	1
sweetened	1 cup	116	1

FOOD	PORTION	CALORIES	IRON

GRAPES

CANNED

Food	Portion	Calories	Iron
Thompson Seedless Premium (S&W)	½ cup	100	tr
thompson seedless in heavy syrup	½ cup	94	1
thompson seedless water pack	½ cup	48	1

FRESH

Food	Portion	Calories	Iron
grapes	10	36	tr

JUICE

Food	Portion	Calories	Iron
S&W Concord Unsweetened	6 oz	100	tr
Tang Fruit Box	8.45 oz	131	tr
Tree Top	6 oz	120	tr
Veryfine 100%	8 oz	153	1
bottled	1 cup	155	1
frzn sweetened, as prep	1 cup	128	tr
frzn sweetened, not prep	6 oz	386	1
grape drink	6 oz	84	tr

GRAVY

CANNED

Food	Portion	Calories	Iron
Bovril	1 heaping tsp	9	1
Gravymaster	¼ tsp	3	tr
Marmite	1 heaping tsp	9	tr
au jus	1 cup	38	1
beef	1 can (10 oz)	155	2
beef	1 cup	124	2
chicken	1 cup	189	1
mushroom	1 cup	120	2
turkey	1 cup	122	2

FOOD	PORTION	CALORIES	IRON
DRY			
Bournvita	2 heaping tsp	34	tr
Brown (Pillsbury)	¼ cup	15	0
Chicken (Pillsbury)	¼ cup	25	0
Home Style (Pillsbury)	¼ cup	15	0
Oil-Less Roux & Gravy Mix (Cajun King)	3.5 oz	394	4
brown, as prep w/ water	1 cup	75	tr

GREAT NORTHERN BEANS

FOOD	PORTION	CALORIES	IRON
CANNED			
Green Giant	½ cup	80	2
Trappey's	½ cup	80	1
great northern	1 cup	300	4
DRIED			
cooked	1 cup	210	4

GREEN BEANS

FOOD	PORTION	CALORIES	IRON
CANNED			
Almondine (Green Giant)	½ cup	45	1
Cut (Green Giant)	½ cup	16	1
Cut Premium Blue Lake (S&W)	½ cup	20	1
Cut Water Pack (S&W)	½ cup	20	1
Dilled (S&W)	½ cup	60	3
French (Green Giant)	½ cup	16	1
French Style Premium Blue Lake (S&W)	½ cup	20	1
Green Beans & Wax Beans (S&W)	½ cup	20	1
Kitchen Sliced (Green Giant)	½ cup	16	1
Whole Fancy Stringless (S&W)	½ cup	20	1
Whole Vertical Pack (S&W)	½ cup	20	1

FOOD	PORTION	CALORIES	IRON
FROZEN			
Cut (Birds Eye)	½ cup	25	1
Cut in Butter Sauce (Green Giant)	½ cup	30	tr
Farm Fresh Whole (Birds Eye)	¾ cup	30	1
French Cut (Birds Eye)	½ cup	25	1
French Green Beans in Sauce w/ Toasted Almonds (Birds Eye)	½ cup	50	tr
Harvest Fresh Cut (Green Giant)	½ cup	16	1
Italian (Birds Eye)	½ cup	30	1
One Serve in Butter Sauce (Green Giant)	1 pkg	60	1
Polybag Cut (Birds Eye)	½ cup	25	1
Polybag French Cut (Birds Eye)	½ cup	25	1
Polybag Deluxe Whole (Birds Eye)	½ cup	20	1
Whole Deluxe (Birds Eye)	½ cup	45	1
SHELF-STABLE			
Cut (Pantry Express)	½ cup	12	tr

GROUND-CHERRIES

Fresh	½ cup	37	1

GROUPER

FRESH			
cooked	3 oz	100	1
fillet, cooked	7.1 oz	238	2
raw	3 oz	78	1

GUAVA

Kern's Nectar	6 oz	110	tr
fresh	1	45	tr
guava sauce	½ cup	43	tr

FOOD	PORTION	CALORIES	IRON

HADDOCK

FRESH

FOOD	PORTION	CALORIES	IRON
cooked	3 oz	95	1
fillet, cooked	5.3 oz	168	2
raw	3 oz	74	1

FROZEN

Crunchy Batter Fillets (Mrs. Paul's)	2	190	1
Fishmarket Fresh (Gorton's)	5 oz	110	tr
Light Fillets (Mrs. Paul's)	1	220	tr
Microwave Entree Haddock in Lemon Butter (Gorton's)	1 pkg	360	tr

SMOKED

smoked	1 oz	33	tr
smoked	3 oz	99	1

HALIBUT

FRESH

atlantic & pacific, cooked	½ fillet (5.6 oz)	223	2
atlantic & pacific, cooked	3 oz	119	1
atlantic & pacific, raw	3 oz	93	1
greenland, baked	3 oz	203	1
greenland, baked	5.6 oz	380	1

HAM

Carl Buddig	1 oz	50	tr
Oscar Mayer Baked Cooked	1 slice (.75 oz)	21	tr
Oscar Mayer Boiled	1 slice (.75 oz)	23	tr
Oscar Mayer Boiled Thin Sliced	1 slice (.4 oz)	13	tr
Oscar Mayer Breakfast Ham	1 slice (1.5 oz)	47	tr
Oscar Mayer Chopped	1 slice (1 oz)	41	tr

FOOD	PORTION	CALORIES	IRON
Oscar Mayer Cracked Black Pepper	1 slice (.75 oz)	22	tr
Oscar Mayer Ham & Cheese Loaf	1 slice (1 oz)	66	tr
Oscar Mayer Honey Ham	1 slice (.75 oz)	23	tr
Oscar Mayer Honey Ham Thin Sliced	1 slice (.4 oz)	13	tr
Oscar Mayer Jubilee Boneless	1 oz	43	tr
Oscar Mayer Jubilee Canned	1 oz	29	tr
Oscar Mayer Jubilee Sliced	1 oz	29	tr
Oscar Mayer Jubilee Steak	2 oz	57	1
Oscar Mayer Lower Salt	1 slice (.75 oz)	23	tr
Oscar Mayer Peppered Chopped	1 slice (1 oz)	55	tr
Oscar Mayer Smoked Cooked	1 slice (.75 oz)	22	tr
canned (13% fat), roasted	3 oz	192	1
canned extra lean (4% fat)	3 oz	116	1
center slice, lean & fat	4 oz	229	1
chopped	1 oz	65	tr
chopped, canned	1 oz	68	tr
ham & cheese loaf	1 oz	73	1
ham & cheese spread	1 oz	69	tr
ham & cheese spread	1 tbsp	37	tr
ham salad spread	1 oz	61	tr
ham salad spread	1 tbsp	32	tr
minced	1 oz	75	tr
sliced extra lean (5% fat)	1 oz	37	tr
sliced regular (11% fat)	1 oz	52	tr
steak boneless extra lean	1 oz	35	tr

HAM DISHES

| HOME RECIPE croquettes | 1 (3.1 oz) | 217 | 2 |

FOOD	PORTION	CALORIES	IRON
salad	½ cup	287	2
TAKE-OUT			
sandwich w/ cheese	1	353	3

HAMBURGER

FOOD	PORTION	CALORIES	IRON
FROZEN			
Kid Cuisine Beef Patty Sandwich w/ Cheese	6.25 oz	430	3
MicroMagic Cheeseburger	1 pkg (4.75 oz)	450	1
MicroMagic Hamburger	1 pkg (4 oz)	350	1
TAKE-OUT			
double patty w/ bun	1 reg	544	5
double patty w/ catsup, cheese, mayonnaise, mustard, pickle, tomato & bun	1 lg	706	6
double patty w/ catsup, mayonnaise, onion, pickle, tomato & bun	1 reg	649	5
double patty w/ catsup, mustard, mayonnaise, onion, pickle, tomato & bun	1 lg	540	6
double patty w/ catsup, mustard, onion, pickle & bun	1 reg	576	6
double patty w/ cheese & bun	1 reg	457	3
double patty w/ cheese & double bun	1 reg	461	4
double patty w/ cheese, catsup mayonnaise, onion, pickle, tomato & bun	1 reg	416	3
single patty w/ bacon, catsup, cheese, mustard, onion, pickle & bun	1 lg	609	5
single patty w/ bun	1 lg	400	4
single patty w/ bun	1 reg	275	2

FOOD	PORTION	CALORIES	IRON
single patty w/ catsup, cheese, ham, mayonnaise, pickle, tomato & bun	1 lg	745	5
single patty w/ catsup, mustard, mayonnaise, onion, pickle, tomato & bun	1 reg	279	3
single patty w/ cheese & bun	1 lg	608	5
single patty w/ cheese & bun	1 reg	320	2
triple patty w/ catsup, mustard, pickle & bun	1 lg	693	8
triple patty w/ cheese & bun	1 lg	769	8

HEART

FOOD	PORTION	CALORIES	IRON
beef, simmered	3 oz	148	6
chicken, simmered	1 cup (5 oz)	268	13
lamb, braised	3 oz	158	5
turkey, simmered	1 cup (5 oz)	257	10
veal, braised	3 oz	158	4

HERBS/SPICES

FOOD	PORTION	CALORIES	IRON
curry powder	1 tsp	6	1
poultry seasoning	1 tsp	5	1
pumpkin pie spice	1 tsp	6	tr

HERRING

FRESH

FOOD	PORTION	CALORIES	IRON
atlantic, cooked	3 oz	172	1
atlantic fillet, cooked	5 oz	290	2
atlantic, raw	3 oz	134	1
pacific, baked	3 oz	213	1
pacific fillet, baked	5.1 oz	360	2

FOOD	PORTION	CALORIES	IRON
READY-TO-USE			
atlantic fillet, kippered	1.4 oz	87	1
atlantic, pickled	½ oz	39	tr

HICKORY NUTS

dried	1 oz	187	1

HOMINY

canned	½ cup	57	tr

HONEY

Burleson's Clover	1 tbsp	60	tr
Burleson's Creamed	1 tbsp	60	tr
Burleson's Natural	1 tbsp	60	tr
Burleson's Pure	1 tbsp	60	tr
Burleson's Raw	1 tbsp	60	tr
Burleson's Rocky Mountain Clover	1 tbsp	60	tr
Golden Blossom	1 tsp	20	tr
honey	1 cup	1030	2
honey	1 tbsp	65	tr

HONEYDEW

cubed	1 cup	60	tr
fresh	1/10	46	tr

HORSE

roasted	3 oz	149	4

HOT DOG

chicken	1 (1.5 oz)	116	1

FOOD	PORTION	CALORIES	IRON
MEAT			
Oscar Mayer			
Bacon & Cheddar Cheese	1 (1.5 oz)	137	tr
Beef Franks	1 (1.5 oz)	144	1
Beef Franks w/ Cheddar	1 (1.5 oz)	136	1
Bun-Length Beef	1 (2 oz)	182	1
Bun-Length Wieners	1 (2 oz)	184	1
Cheese Hot Dogs	1 (1.5 oz)	143	tr
Light Beef Franks	1 (2 oz)	131	1
Light Wieners	1 (2 oz)	127	1
Little Wieners	1 (.33 oz)	28	tr
Wieners	1 (1.5 oz)	144	tr
beef	1 (1.5)	142	1
beef	1 (2 oz)	180	1
beef & pork	1 (1.5 oz)	144	1
beef & pork	1 (2 oz)	183	1
pork cheesefurter smokie	1 (1.5 oz)	141	tr
TAKE-OUT			
corn dog	1	460	6
w/ bun & chili	1	297	3
w/ bun, plain	1	242	2
TURKEY			
Louis Rich	1 (1.5 oz)	101	1
Louis Rich Bun Length	2 oz	128	1
Louis Rich Turkey Cheese Franks	1 (1.5 oz)	109	1
turkey	1 (1.5 oz)	102	1

HUMMUS

hummus	1 cup	420	4
hummus	⅓ cup	140	1

FOOD	PORTION	CALORIES	IRON

HYACINTH BEANS

FOOD	PORTION	CALORIES	IRON
dried, cooked	1 cup	228	9

ICE CREAM AND FROZEN DESSERTS

FOOD	PORTION	CALORIES	IRON
Berry Berry Berry (Mocha Mix)	3.5 oz	209	1
Black Cherry Fat Free (Borden)	½ cup	90	0
Butter Pecan (Haagen-Dazs)	4 oz	390	tr
Caramel Almond Crunch Bar (Haagen-Dazs)	1	240	tr
Caramel Nut Sundae (Haagen-Dazs)	4 oz	310	tr
Chocolate (Haagen-Dazs)	4 oz	270	tr
Chocolate (Ultra Slim-Fast)	4 oz	100	3
Chocolate Chocolate Chip (Haagen-Dazs)	4 oz	290	2
Chocolate Chocolate Mint (Haagen-Dazs)	4 oz	300	1
Chocolate Dark Chocolate Bar (Haagen-Dazs)	1	390	1
Chocolate Fat Free (Borden)	½ cup	100	0
Chocolate Fudge (Ultra Slim-Fast)	4 oz	120	3
Coffee (Haagen-Dazs)	4 oz	270	tr
Cool 'n Creamy Amaretto w/ Chocolate Swirl	1 bar	62	tr
Cool 'n Creamy Chocolate/Vanilla	1 bar	54	tr
Cool 'n Creamy Double Chocolate Fudge	1 bar	55	tr
Deep Chocolate (Haagen-Dazs)	4 oz	290	1
Deep Chocolate Fudge (Haagen-Dazs)	4 oz	290	1
Dutch Chocolate (Mocha Mix)	3.5 oz	210	1
Fudge Bar (Ultra Slim-Fast)	1	90	2

FOOD	PORTION	CALORIES	IRON
Fudge Pop Bar (Haagen-Dazs)	1	210	1
Heavenly Hash (Mocha Mix)	3.5 oz	244	1
Macadamia Brittle (Haagen-Dazs)	4 oz	280	tr
Mocha Almond Fudge (Mocha Mix)	3.5 oz	229	1
Neapolitan (Mocha Mix)	3.5 oz	208	1
Orange & Cream Pop (Haagen-Dazs)	1	130	1
Peach (Mocha Mix)	3.5 oz	198	1
Peach (Ultra Slim-Fast)	4 oz	100	3
Peach Fat Free (Borden)	½ cup	90	0
Peanut Butter Crunch Bar (Haagen-Dazs)	1	270	1
Pralines & Caramel (Ultra Slim-Fast)	4 oz	120	3
Rum Raisin (Haagen-Dazs)	4 oz	250	tr
Strawberry (Haagen-Dazs)	4 oz	250	1
Strawberry Fat Free (Borden)	½ cup	90	0
Strawberry Swirl (Mocha Mix)	3.5 oz	209	1
Toasted Almond (Mocha Mix)	3.5 oz	229	1
Vanilla (Mocha Mix)	3.5 oz	209	1
Vanilla (Ultra Slim-Fast)	4 oz	90	3
Vanilla Chocolate Sandwich (Ultra Slim-Fast)	1	140	2
Vanilla Cookie Crunch Bar (Ultra Slim-Fast)	1	90	2
Vanilla Crunch Bar (Haagen-Dazs)	1	220	tr
Vanilla Fat Free (Borden)	½ cup	90	0
Vanilla Fudge (Haagen-Dazs)	4 oz	270	tr
Vanilla Fudge Cookie (Ultra Slim-Fast)	4 oz	110	3
Vanilla Milk Chocolate Almond Bar (Haagen-Dazs)	1	370	1

FOOD	PORTION	CALORIES	IRON
Vanilla Milk Chocolate Bar (Haagen-Dazs)	1	360	1
Vanilla Milk Chocolate Brittle Bar (Haagen-Dazs)	1	370	1
Vanilla Oatmeal Sandwich (Ultra Slim-Fast)	1	150	2
Vanilla Peanut Butter Swirl (Haagen-Dazs)	4 oz	280	tr
Vanilla Sandwich (Ultra Slim-Fast)	1	140	2
Vanilla Swiss Almond (Haagen-Dazs)	4 oz	290	tr
french vanilla soft serve	1 cup	377	tr
french vanilla soft serve	½ gal	3014	3
vanilla (10% fat)	1 cup	269	tr
vanilla (10% fat)	½ gal	2153	1
vanilla (16% fat)	1 cup	349	tr
vanilla (16% fat)	½ gal	2805	1
vanilla ice milk	1 cup	184	tr
vanilla ice milk	½ gal	1469	1
vanilla ice milk soft serve	1 cup	223	tr
vanilla ice milk soft serve	½ gal	1787	2
TAKE-OUT			
cone, vanilla ice milk soft serve	1 (4.6 oz)	164	tr
sundae, caramel	1 (5.4 oz)	303	tr
sundae, hot fudge	1 (5.4 oz)	284	tr
sundae, strawberry	1 (5.4 oz)	269	tr

ICE CREAM CONES AND CUPS

Keebler Sugar Cones	1	45	tr
sugar cone	1	40	tr
wafer cone	1	17	tr

FOOD	PORTION	CALORIES	IRON

ICE CREAM TOPPINGS

FOOD	PORTION	CALORIES	IRON
Chocolate (Smucker's)	2 tbsp	130	tr
Chocolate Fudge (Hershey)	2 tbsp	100	tr
Hot Fudge Light (Smucker's)	2 tbsp	70	1
Pecans in Syrup (Smucker's)	2 tbsp	130	tr
Walnuts in Syrup (Smucker's)	2 tbsp	130	4

ICES AND ICE POPS

FOOD	PORTION	CALORIES	IRON
Crystal Light			
Berry Blend	1	13	tr
Cherry	1	13	tr
Fruit Punch	1	14	tr
Orange	1	13	tr
Pina Colada	1	14	tr
Pineapple	1	14	tr
Pink Lemonade	1	14	tr
Raspberry	1	13	tr
Strawberry	1	13	tr
Strawberry Daiquiri	1	14	tr
Dole Fruit 'n Cream Bar Peach	1	90	tr
Dole Fruit 'n Cream Bar Raspberry	1	90	tr
Dole Fruit 'n Cream Bar Strawberry	1	90	tr
Dole Fruit 'n Juice Bar Pineapple	1	70	tr
Dole Fruit 'n Juice Bar Pineapple Orange Banana	1	70	tr
Dole Fruit 'n Juice Bar Raspberry	1	70	tr
Dole Fruit 'n Juice Bar Strawberry	1	70	tr
Dole Sorbet Mandarin Orange	4 oz	110	tr
Dole Sorbet Peach	4 oz	110	1
Dole Sorbet Pineapple	4 oz	110	tr

FOOD	PORTION	CALORIES	IRON
Dole Sorbet Raspberry	4 oz	110	tr
Dole Sorbet Strawberry	4 oz	100	tr
Haagen-Dazs Sorbet & Cream Keylime	4 oz	190	1
Haagen-Dazs Sorbet & Cream Blueberry	4 oz	190	1
Haagen-Dazs Sorbet & Cream Orange	4 oz	190	1
Haagen-Dazs Sorbet & Cream Raspberry	4 oz	180	1

JACKFRUIT

fresh	3.5 oz	70	1

JAM/JELLY/PRESERVES

Blueberry Jam (Whistling Wings)	1 oz	50	tr
Raspberry Jam (Whistling Wings)	1 oz	60	tr

JAVA PLUM

fresh	1	5	tr
fresh	1 cup	82	tr

JEW'S-EAR

pepeao, dried	½ cup	36	1
pepeao, raw, sliced	1 cup	25	1

JUJUBE

fresh	3.5 oz	105	1

KALE

FRESH

chopped, cooked	½ cup	21	1

FOOD	PORTION	CALORIES	IRON
raw, chopped	½ cup	21	1
scotch, chopped, cooked	½ cup	18	1
FROZEN chopped, cooked	½ cup	20	1

KEFIR
kefir	3.5 oz	66	tr

KIDNEY
beef, simmered	3 oz	122	6
lamb, braised	3 oz	117	11
veal, braised	3 oz	139	3

KIDNEY BEANS
CANNED Goya Spanish Style	7.5 oz	140	4
Green Giant Dark Red	½ cup	90	2
Green Giant Light Red	½ cup	90	2
Hunt's Red	4 oz	100	2
S&W Dark Red Lite 50% Less Salt	½ cup	120	2
S&W Water Pack	½ cup	90	1
Trappey's New Orleans Style	½ cup	100	1
Van Camp's Dark Red	1 cup	182	3
Van Camp's Light Red	1 cup	184	3
Van Camp's New Orleans Style Red	1 cup	178	3
kidney beans	1 cup	208	3
red	1 cup	216	3
DRIED california red, cooked	1 cup	219	5

FOOD	PORTION	CALORIES	IRON
cooked	1 cup	225	5
red, cooked	1 cup	225	5
royal red, cooked	1 cup	218	5
SPROUTS			
cooked	1 lb	152	4
raw	½ cup	27	1

KIWIFRUIT

fresh	1 med	46	tr

KOHLRABI

FRESH			
raw, sliced	½ cup	19	tr
sliced, cooked	½ cup	24	tr

KUMQUATS

fresh	1	12	tr

LAMB

FRESH			
cubed, lean only, braised	3 oz	190	2
cubed, lean only, broiled	3 oz	158	2
ground, broiled	3 oz	240	2
leg, lean & fat, Choice, roasted	3 oz	219	2
loin chop w/ bone, lean & fat, Choice, broiled	1 chop (2.3 oz)	201	1
loin chop w/ bone, lean only, Choice, broiled	1 chop (1.6 oz)	100	tr
rib chop, lean & fat, Choice, broiled	3 oz	307	2
rib chop, lean only, Choice, broiled	3 oz	200	2

FOOD	PORTION	CALORIES	IRON
shank, lean & fat, Choice, braised	3 oz	206	2
shank, lean & fat, Choice, roasted	3 oz	191	2
shoulder chop w/ bone, lean & fat, Choice, braised	1 chop (2.5 oz)	244	2
shoulder chop w/ bone, lean only, Choice, braised	1 chop (1.9 oz)	152	1
sirloin, lean & fat, Choice, roasted	3 oz	248	2
FROZEN New Zealand, lean & fat, cooked	3 oz	259	2
New Zealand, lean only, cooked	3 oz	175	2

LAMB DISHES

TAKE-OUT curry	¾ cup	345	3
moussaka	5.6 oz	312	2
stew	¾ cup	124	1

LAMB'S-QUARTERS

fresh, chopped, cooked	½ cup	29	1

LEEKS

DRIED freeze dried	1 tbsp	1	tr
FRESH chopped, cooked	¼ cup	8	tr
cooked	1 (4.4 oz)	38	1
raw	1 (4.4 oz)	76	3
raw, chopped	¼ cup	16	1

LEMON

lemon	1 med	22	1

FOOD	PORTION	CALORIES	IRON
peel	1 tbsp	0	tr
wedge	1	5	tr
JUICE			
bottled	1 tbsp	3	tr
fresh	1 tbsp	4	0
frzn	1 tbsp	3	tr

LEMON CURD

lemon curd made w/ egg	2 tsp	29	tr
lemon curd made w/ starch	2 tsp	28	tr

LENTILS

CANNED			
Health Valley Fast Menu Hearty Lentils w/ Garden Vegetables	7.5 oz	150	15
Health Valley Fat Menu Organic Lentils w/ Tofu Wieners	7.5 oz	170	9
DRIED			
cooked	1 cup	231	7
SPROUTS			
raw	½ cup	40	1

LETTUCE

bibb	1 head (6 oz)	21	tr
boston	1 head (6 oz)	21	tr
boston	2 leaves	2	tr
iceberg	1 head (19 oz)	70	3
iceberg	1 leaf	3	tr
looseleaf, shredded	½ cup	5	tr
romaine, shredded	½ cup	4	tr

FOOD	PORTION	CALORIES	IRON

LIMA BEANS

CANNED

FOOD	PORTION	CALORIES	IRON
S&W Small Fancy	½ cup	80	1
Trappey's Baby Green	½ cup	90	1
Trappey's Baby White	½ cup	90	1
large	1 cup	191	4
lima beans	½ cup	93	2

DRIED

FOOD	PORTION	CALORIES	IRON
baby, cooked	1 cup	229	4
cooked	½ cup	104	2
large, cooked	1 cup	217	5

FROZEN

FOOD	PORTION	CALORIES	IRON
Birds Eye Baby	½ cup	130	2
Birds Eye Fordhook	½ cup	100	1
Green Giant Harvest Fresh	½ cup	80	1
Green Giant in Butter Sauce	½ cup	100	1
cooked	½ cup	94	2
fordhook, cooked	½ cup	85	1

LIME

FRESH

FOOD	PORTION	CALORIES	IRON
lime	1	20	tr

JUICE

FOOD	PORTION	CALORIES	IRON
bottled	1 tbsp	3	tr
fresh	1 tbsp	4	0

LING

FOOD	PORTION	CALORIES	IRON
fresh, baked	3 oz	95	1
fresh fillet, baked	5.3 oz	168	1

FOOD	PORTION	CALORIES	IRON

LINGCOD

baked	3 oz	93	tr
fillet, baked	5.3 oz	164	1

LIQUOR/LIQUEUR

bloody mary	5 oz	116	1
coffee liqueur	1.5 oz	174	tr
coffee w/ cream liqueur	1.5 oz	154	tr
creme de menthe	1.5 oz	186	tr
daiquiri	2 oz	111	tr
gin	1.5 oz	110	0
manhattan	2 oz	128	tr
martini	2.5 oz	156	tr
pina colada	4.5 oz	262	tr
rum	1.5 oz	97	tr
screwdriver	7 oz	174	tr
sloe gin fizz	2.5 oz	132	0
tequila sunrise	5.5 oz	189	tr
vodka	1.5 oz	97	tr
whiskey	1.5 oz	105	tr
whiskey sour	3 oz	123	tr
whiskey sour mix, as prep	3.6 oz	169	tr
whiskey sour mix, not prep	1 pkg (.6 oz)	64	tr

LIVER

beef, braised	3 oz	137	6
beef, pan fried	3 oz	184	5
chicken, stewed	1 cup (5 oz)	219	12
duck, raw	1 (1.5 oz)	60	13
lamb, braised	3 oz	187	7

FOOD	PORTION	CALORIES	IRON
lamb, fried	3 oz	202	9
pork, braised	3 oz	141	15
sheep, raw	3.5 oz	131	12
turkey, simmered	1 cup (5 oz)	237	11
veal, braised	3 oz	140	2
veal, fried	3 oz	208	4

LOBSTER

FRESH			
northern, cooked	1 cup	142	1
northern, cooked	3 oz	83	tr
spiny, steamed	1 (5.7 oz)	233	2
spiny, steamed	3 oz	122	1
TAKE-OUT			
newburg	1 cup	485	1

LOGANBERRIES

| frzn | 1 cup | 80 | 1 |

LONGANS

| fresh | 1 | 2 | 0 |

LOQUATS

| fresh | 1 | 5 | tr |

LOTUS

root, raw, sliced	10 slices	45	1
root, sliced, cooked	10 slices	59	1
seeds, dried	1 oz	94	1

FOOD	PORTION	CALORIES	IRON

LUNCHEON MEATS/COLD CUTS

FOOD	PORTION	CALORIES	IRON
Carl Buddig Beef	1 oz	40	1
Carl Buddig Corned Beef	1 oz	40	1
Carl Buddig Pastrami	1 oz	40	1
Oscar Mayer Bar-B-Q Loaf	1 slice (1 oz)	46	tr
Oscar Mayer Bologna	1 slice (1 oz)	90	tr
Oscar Mayer Bologna Beef	1 slice (1 oz)	90	tr
Oscar Mayer Bologna Beef Lebanon	1 slice	46	1
Oscar Mayer Bologna Beef Light	1 slice (1 oz)	64	tr
Oscar Mayer Bologna Garlic Beef	1 slice (1 oz)	90	tr
Oscar Mayer Bologna Light	1 slice (1 oz)	64	tr
Oscar Mayer Bologna w/ Cheese	1 slice	74	tr
Oscar Mayer Braunschweiger German Brand	1 oz	96	3
Oscar Mayer Braunschweiger Sliced	1 slice (1 oz)	96	3
Oscar Mayer Braunschweiger Tube	1 oz	97	3
Oscar Mayer Corned Beef	1 slice (.5 oz)	17	tr
Oscar Mayer Cotto Salami	1 slice	45	1
Oscar Mayer Genoa Salami	1 slice	34	tr
Oscar Mayer Hard Salami	1 slice	33	tr
Oscar Mayer Head Cheese	1 slice (1 oz)	54	tr
Oscar Mayer Honey Loaf	1 slice (1 oz)	34	tr
Oscar Mayer Liver Cheese	1 slice	116	4
Oscar Mayer Luncheon Meat	1 slice (1 oz)	94	tr
Oscar Mayer New England Brand Sausage	1 slice	29	tr
Oscar Mayer Old Fashioned Loaf	1 slice (1 oz)	62	tr
Oscar Mayer Olive Loaf	1 slice (1 oz)	63	tr
Oscar Mayer Pastrami	1 slice (.5 oz)	16	tr

FOOD	PORTION	CALORIES	IRON
Oscar Mayer Peppered Loaf	1 slice (1 oz)	39	tr
Oscar Mayer Pickle & Pimiento Loaf	1 slice (1 oz)	66	tr
Oscar Mayer Picnic Loaf	1 slice (1 oz)	61	tr
Oscar Mayer Salami for Beer	1 slice	50	tr
Oscar Mayer Salami for Beer Beef	1 slice	63	tr
Oscar Mayer Sandwich Spread	1 oz	67	tr
Oscar Mayer Smoked Beef	1 slice (.5 oz)	14	tr
Oscar Mayer Summer Sausage	1 slice	69	1
Oscar Mayer Summer Sausage Beef	1 slice	70	1
barbecue loaf pork & beef	1 oz	49	tr
beerwurst beef	1 slice (1/16" x 2¾")	20	tr
beerwurst beef	1 slice (4" x 1/8")	75	tr
beerwurst pork	1 slice (2¾" x 1/16")	14	tr
beerwurst pork	1 slice (4" x 1/8")	55	tr
berliner pork & beef	1 oz	65	tr
bologna beef	1 oz	88	tr
bologna beef & pork	1 oz	89	tr
bologna pork	1 oz	70	tr
braunschweiger pork	1 oz	102	3
braunschweiger pork	1 slice (2½" x ¼")	65	2
corned beef loaf	1 oz	43	1
dutch brand loaf pork & beef	1 oz	68	tr
headcheese pork	1 oz	60	tr
honey loaf pork & beef	1 oz	36	tr
honey roll sausage beef	1 oz	42	1

FOOD	PORTION	CALORIES	IRON
lebanon bologna beef	1 oz	60	1
liver cheese pork	1 oz	86	3
liverwurst pork	1 oz	92	2
luncheon meat beef	1 oz	87	1
luncheon meat pork & beef	1 oz	100	tr
luncheon meat pork, canned	1 oz	95	tr
luncheon sausage pork & beef	1 oz	74	tr
luxury loaf pork	1 oz	40	tr
mortadella beef & pork	1 oz	88	tr
mother's loaf pork	1 oz	80	tr
new england sausage pork & beef	1 oz	46	tr
olive loaf pork	1 oz	67	tr
peppered loaf pork & beef	1 oz	42	tr
pepperoni pork & beef	1 slice (.2 oz)	27	tr
pepperoni pork & beef	1 (9 oz)	1248	4
pickle & pimiento loaf pork	1 oz	74	tr
picnic loaf pork & beef	1 oz	66	tr
salami, cooked, beef & pork	1 oz	71	1
salami, hard, pork	1 pkg (4 oz)	460	1
salami, hard, pork	1 slice (.33 oz)	41	tr
salami, hard, pork & beef	1 pkg (4 oz)	472	2
salami, hard, pork & beef	1 slice (.33 oz)	42	tr
sandwich spread pork & beef	1 oz	67	tr
sandwich spread pork & beef	1 tbsp	35	tr
summer sausage thuringer cervelat	1 oz	98	1
TAKE-OUT			
submarine w/ salami, ham, cheese, lettuce, tomato, onion & oil	1	456	3

FOOD	PORTION	CALORIES	IRON

LUPINES

dried, cooked	1 cup	197	2

LYCHEES

fresh	1	6	tr

MACADAMIA NUTS

Candy Glazed (Mauna Loa)	1 oz	170	tr
Chocolate Covered (Mauna Loa)	1 oz	170	tr
Honey Roasted (Mauna Loa)	1 oz	200	tr
Macadamia Nut Brittle (Mauna Loa)	1 oz	150	tr
Roasted & Salted (Mauna Loa)	1 oz	210	1
dried	1 oz	199	1
oil roasted	1 oz	204	1

MACE

ground	1 tsp	8	tr

MACKEREL

CANNED			
Jack (Empress)	4 oz	140	1
jack	1 can (12.7 oz)	563	7
jack	1 cup	296	4
FRESH			
atlantic, cooked	3 oz	223	1
atlantic, raw	3 oz	174	1
jack, baked	3 oz	171	1
jack fillet, baked	6.2 oz	354	3
king, baked	3 oz	114	2
king fillet, baked	5.4 oz	207	4

FOOD	PORTION	CALORIES	IRON
pacific, baked	3 oz	171	1
pacific fillet, baked	6.2 oz	354	3
spanish, cooked	3 oz	134	1
spanish fillet, cooked	5.1 oz	230	1
spanish, raw	3 oz	118	tr

MALT

nonalcoholic	12 oz	32	tr

MALTED MILK

Kraft Instant Chocolate	3 tsp	90	tr
chocolate, as prep w/ milk	1 cup	229	1
chocolate flavor powder	3 heaping tsp (.75 oz)	79	tr
natural flavor, as prep w/ milk	1 cup	237	tr
natural flavor powder	3 heaping tsp (.75 oz)	87	tr

MAMMY-APPLE

fresh	1	431	6

MANGO

fresh	1	135	tr
JUICE Kern's Nectar	6 oz	110	tr

MARGARINE

regular, salted	1 stick (4 oz)	815	tr
regular, salted	1 tsp	39	0

MARJORAM

dried	1 tsp	2	1

FOOD	PORTION	CALORIES	IRON

MARSHMALLOW

FOOD	PORTION	CALORIES	IRON
Marshmallow Fluff	1 heaping tsp	59	tr
marshmallow	1 oz	90	1

MATZO

FOOD	PORTION	CALORIES	IRON
Daily Tea Thins (Manischewitz)	1	103	1
Dietetic Thins (Manischewitz)	1	91	3
Egg 'n Onion (Manischewitz)	1	112	1
Matzo Cracker Miniatures (Manischewitz)	10	90	1
Matzo Farfel (Manischewitz)	1 cup	180	2
Matzo Meal (Manischewitz)	1 cup	514	4
Passover Egg Matzo Crackers (Manischewitz)	10	108	1
Salted Thins (Manischewitz)	1	100	1
Unsalted (Manischewitz)	1	110	1
Wheat Matzo Crackers (Manischewitz)	10	90	1
Whole Wheat w/ Bran (Manischewitz)	1	110	2

MAYONNAISE

FOOD	PORTION	CALORIES	IRON
regular	1 cup	1577	1
regular	1 tbsp	99	tr

MAYONNAISE-TYPE SALAD DRESSING

FOOD	PORTION	CALORIES	IRON
home recipe	1 cup	400	1
home recipe	1 tbsp	25	tr
salad dressing	1 cup	916	1

FOOD	PORTION	CALORIES	IRON

MEAT SUBSTITUTES

FOOD	PORTION	CALORIES	IRON
Spring Creek Soysage	1 patty (1.6 oz)	63	1
simulated meat product	1 oz	88	3
simulated sausage	1 link (.9 oz)	64	1
simulated sausage	1 patty (1.36 oz)	97	1

MELON

melon balls, frzn	1 cup	55	1

MILK
(*see also* MILK DRINKS, MILK SUBSTITUTES)

CANNED			
condensed sweetened	1 cup	982	1
condensed sweetened	1 oz	123	tr
evaporated	½ cup	169	tr
evaporated skim	½ cup	99	tr
DRIED			
buttermilk	1 tbsp	25	tr
nonfat instant	1 pkg (3.2 oz)	244	tr
LIQUID, LOWFAT			
1%	1 cup	102	tr
1%	1 qt	409	tr
1% protein fortified	1 cup	119	tr
1% protein fortified	1 qt	477	1
2%	1 cup	121	tr
2%	1 qt	485	tr
CalciMilk	1 cup	102	tr
Lactaid 1%	1 cup	102	tr
buttermilk	1 cup	99	tr

FOOD	PORTION	CALORIES	IRON
buttermilk	1 qt	396	tr
LIQUID, REGULAR			
buffalo	3.5 oz	112	tr
donkey	3.5 oz	43	tr
goat	1 cup	168	tr
goat	1 qt	672	tr
human	1 cup	171	tr
indian buffalo	1 cup	236	tr
mare	3.5 oz	49	tr
sheep	1 cup	264	tr
whole	1 cup	150	tr
LIQUID, SKIM			
Lactaid Nonfat	1 cup	86	tr
skim	1 cup	86	tr
skim	1 qt	342	1
skim, protein fortified	1 cup	100	tr
skim, protein fortified	1 qt	400	1

MILK DRINKS

FOOD	PORTION	CALORIES	IRON
Chocolate Milk 1% (Lactaid)	1 cup	158	1
Quik Chocolate (Nestle)	.75 oz	90	tr
Quik Chocolate, as prep w/ 2% milk (Nestle)	8 oz	210	1
Quik Chocolate, as prep w/ skim milk (Nestle)	8 oz	170	1
Quik Chocolate, as prep w/ whole milk (Nestle)	8 oz	230	1
Quik Chocolate Lowfat (Nestle)	8 oz	200	1
Quik Lite Ready to Drink Chocolate Lowfat (Nestle)	8 oz	130	tr
Quik Sugar Free Chocolate, as prep w/ 2% milk (Nestle)	8 oz	140	1

FOOD	PORTION	CALORIES	IRON
Quik Syrup Chocolate (Nestle)	1⅔ tbsp	100	2
Quik Syrup Chocolate, as prep w/ 2% milk (Nestle)	8 oz	220	1
Quik Syrup Chocolate, as prep w/ skim milk (Nestle)	8 oz	220	1
Quik Syrup Chocolate, as prep w/ whole milk (Nestle)	8 oz	240	1
chocolate milk	1 cup	208	1
chocolate milk	1 qt	833	2
chocolate milk 1%	1 cup	158	1
chocolate milk 1%	1 qt	630	2
chocolate milk 2%	1 cup	179	1
strawberry flavor mix, as prep w/ whole milk	9 oz	234	tr

MILK SUBSTITUTES

FOOD	PORTION	CALORIES	IRON
imitation milk	1 cup	150	1
imitation milk	1 qt	600	4

MILKFISH

FOOD	PORTION	CALORIES	IRON
baked	3 oz	162	tr

MILKSHAKE

FOOD	PORTION	CALORIES	IRON
chocolate	10 oz	360	1
strawberry	10 oz	319	tr
thick shake, chocolate	10.6 oz	356	1
thick shake, vanilla	11 oz	350	tr
vanilla	10 oz	314	tr

MILLET

FOOD	PORTION	CALORIES	IRON
cooked	½ cup	143	tr

FOOD	PORTION	CALORIES	IRON

MINERAL WATER/BOTTLED WATER

FOOD	PORTION	CALORIES	IRON
San Pellegrino	1 liter	0	tr

MISO

miso	½ cup	284	4

MOLASSES

Brer Rabbit Dark	2 tbsp	110	4
Brer Rabbit Light	2 tbsp	110	3
blackstrap	2 tbsp	85	10
molasses	2 tbsp	85	10

MONKFISH

baked	3 oz	82	tr

MOOSE

roasted	3 oz	114	4

MOTH BEANS

dried, cooked	1 cup	207	6

MOUSSE

FROZEN

Chocolate (Sara Lee)	1 slice (2.7 oz)	260	1
Chocolate Light (Sara Lee)	1 (3 oz)	170	1
San Francisco Chocolate Mousse (Pepperidge Farm)	1	490	1

HOME RECIPE

orange	½ cup	87	tr

MIX

Chocolate No-Bake (Royal)	⅛ pie	130	tr

FOOD	PORTION	CALORIES	IRON
Chocolate Rich & Luscious (Jell-O)	½ cup	145	1
Chocolate Fudge Rich & Luscious (Jell-O)	½ cup	143	1
Dark Chocolate, as prep (Knorr)	½ cup	90	tr
Milk Chocolate, as prep (Knorr)	½ cup	90	tr

MUFFIN

FROZEN

FOOD	PORTION	CALORIES	IRON
Almond & Date Oat Bran Fancy Fruit (Health Valley)	1	180	4
Apple Oat Bran (Sara Lee)	1	190	5
Apple Spice (Healthy Choice)	1 (2.5 oz)	190	2
Apple Spice (Sara Lee)	1	220	5
Apple Spice Fat Free (Health Valley)	1	140	1
Banana Fat Free (Health Valley)	1	130	1
Banana Nut (Healthy Choice)	1 (2.5 oz)	180	2
Banana Nut (Pepperidge Farm)	1	170	1
Blueberry (Healthy Choice)	1 (2.5 oz)	190	1
Blueberry (Pepperidge Farm)	1	170	tr
Blueberry (Sara Lee)	1	200	5
Blueberry Free & Light (Sara Lee)	1	120	5
Cheese Streusel (Sara Lee)	1	220	1
Chocolate Chunk (Sara Lee)	1	220	2
Cholesterol Free Multi Grain Muesli (Pepperidge Farm)	1	200	1
Cholesterol Free Oat Bran w/ Apple (Pepperidge Farm)	1	190	1
Cholesterol Free Raisin Bran (Pepperidge Farm)	1	170	2
Cinnamon Swirl (Pepperidge Farm)	1	190	tr
Corn (Pepperidge Farm)	1	180	tr

FOOD	PORTION	CALORIES	IRON
Golden Corn (Sara Lee)	1	240	5
Oat Bran (Sara Lee)	1	210	5
Oat Bran Fancy Fruit Blueberry (Health Valley)	1	140	5
Oat Bran Francy Fruit Raisin (Health Valley)	1	180	3
Raisin Bran (Sara Lee)	1	220	5
Raisin Spice Fat Free (Health Valley)	1	140	1
Rice Bran Fancy Fruit Raisin (Health Valley)	1	210	3
HOME RECIPE			
blueberry, as prep w/ 2% milk	1 (2 oz)	163	1
blueberry, as prep w/ whole milk	1 (2 oz)	165	1
corn, as prep w/ 2% milk	1 (2 oz)	180	1
corn, as prep w/ whole milk	1 (2 oz)	183	1
plain, as prep w/ 2% milk	1 (2 oz)	169	1
plain, as prep w/ whole milk	1 (2 oz)	172	1
wheat bran, as prep w/ 2% milk	1 (2 oz)	161	2
wheat bran, as prep w/ whole milk	1 (2 oz)	164	2
MIX			
Apple Cinnamon (Betty Crocker)	1	120	tr
Apple Cinnamon No Cholesterol Recipe (Betty Crocker)	1	110	tr
Banana Nut (Betty Crocker)	1	120	tr
Banana Nut No Cholesterol Recipe (Betty Crocker)	1	110	tr
Blueberry Streusel Bake Shop (Betty Crocker)	1	210	1
Cinnamon Streusel (Betty Crocker)	1	200	tr
Corn Muffin (Dromedary)	1	120	1
Corn Muffin (Flako)	1	120	tr

FOOD	PORTION	CALORIES	IRON
Oat Bran (Betty Crocker)	1	190	1
Oat Bran No Cholesterol Recipe (Betty Crocker)	1	180	1
Twice the Blueberries (Betty Crocker)	1	120	tr
Twice the Blueberries No Cholesterol Recipe (Betty Crocker)	1	110	tr
Wild Blueberry (Betty Crocker)	1	120	tr
Wild Blueberry Light (Betty Crocker)	1	70	tr
Wild Blueberry Light No Cholesterol Recipe (Betty Crocker)	1	70	tr
Wild Blueberry No Cholesterol Recipe (Betty Crocker)	1	110	tr
blueberry	1 (1.75 oz)	149	1
corn	1 (1.75 oz)	160	1
wheat bran, as prep	1 (1.75 oz)	138	1
READY-TO-EAT Bran'nola (Arnold)	1	138	2
Extra Crisp (Arnold)	1	122	1
Raisin (Arnold)	1	149	2
Sourdough (Arnold)	1	124	2
blueberry	1 (2 oz)	158	1
corn	1 (2 oz)	174	2
oat bran wheat free	1 (2 oz)	154	2
toaster-type blueberry	1	103	tr
toaster-type corn	1	114	tr
toaster-type wheat bran	1	106	1

MULBERRIES

FOOD	PORTION	CALORIES	IRON
fresh	1 cup	61	3

FOOD	PORTION	CALORIES	IRON

MULLET

FOOD	PORTION	CALORIES	IRON
striped, cooked	3 oz	127	1
striped, raw	3 oz	99	1

MUNG BEANS

dried, cooked	1 cup	213	3
SPROUTS canned	½ cup	8	tr
cooked	½ cup	13	tr
raw	½ cup	16	tr
stir fried	½ cup	31	1

MUNGO BEANS

dried, cooked	1 cup	190	3

MUSHROOMS

CANNED Mushrooms (B In B)	¼ cup	12	tr
Mushrooms w/ Garlic (B In B)	¼ cup	12	0
Oriental Straw Mushrooms (Green Giant)	¼ cup	12	0
Pieces & Stems (Green Giant)	¼ cup	12	0
Sliced (Green Giant)	¼ cup	12	0
Straw Mushrooms Broken (Empress)	2 oz	10	1
Whole (Green Giant)	¼ cup	12	0
chanterelle	3.5 oz	12	1
pieces	½ cup	19	1
whole	1 (.4 oz)	3	tr
DRIED chanterelle	3.5 oz	89	17

FOOD	PORTION	CALORIES	IRON
shiitake	4 (.5 oz)	44	tr
FRESH			
chanterelle	3.5 oz	11	7
morel	3.5 oz	9	1
raw	1 (.5 oz)	5	tr
raw, sliced	½ cup	9	tr
shiitake, cooked	4 (2.5 oz)	40	tr
sliced, cooked	½ cup	21	1
whole, cooked	1 (.4 oz)	3	tr
FROZEN			
Breaded Mushrooms (Ore Ida)	2.67 oz	120	1

MUSSELS

FRESH			
blue, cooked	3 oz	147	6
blue, raw	1 cup	129	6
blue, raw	3 oz	73	3

MUSTARD

dry mustard seed, yellow	1 tsp	15	tr
yellow ready-to-use	1 tsp	5	tr

MUSTARD GREENS

FRESH			
chopped, cooked	½ cup	11	tr
raw, chopped	½ cup	7	tr
FROZEN			
chopped, cooked	½ cup	14	1

NATTO

natto	½ cup	187	8

FOOD	PORTION	CALORIES	IRON

NAVY BEANS

CANNED

Trappey's	½ cup	90	1
Trappey's Jalapeno	½ cup	90	1
navy	1 cup	296	5

DRIED

cooked	1 cup	259	5

NECTARINE

fresh	1	67	tr

NOODLES

CANNED

Van Camp's Noodle Weenee	1 cup	245	6

DRY

Chinese (Azumaya)	4 oz	293	2
Chow Mein Narrow (La Choy)	½ cup	150	2
Chow Mein Wide (La Choy)	½ cup	150	2
Egg (Golden Grain)	2 oz	210	3
Egg (Mueller's)	2 oz	220	2
Japanese (Azumaya)	4 oz	289	2
Noodle Trio (Mueller's)	2 oz	220	2
Rice (La Choy)	½ cup	130	1
cellophane	1 cup	492	3
chow mein	1 cup	237	2
egg	½ cup	145	2
egg, cooked	1 cup	212	3
japanese soba	2 oz	192	2
japanese soba, cooked	½ cup	56	tr
japanese somen	2 oz	203	tr

FOOD	PORTION	CALORIES	IRON
japanese somen, cooked	½ cup	115	tr
spinach/egg	1 cup	145	2
spinach/egg, cooked	1 cup	211	2
DRY MIX			
Kraft Egg Noodle w/ Chicken Dinner	¾ cup	240	2
La Choy Ramen Noodles Beef, as prep	1 cup	200	2
La Choy Ramen Noodles Chicken, as prep	1 cup	200	2
Lipton Noodles & Sauce			
Alfredo	½ cup	131	1
Beef	½ cup	120	1
Butter	½ cup	142	1
Butter & Herb	½ cup	136	1
Carbonara Alfredo	½ cup	126	1
Cheese	½ cup	136	1
Chicken	½ cup	125	1
Chicken Broccoli	½ cup	124	1
Creamy Chicken	½ cup	125	1
Parmesan	½ cup	138	1
Romanoff	½ cup	136	1
Sour Cream & Chives	½ cup	142	1
Stroganoff	½ cup	110	1
Tomato Alfredo	½ cup	126	1
Minute Microwave Chicken Flavored	½ cup	157	1
Minute Microwave Parmesan	½ cup	178	1
Noodle Roni			
Chicken & Mushroom	½ cup	160	1
Fettucini	½ cup	300	1
Herb & Butter	½ cup	160	1

FOOD	PORTION	CALORIES	IRON
Parmesano	½ cup	240	1
Romanoff	½ cup	240	1
Stroganoff	½ cup	350	2
Ultra Slim-Fast			
Noodles & Alfredo Sauce	2.3 oz	240	5
Noodles & Beef	2.3 oz	230	5
Noodles & Cheese	2.3 oz	230	5
Noodles & Chicken Sauce	2.3 oz	220	5
Noodles & Tomato Herb Sauce	2.3 oz	220	5
TAKE-OUT			
noodle pudding	½ cup	132	1

NUTMEG

ground	1 tsp	12	tr

NUTRITIONAL SUPPLEMENTS

DIET			
Dynatrim Dutch Chocolate, as prep w/ 1% milk	8 oz	220	6
Dynatrim Strawberry Royale, as prep w/ 1% milk	8 oz	220	6
Dynatrim Vanilla, as prep w/ 1% milk	8 oz	220	6
Figurines Chocolate	1 bar	100	3
Figurines Chocolate Caramel	1 bar	100	2
Figurines Chocolate Peanut Butter	1 bar	100	2
Figurines S'Mores	1 bar	100	2
Figurines Vanilla	1 bar	100	2
Slim-Fast Nutrition Bar Dutch Chocolate	1	130	6
Slim-Fast Nutrition Bar Peanut Butter	1	140	6

FOOD	PORTION	CALORIES	IRON
Slim-Fast Powder			
Chocolate, as prep w/ skim milk	8 oz	190	6
Chocolate Malt, as prep w/ skim milk	8 oz	190	6
Strawberry, as prep w/ skim milk	8 oz	190	6
Vanilla, as prep w/ skim milk	8 oz	190	6
Ultra Slim-Fast			
Cafe Mocha, as prep w/ skim milk	8 oz	200	6
Chocolate Royale, as prep w/ skim milk	8 oz	200	6
Crunch Bar Cocoa Almond	1	110	3
Crunch Bar Cocoa Raspberry	1	100	3
Crunch Bar Vanilla Almond	1	110	3
Dutch Chocolate, as prep w/ water	8 oz	220	6
French Vanilla, as prep w/ skim milk	8 oz	190	6
French Vanilla, as prep w/ water	8 oz	220	6
Fruit Juice Mix, as prep w/ fruit juice	8 oz	200	6
Pina Colada, as prep w/ skim milk	8 oz	180	6
Ready-to-Drink Chocolate Royale	11 oz	230	6
Ready-to-Drink Chocolate Royale	12 oz	250	6
Ready-to-Drink French Vanilla	11 oz	230	6
Ready-to-Drink French Vanilla	12 oz	220	6
Ready-to-Drink Strawberry Supreme	12 oz	220	6
Strawberry, as prep w/ skim milk	8 oz	190	6

FOOD	PORTION	CALORIES	IRON
Strawberry Supreme, as prep w/ water	8 oz	220	6
REGULAR EggPro	4 oz	200	2

NUTS, MIXED

FOOD	PORTION	CALORIES	IRON
Cashews & Peanuts Honey Roasted (Eagle)	1 oz	170	tr
Cashews & Peanuts Honey Roasted (Planters)	1 oz	170	1
Mixed (Eagle)	1 oz	180	tr
Mixed Deluxe (Eagle)	1 oz	180	tr
Mixed Lightly Salted (Planters)	1 oz	170	1
Peanuts & Cashews Honey Roasted (Planters)	1 oz	170	tr
dry roasted w/ peanuts	1 oz	169	1
dry roasted w/ peanuts, salted	1 oz	169	1
oil roasted w/ peanuts	1 oz	175	1
oil roasted w/ peanuts, salted	1 oz	175	1
oil roasted w/o peanuts	1 oz	175	1
oil roasted w/o peanuts, salted	1 oz	175	1

OCTOPUS

FOOD	PORTION	CALORIES	IRON
fresh, steamed	3 oz	140	8

OHELO BERRIES

FOOD	PORTION	CALORIES	IRON
fresh	1 cup	39	tr

OIL

FOOD	PORTION	CALORIES	IRON
Wesson Canola	1 tbsp	120	0
Wesson Corn	1 tbsp	120	0
Wesson Lite Cooking Spray	.5-sec spray	0	0

FOOD	PORTION	CALORIES	IRON
Wesson Olive	1 tbsp	120	0
Wesson Sunflower	1 tbsp	120	0
Wesson Vegetable	1 tbsp	120	0
coconut	1 tbsp	117	tr
olive	1 cup	1909	1
olive	1 tbsp	119	tr
palm	1 cup	1927	tr
palm	1 tbsp	120	0
peanut	1 cup	1909	tr
peanut	1 tbsp	119	0
rice bran	1 tbsp	120	tr
soybean	1 cup	1927	tr
soybean	1 tbsp	120	0

OKRA

FOOD	PORTION	CALORIES	IRON
FRESH			
raw	8 pods	36	1
raw, sliced	½ cup	19	tr
sliced, cooked	8 pods	27	tr
sliced, cooked	½ cup	25	tr
FROZEN			
Breaded Okra (Ore Ida)	3 oz	170	1
sliced, cooked	1 pkg (10 oz)	94	2
sliced, cooked	½ cup	34	1

OLIVES

FOOD	PORTION	CALORIES	IRON
California Ripe	3 sm	4	tr
Ripe Extra Large (S&W)	3.5 oz	163	1
Ripe Pitted Large (S&W)	3.5 oz	163	1
green	3 extra lg	15	tr

FOOD	PORTION	CALORIES	IRON
green	4 med	15	tr
ripe	1 colossal	12	1
ripe	1 jumbo	7	tr
ripe	1 lg	5	tr
ripe	1 sm	4	tr

ONION

FOOD	PORTION	CALORIES	IRON
CANNED			
Whole Small (S&W)	½ cup	35	1
chopped	½ cup	21	tr
whole	1 (2.2 oz)	12	tr
DRIED			
flakes	1 tbsp	16	tr
powder	1 tsp	7	tr
FRESH			
Antioch Farms Vidalia	1 med	60	tr
chopped, cooked	½ cup	47	tr
raw, chopped	1 tbsp	4	tr
raw, chopped	½ cup	30	tr
scallions, raw, chopped	1 tbsp	2	tr
scallions, raw, sliced	½ cup	16	1
FROZEN			
Crispy Onion Rings (Mrs. Paul's)	2.5 oz	190	tr
Onion Ringers (Ore Ida)	2 oz	150	tr
Polybag Whole Small (Birds Eye)	½ cup	30	tr
Small w/ Cream Sauce (Birds Eye)	½ cup	100	1
chopped, cooked	1 tbsp	4	tr
chopped, cooked	½ cup	30	tr
rings	7 (2.5 oz)	285	1
rings, cooked	2 (.7 oz)	81	tr

FOOD	PORTION	CALORIES	IRON
whole, cooked	3.5 oz	28	tr
TAKE-OUT			
rings, breaded & fried	8–9	275	tr

ORANGE

CANNED			
Mandarin (Empress)	5.5 oz	100	tr
Mandarin Unsweetened (S&W)	½ cup	28	tr
Pineapple Mandarin Segments (Dole)	½ cup	60	tr
FRESH			
california navel	1	65	tr
california valencia	1	59	tr
florida	1	69	tr
peel	1 tbsp	6	tr
sections	1 cup	85	tr
JUICE			
Kool-Aid Koolers	1 (8.45 oz)	115	tr
Tree Top	6 oz	90	tr
Veryfine 100%	8 oz	121	1
canned	1 cup	104	1
chilled	1 cup	110	tr
fresh	1 cup	111	1
frzn, as prep	1 cup	112	tr
frzn, not prep	6 oz	339	1
mandarin orange	3.5 oz	47	tr
orange drink	6 oz	94	1

OREGANO

ground	1 tsp	5	1

FOOD	PORTION	CALORIES	IRON

ORIENTAL FOOD

CANNED
La Choy Bi-Pack

FOOD	PORTION	CALORIES	IRON
Beef Pepper	¾ cup	80	2
Chow Mein Chicken	¾ cup	80	1
Chow Mein Pork	¾ cup	80	1
Chow Mein Shrimp	¾ cup	70	1
Sweet & Sour Chicken	¾ cup	120	2
Teriyaki Chicken	¾ cup	85	1
La Choy Dinner Chow Mein Chicken	½ pkg	300	4

La Choy Entree

FOOD	PORTION	CALORIES	IRON
Beef Pepper Oriental	¾ cup	100	2
Chow Mein Beef	¾ cup	40	1
Chow Mein Chicken	¾ cup	70	1
Chow Mein Meatless	¾ cup	25	1
Chow Mein Shrimp	¾ cup	35	1
Sweet & Sour Chicken	¾ cup	240	2
Sweet & Sour Pork	¾ cup	250	1
chow mein chicken	1 cup	95	1

FRESH

FOOD	PORTION	CALORIES	IRON
Won Ton Wraps (Azumaya)	1	23	tr
egg roll wrapper	1	83	1
wonton wrapper	1	23	tr

FROZEN

FOOD	PORTION	CALORIES	IRON
Birds Eye Chicken Teriyaki Easy Recipe, not prep	½ pkg	160	3
Birds Eye Chinese Stir Fry Internationals, not prep	3.3 oz	35	1
Birds Eye Oriental Beef Easy Recipe, not prep	½ pkg	100	1

FOOD	PORTION	CALORIES	IRON
Chun King			
Beef Pepper Oriental	13 oz	319	4
Chicken Chow Mein	13 oz	370	2
Crunchy Walnut Chicken	13 oz	310	2
Fried Rice w/ Chicken	8 oz	260	2
Fried Rice w/ Pork	8 oz	270	2
Imperial Chicken	13 oz	300	2
Sweet & Sour Pork	13 oz	400	2
Dining Light Chicken Chow Mein	9 oz	180	1
Healthy Choice Chicken Chow Mein	8.5 oz	220	1
Japanese Stir Fry International, not prep (Birds Eye)	3.3 oz	30	tr
La Choy			
Restaurant Style Egg Roll Almond Chicken	1 (3 oz)	120	1
Restaurant Style Egg Roll Pork	1 (3 oz)	150	2
Restaurant Style Egg Roll Shrimp	1 (3 oz)	130	1
Restaurant Style Egg Roll Sweet & Sour Chicken	1 (3 oz)	150	1
Snack Egg Roll Chicken	2	90	1
Snack Egg Roll Lobster	1 (1.45 oz)	75	1
Snack Egg Roll Meat & Shrimp	1 (1.45 oz)	80	1
Snack Egg Roll Shrimp	1 (1.45 oz)	75	1
Lean Cuisine Chicken Chow Mein w/ Rice	9 oz	240	1
HOME RECIPE			
chop suey w/ beef & pork	1 cup	300	5
chow mein chicken	1 cup	255	3
MIX			
La Choy Dinner Classics			
Egg Foo Yong	2 patties + 3 oz sauce	170	1

FOOD	PORTION	CALORIES	IRON
Pepper Steak	¾ cup	180	2
Sweet & Sour	¾ cup	310	3
TAKE-OUT			
chicken teriyaki	¾ cup	399	3
chop suey w/ pork	1 cup	375	3
chow mein pork	1 cup	425	5
chow mein shrimp	1 cup	221	3
fried rice	6.6 oz	249	1
fried rice w/ egg	6.7 oz	395	1
wonton	1 cup	205	3
wonton, fried	½ cup (1 oz)	111	1

OYSTERS

CANNED			
Bumble Bee Whole	½ cup (3.5 oz)	100	3
Empress Whole	4 oz	100	3
S&W Fancy Whole	2 oz	95	7
eastern	1 cup	170	17
eastern	3 oz	58	6
FRESH			
eastern, cooked	3 oz	117	11
eastern, cooked	6 med	58	6
eastern, raw	1 cup	170	17
eastern, raw	6 med	58	6
pacific, raw	3 oz	69	4
pacific, raw	1 med	41	3
steamed	3 oz	138	8
steamed	1 med	41	2
TAKE-OUT			
battered & fried	6 (4.9 oz)	368	4

FOOD	PORTION	CALORIES	IRON
eastern, breaded & fried	3 oz	167	6
eastern, breaded & fried	6 med	173	6
oysters rockefeller	3 oysters	66	5
stew	1 cup	278	6

PANCAKE/WAFFLE SYRUP

Brer Rabbit Dark	2 tbsp	120	tr
Brer Rabbit Light	2 tbsp	120	tr
maple	2 tbsp	122	tr

PANCAKES

FROZEN

Blueberry (Aunt Jemima)	3.48 oz	220	2
Blueberry Microwave (Pillsbury)	3	250	1
Buttermilk (Aunt Jemima)	3.48 oz	210	2
Buttermilk Batter, as prep (Aunt Jemima)	3.6 oz	180	2
Buttermilk Microwave (Pillsbury)	3	260	1
Harvest Wheat Microwave (Pillsbury)	3	240	1
Lite Buttermilk (Aunt Jemima)	3.48 oz	140	2
Lite Pancakes & Lite Links (Quaker)	1 pkg (6 oz)	310	4
Lite Pancakes & Lite Syrup (Quaker)	1 pkg (6 oz)	260	4
Original (Aunt Jemima)	3.48 oz	211	2
Original Batter, as prep (Aunt Jemima)	3.6 oz	183	2
Original Microwave (Pillsbury)	3	240	1
Pancakes & Sausages (Great Starts)	6 oz	460	3
Pancakes & Sausages (Quaker)	1 pkg (6 oz)	420	4

FOOD	PORTION	CALORIES	IRON
Pancakes w/ Bacon (Great Starts)	4.5 oz	400	2
Silver Dollar Pancakes & Sausages (Great Starts)	3.75 oz	310	2
Whole Wheat Pancakes w/ Lite Links (Great Starts)	5½ oz	350	3
buttermilk	1 (4″ diam)	83	1
plain	1 (4″ diam)	83	1
HOME RECIPE			
blueberry	1 (4″ diam)	84	1
plain	1 (4″ diam)	86	1
MIX			
Apple Cinnamon Shake 'n Pour (Bisquick)	3 (4″ diam)	240	2
Blueberry (Hungry Jack)	3 (4″ diam)	320	1
Blueberry Shake 'n Pour (Bisquick)	3 (4″ diam)	270	2
Buckwheat Pancake & Waffle Mix (Aunt Jemima)	3 (4″ diam)	230	3
Buttermilk (Betty Crocker)	3 (4″ diam)	280	2
Buttermilk (Hungry Jack)	3 (4″ diam)	240	1
Buttermilk Complete (Hungry Jack)	3 (4″ diam)	180	3
Buttermilk Complete Packets (Hungry Jack)	3 (4″ diam)	180	2
Buttermilk Complete Pancake & Waffle Mix (Aunt Jemima)	3 (4″ diam)	230	2
Buttermilk Pancake & Waffle Mix (Aunt Jemima)	3 (4″ diam)	220	2
Buttermilk Shake 'n Pour (Bisquick)	3 (4″ diam)	250	2
Complete Pancake & Waffle Mix (Aunt Jemima)	3 (4″ diam)	250	2
Extra Lights (Hungry Jack)	3 (4″ diam)	210	1
Extra Lights Complete (Hungry Jack)	3 (4″ diam)	190	3

FOOD	PORTION	CALORIES	IRON
Original Pancake & Waffle Mix (Aunt Jemima)	3 (4″ diam)	200	1
Original Shake 'n Pour (Bisquick)	3 (4″ diam)	250	2
Pancake Mix, not prep (Health Valley)	1 oz	100	1
Panshakes (Hungry Jack)	3 (4″ diam)	250	2
Whole Wheat Pancake & Waffle Mix (Aunt Jemima)	3 (4″ diam)	270	5
buckwheat	1 (4″ diam)	62	1
buttermilk	1 (4″ diam)	74	1
plain	1 (4″ diam)	74	1
sugar free, low sodium	1 (3″ diam)	44	tr
whole wheat	1 (4″ diam)	92	1
TAKE-OUT			
buckwheat	1 (4″ diam)	55	tr
potato	1 (4″ diam)	78	tr
w/ butter & syrup	3	519	3

PAPAYA

FRESH			
cubed	1 cup	54	tr
papaya	1	117	tr
JUICE			
Goya Nectar	6 oz	110	1
Kern's Nectar	6 oz	110	tr
Libby's Nectar	6 oz	110	tr
nectar	1 cup	142	1

PAPRIKA

paprika	1 tsp	6	1

FOOD	PORTION	CALORIES	IRON
PARSLEY			
dry	1 tbsp	1	tr
dry	1 tsp	1	tr
fresh, chopped	½ cup	11	2
PARSNIPS			
FRESH			
cooked	1 (5.6 oz)	130	1
cooked, sliced	½ cup	63	tr
raw, sliced	½ cup	50	tr
PASSION FRUIT			
purple	1	18	tr
JUICE			
purple	1 cup	126	1
yellow	1 cup	149	1
PASTA			
DRY			
Dinosaurs (Mueller's)	2 oz	210	2
Egg (Prince)	2 oz	221	2
Jungle Animals (Mueller's)	2 oz	210	2
Lasagna Spinach Whole Wheat (Health Valley)	2 oz	170	5
Lasagna Whole Wheat (Health Valley)	2 oz	170	5
Lasagne (Mueller's)	2 oz	210	2
Monsters (Mueller's)	2 oz	210	2
Outer Space (Mueller's)	2 oz	210	2
Pasta (Anthony)	2 oz	210	2

FOOD	PORTION	CALORIES	IRON
Pasta (Gioia)	2 oz	210	2
Pasta (Golden Grain)	2 oz	203	2
Pasta (Luxury)	2 oz	210	2
Pasta (Merlino's)	2 oz	210	2
Pasta (Penn Dutch)	2 oz	210	2
Pasta (Prince)	2 oz	210	2
Pasta (Red Cross)	2 oz	210	2
Pasta (Ronco)	2 oz	210	2
Pasta (Vimco)	2 oz	210	2
Rainbow (Prince)	2 oz	210	2
Spaghetti (Mueller's)	2 oz	210	2
Spaghetti Amaranth (Health Valley)	2 oz	170	3
Spaghetti Oat Bran (Health Valley)	2 oz	120	1
Spaghetti Spinach Whole Wheat (Health Valley)	2 oz	170	5
Spaghetti Whole Wheat (Health Valley)	2 oz	170	5
Spinach Egg (Prince)	2 oz	220	2
Teddy Bears (Mueller's)	2 oz	210	2
Twists Tri Color (Mueller's)	2 oz	210	2
corn, cooked	1 cup	176	tr
elbows	1 cup	389	4
elbows, cooked	1 cup	197	2
protein fortified, cooked	1 cup	188	tr
shells	1 cup	389	4
shells, cooked	1 cup	197	2
spaghetti	2 oz	211	2
spaghetti, cooked	1 cup	197	2
spaghetti, protein fortified, cooked	1 cup	229	1
spinach spaghetti	2 oz	212	1

FOOD	PORTION	CALORIES	IRON
spinach spaghetti, cooked	1 cup	183	1
spirals	1 cup	389	4
spirals, cooked	1 cup	197	2
vegetable	1 cup	308	4
vegetable, cooked	1 cup	171	tr
whole wheat spaghetti	2 oz	198	2
whole wheat spaghetti, cooked	1 cup	174	1
FRESH			
plain made w/ egg, cooked	2 oz	75	tr
spinach made w/ egg, cooked	2 oz	74	tr
HOME RECIPE			
made w/ egg, cooked	2 oz	74	tr
made w/o egg, cooked	2 oz	71	tr

PASTA DISHES

CANNED			
Franco-American			
Beef RavioliO's in Meat Sauce	½ can (7.5 oz)	250	2
CircusO's Pasta in Tomato & Cheese Sauce	½ can (7⅜ oz)	170	1
CircusO's Pasta w/ Meatballs in Tomato Sauce	½ can (7⅜ oz)	210	2
Macaroni & Cheese	½ can (7⅜ oz)	170	1
Spaghetti in Tomato Sauce w/ Cheese	½ can (7⅜ oz)	180	1
Spaghetti w/ Meatballs in Tomato Sauce	½ can (7⅜ oz)	220	2
SpaghettiO's in Tomato & Cheese Sauce	½ can (7⅜ oz)	170	1
SpaghettiO's w/ Meatballs	½ can (7⅜ oz)	220	2
SpaghettiO's w/ Sliced Franks	½ can (7⅜ oz)	220	1

FOOD	PORTION	CALORIES	IRON
Franco-American *(cont.)*			
SportyO's in Tomato & Cheese Sauce	½ can (7.5 oz)	170	1
SportyO's Pasta w/ Meatballs in Tomato Sauce	½ can (7⅜ oz)	210	2
TeddyO's in Tomato & Cheese Sauce	½ can (7.5 oz)	170	1
TeddyO's Pasta w/ Meatballs	½ can (7⅜ oz)	210	2
Healthy Choice Lasagne w/ Meat Sauce	½ can (7.5 oz)	220	2
Healthy Choice Spaghetti Rings	½ can (7.5 oz)	140	3
Healthy Choice Spaghetti w/ Meat Sauce	½ can (7.5 oz)	150	2
Van Camp's Spaghetti Weenee	1 cup	243	6
DRY MIX Golden Grain Macaroni & Cheese	½ cup	310	1
Kraft Dinomac Macaroni & Cheese Dinner	¾ cup	310	2
Kraft Egg Noodle & Cheese Dinner	¾ cup	340	2
Kraft Macaroni & Cheese Deluxe Dinner	¾ cup	260	2
Kraft Macaroni & Cheese Dinner	¾ cup	290	2
Kraft Macaroni & Cheese Dinner Family Size	¾ cup	290	2
Kraft Mild American Style Spaghetti Dinner	1 cup	300	3
Kraft Pasta & Cheese 3-Cheese w/ Vegetables	½ cup	180	1
Kraft Pasta & Cheese Cheddar Broccoli	½ cup	180	1
Kraft Pasta & Cheese Chicken w/ Herbs	½ cup	170	1
Kraft Pasta & Cheese Fettuccini Alfredo	½ cup	180	1
Kraft Pasta & Cheese Parmesan	½ cup	180	1

FOOD	PORTION	CALORIES	IRON
Kraft Pasta & Cheese Sour Cream w/ Chives	½ cup	180	1
Kraft Spaghetti w/ Meat Sauce Dinner	1 cup	360	3
Kraft Spirals Macaroni & Cheese Dinner	¾ cup	340	2
Kraft Tangy Italian Style Spaghetti Dinner	1 cup	310	3
Kraft Teddy Bears Macaroni & Cheese Dinner	¾ cup	310	2
Kraft Wild Wheels Macaroni & Cheese Dinner	¾ cup	310	2
Lipton Pasta & Sauce			
Cheddar Broccoli	½ cup	132	1
Creamy Garlic	½ cup	146	1
Creamy Mushroom	½ cup	143	1
Herb Tomato	½ cup	130	1
Minute Microwave Cheddar Cheese, Broccoli & Pasta, as prep	½ cup	160	1
Ultra Slim-Fast Macaroni & Cheese	2.3 oz	230	5
Velveeta Bits of Bacon Shells & Cheese Dinner	½ cup	240	2
Velveeta Shells & Cheese Dinner	¾ cup	210	1
Velveeta Touch of Mexico Shells & Cheese Dinner	½ cup	210	1
FROZEN			
Banquet Macaroni & Cheese	6.5 oz	290	1
Banquet Macaroni & Cheese	9 oz	240	2
Birds Eye Easy Recipe Chicken Alfredo, not prep	½ pkg	160	2
Birds Eye Easy Recipe Chicken Primavera, not prep	½ pkg	80	3
Budget Gourmet			
Cheese Lasagna w/ Vegetables	1 pkg	290	2

FOOD	PORTION	CALORIES	IRON
Budget Gourmet *(cont.)*			
Cheese Manicotti	1 pkg	430	2
Cheese Ravioli	1 pkg	290	2
Cheese Tortellini	1 pkg	210	1
Italian Sausage Lasagna	1 pkg	430	2
Lasagna w/ Meat Sauce	1 pkg	300	1
Linguini w/ Scallops & Clams	1 pkg	290	2
Linguini w/ Shrimp & Clams	1 pkg	270	4
Macaroni & Cheese	1 pkg	240	1
Pasta Alfredo w/ Broccoli	1 pkg	230	1
Shrimp w/ Fettucini	1 pkg	370	1
Three Cheese Lasagna	1 pkg	390	2
Ziti in Marinara Sauce	1 pkg	200	1
Dining Light Cheese Cannelloni	9 oz	310	3
Dining Light Cheese Lasagna	9 oz	260	3
Dining Light Fettucini	9 oz	290	3
Dining Light Lasagna	9 oz	240	4
Dining Light Spaghetti	9 oz	220	3
Green Giant			
Garden Gourmet Creamy Mushroom	1 pkg	220	2
Garden Gourmet Pasta Dijon	1 pkg	260	1
Garden Gourmet Pasta Florentine	1 pkg	230	2
Garden Gourmet Rotini Cheddar	1 pkg	230	1
One Serve Cheese Tortellini	1 pkg	260	1
One Serve Macaroni & Cheese	1 pkg	230	1
One Serve Pasta Marinara	1 pkg	180	1
One Serve Pasta Parmesan w/ Green Peas	1 pkg	170	1
Pasta Accents Creamy Cheddar	½ cup	100	1

FOOD	PORTION	CALORIES	IRON
Pasta Accents Garden Herb	½ cup	80	1
Pasta Accents Garlic Seasoning	½ cup	110	1
Pasta Accents Pasta Primavera	½ cup	110	1
Healthy Choice			
Baked Cheese Ravioli	9 oz	240	3
Cheese Manicotti	9.25 oz	230	3
Chicken Fettucini	8.5 oz	240	2
Fettucini Alfredo	8 oz	240	2
Fettucini w/ Turkey & Vegetables	12.5 oz	350	3
Lasagna w/ Meat Sauce	10 oz	260	3
Linguini w/ Shrimp	9.5 oz	230	2
Macaroni & Cheese	9 oz	280	2
Pasta Primavera	11 oz	280	2
Pasta w/ Shrimp	12.5 oz	270	2
Rigatoni in Meat Sauce	9.5 oz	240	4
Rigatoni w/ Chicken	12.5 oz	360	2
Spaghetti w/ Meat Sauce	10 oz	280	4
Stuffed Pasta Shells in Tomato Sauce	12 oz	330	3
Teriyaki Pasta w/ Chicken	12.6 oz	350	3
Zesty Tomato Sauce & Ziti Pasta	12 oz	350	4
Zucchini Lasagna	11.5 oz	240	3
Kid Cuisine Macaroni & Cheese w/ Mini Franks	9 oz	360	2
Kid Cuisine Mini Cheese Ravioli	8.75 oz	290	1
Kid Cuisine Spaghetti w/ Meat Sauce	9.25 oz	310	3
Le Menu Entree LightStyle			
Garden Vegetables Lasagna	10.5 oz	260	2
Lasagna w/ Meat Sauce	10 oz	290	4
Meat Sauce & Cheese Tortellini	8 oz	250	3

FOOD	PORTION	CALORIES	IRON
Le Menu Entree LightStyle *(cont.)*			
Spaghetti w/ Beef Sauce & Mushrooms	9 oz	280	tr
Le Menu LightStyle 3-Cheese Stuffed Shells	10 oz	280	2
Le Menu LightStyle Cheese Tortellini	10 oz	230	3
Le Menu Manicotti w/ Three Cheeses	11.75 oz	390	3
Lean Cuisine			
Beef Cannelloni w/ Mornay Sauce	9⅝ oz	210	3
Cheese Cannelloni w/ Tomato Sauce	9⅛ oz	270	1
Cheese Ravioli	8.5 oz	240	1
Chicken Fettucini	9 oz	280	1
Lasagna w/ Meat Sauce	10.25 oz	260	2
Linguini w/ Clam Sauce	9⅝ oz	280	3
Macaroni & Beef in Tomato Sauce	10 oz	240	2
Macaroni & Cheese	9 oz	290	1
Rigatoni w/ Meat Sauce & Cheese	9.75 oz	250	3
Spaghetti & Meatballs	9.5 oz	280	2
Spaghetti w/ Meat Sauce	11.5 oz	290	4
Tuna Lasagna w/ Spinach Noodles & Vegetables	9.75 oz	240	1
Zucchini Lasagna	11 oz	260	1
Morton Macaroni & Cheese	6.5 oz	290	1
Morton Spaghetti & Meat Sauce	8.5 oz	170	1
Mrs. Paul's Light Seafood Entree Seafood Lasagna	9.5 oz	290	1
Mrs. Paul's Light Seafood Entree Seafood Rotini	9 oz	240	2

FOOD	PORTION	CALORIES	IRON
Mrs. Paul's Seafood Rotini	9 oz	240	2
Swanson			
Homestyle Lasagne w/ Meat Sauce	10.5 oz	400	3
Homestyle Macaroni & Cheese	10 oz	390	2
Homestyle Spaghetti w/ Italian Style Meatballs	13 oz	490	5
Macaroni & Cheese	12.25 oz	370	3
Macaroni & Cheese	7 oz	200	1
Spaghetti & Meatballs	12.5 oz	390	3
Ultra Slim-Fast Pasta Primavera	12 oz	340	3
Ultra Slim-Fast Spaghetti w/ Beef & Mushroom Sauce	12 oz	370	4
HOME RECIPE			
macaroni & cheese	1 cup	430	2
spaghetti w/ meatballs & tomato sauce	1 cup	330	4
SHELF-STABLE			
Healthy Choice Lasagna w/ Meat Sauce	7.5-oz cup	220	2
Healthy Choice Spaghetti Rings	7.5-oz cup	140	3
Healthy Choice Spaghetti w/ Meat Sauce	7.5-oz cup	150	1
TAKE-OUT			
Lasagna	1 piece (2.5" x 2.5")	374	3
lasagna	8 oz	347	2
macaroni & cheese	1 cup	230	1
manicotti	¾ cup (6.4 oz)	273	3
rigatoni w/ sausage sauce	¾ cup	260	3
spaghetti w/ meatballs & cheese	1 cup	407	5

FOOD	PORTION	CALORIES	IRON

PASTA SALAD

MIX
Kraft Pasta Salad & Dressing

Broccoli & Vegetables	½ cup	210	1
Garden Primavera	½ cup	170	1
Homestyle	½ cup	240	1
Light Italian	½ cup	130	1
Light Rancher's Choice	½ cup	170	1
Lipton Robust Italian	½ cup	126	1
Suddenly Salad			
Classic Pasta, as prep	½ cup	160	1
Creamy Macaroni, as prep	½ cup	200	1
Creamy Macaroni, as prep lowfat recipe	½ cup	140	1
Italian Pasta, as prep	½ cup	160	1
Pasta Primavera, as prep	½ cup	190	1
Pasta Primavera, as prep lowfat recipe	½ cup	150	1
Tortellini Italiano, as prep	½ cup	160	1

TAKE-OUT

elbow macaroni salad	3.5 oz	160	1
italian style	3.5 oz	140	1
mustard macaroni salad	3.5 oz	190	1
w/ vegetables	3.5 oz	140	1

PÂTÉ

CANNED

chicken liver	1 oz	238	3
chicken liver	1 tbsp	109	1
liver	1 oz	90	2
liver	1 tbsp	41	1

FOOD	PORTION	CALORIES	IRON

PEACH

FOOD	PORTION	CALORIES	IRON
Halves (Hunt's)	4 oz	90	tr
Sliced Yellow Cling Natural Style (S&W)	½ cup	90	1
Slices (Hunt's)	4 oz	90	tr
Yellow Cling Natural Lite (S&W)	½ cup	50	tr
halves in heavy syrup	1	60	tr
halves in light syrup	1	44	tr
halves juice pack	1	34	tr
halves water pack	1	18	tr
spiced in heavy syrup	1 cup	180	1
spiced in heavy syrup	1 fruit	66	tr
DRIED			
halves	1 cup	383	7
halves	10	311	5
halves, cooked w/ sugar	½ cup	139	2
halves, cooked w/o sugar	½ cup	99	2
FRESH			
peach	1	37	tr
sliced	1 cup	73	tr
FROZEN			
slices sweetened	1 cup	235	1
JUICE			
Dole Pure & Light	6 oz	100	tr
Goya Nectar	6 oz	110	1
Kern's Nectar	6 oz	110	1
Libby's Nectar	6 oz	100	tr
Smucker's	8 oz	120	tr
nectar	1 cup	134	tr

FOOD	PORTION	CALORIES	IRON

PEANUT BUTTER

FOOD	PORTION	CALORIES	IRON
Health Valley Chunky No Salt	2 tbsp	170	1
Health Valley Creamy No Salt	2 tbsp	170	1
Peter Pan Creamy	2 tbsp	190	1
Peter Pan Creamy Salt Free	2 tbsp	190	1
Peter Pan Crunchy	2 tbsp	190	1
Peter Pan Crunchy Salt Free	2 tbsp	190	1
Reese's Peanut Butter Flavored Chips	¼ cup	230	1
Skippy Creamy	1 cup	1540	4
Skippy Creamy w/ 2 slices white bread	1 sandwich	340	2
Skippy Super Chunk	1 cup	1540	4
Skippy Super Chunk	2 tbsp	190	1
Skippy Super Chunk, w/ 2 slices white bread	1 sandwich	340	2
Smucker's Goober Grape	2 tbsp	180	tr
Smucker's Honey Sweetened	2 tbsp	200	1
Smucker's Natural	2 tbsp	200	1
Smucker's Natural No-Salt Added	2 tbsp	200	1
chunky	1 cup	1520	5
chunky	2 tbsp	188	1
chunky w/o salt	1 cup	1520	5
chunky w/o salt	2 tbsp	188	1
smooth	1 cup	1517	4
smooth	2 tbsp	188	1
smooth w/o salt	1 cup	1517	4
smooth w/o salt	2 tbsp	188	1

FOOD	PORTION	CALORIES	IRON

PEANUTS

FOOD	PORTION	CALORIES	IRON
Cocktail Lightly Salted (Planters)	1 oz	170	tr
Cocktail Unsalted (Planters)	1 oz	170	tr
Dry Roasted Lightly Salted (Planters)	1 oz	160	tr
Dry Roasted Unsalted (Planters)	1 oz	170	tr
Fresh Roast Lightly Salted (Planters)	1 oz	160	1
Fresh Roast Salted (Planters)	1 oz	170	tr
Honey Roasted (Eagle)	1 oz	170	tr
Honey Roasted Cinnamon (Eagle)	1 oz	170	tr
Honey Roasted Dry Roasted (Planters)	1 oz	160	1
Honey Roasted Maple (Eagle)	1 oz	170	tr
Low Salt (Eagle)	1 oz	170	tr
Spanish (Planters)	1 oz	170	tr
Spanish Raw (Planters)	1 oz	160	tr
cooked	½ cup	102	tr
dry roasted	1 cup	855	3
dry roasted	1 oz	164	1
oil roasted	1 cup	837	3
oil roasted	1 oz	163	1
oil roasted, w/o salt	1 cup	837	3
oil roasted, w/o salt	1 oz	163	1
spanish, oil roasted	1 oz	162	1
spanish, oil roasted, w/o salt	1 oz	162	1
unroasted	1 oz	159	1
valencia, oil roasted	1 cup	848	2
valencia, oil roasted	1 oz	165	tr
valencia, oil roasted, w/o salt	1 cup	848	2

FOOD	PORTION	CALORIES	IRON
valencia, oil roasted, w/o salt	1 oz	165	tr
virginia, oil roasted	1 cup	826	2
virginia, oil roasted	1 oz	161	tr

PEAR

CANNED

FOOD	PORTION	CALORIES	IRON
Halves (Hunt's)	4 oz	90	tr
Sliced Natural Light Bartlett (S&W)	½ cup	60	tr
Sliced Natural Style (S&W)	½ cup	80	tr
halves in heavy syrup	1 cup	188	1
halves in heavy syrup	1	68	tr
halves in light syrup	1	45	tr
halves juice pack	1 cup	123	1
halves water pack	1	22	3

DRIED

FOOD	PORTION	CALORIES	IRON
halves	1 cup	472	4
halves	10	459	4
halves, cooked w/ sugar	½ cup	196	1
halves, cooked w/o sugar	½ cup	163	1

FRESH

FOOD	PORTION	CALORIES	IRON
pear	1	98	tr
sliced w/ skin	1 cup	97	tr

JUICE

FOOD	PORTION	CALORIES	IRON
Goya Nectar	6 oz	120	1
Kern's Nectar	6 oz	110	1
Libby's Nectar	6 oz	110	tr
nectar	1 cup	149	1

FOOD	PORTION	CALORIES	IRON

PEAS

CANNED

FOOD	PORTION	CALORIES	IRON
Field Peas (Trappey's)	½ cup	90	1
Field Peas w/ Snaps (Trappey's)	½ cup	90	1
Petit Pois (S&W)	½ cup	70	1
Sweet (Green Giant)	½ cup	50	1
Sweet (S&W)	½ cup	70	1
Sweet Water Pack (S&W)	½ cup	40	1
Veri-Green Sweet (S&W)	½ cup	70	1
green	½ cup	59	1
green low sodium	½ cup	59	1

DRIED

split, cooked	1 cup	231	3

FRESH

edible pod, cooked	½ cup	34	2
edible pod, raw	½ cup	30	2
green, cooked	½ cup	67	1
green, raw	½ cup	58	1

FROZEN

Big Valley	3.3 oz	80	1
Chinese Pea Pods (Chun King)	1.5 oz	20	tr
Green (Birds Eye)	½ cup	80	1
Harvest Fresh Early June (Green Giant)	½ cup	60	1
Harvest Fresh Sugar Snap (Green Giant)	½ cup	30	tr
Harvest Fresh Sweet (Green Giant)	½ cup	50	1
In Butter Sauce (Birds Eye)	½ cup	80	1
Le Suer Early (Green Giant Select)	½ cup	60	1

FOOD	PORTION	CALORIES	IRON
Le Suer Early in Butter Sauce (Green Giant)	½ cup	80	1
One Serve in Butter Sauce (Green Giant)	1 pkg	90	1
Polybag Green (Birds Eye)	½ cup	70	1
Polybag Deluxe Tender Tiny (Birds Eye)	½ cup	60	1
Snow Pea Pods (La Choy)	½ pkg (3 oz)	35	2
Sugar Snap Deluxe (Birds Eye)	½ cup	45	1
Sugar Snap Sweet (Green Giant Select)	½ cup	30	tr
Sweet (Green Giant)	½ cup	50	1
Tender Tiny Deluxe (Birds Eye)	½ cup	60	1
edible pod, cooked	1 pkg (10 oz)	132	6
edible pod, cooked	½ cup	42	2
green, cooked	½ cup	63	1
SHELF-STABLE Mini Sweet (Green Giant)	½ cup	60	1
SPROUTS raw	½ cup	77	1
TAKE-OUT pea & potato curry	1 serv (7 oz)	284	2
pea curry	1 serv (4.4 oz)	438	3

PECANS

FOOD	PORTION	CALORIES	IRON
Halves (Planters)	1 oz	190	tr
Honey Roasted (Eagle)	1 oz	200	tr
Pieces (Planters)	1 oz	190	tr
dried	1 oz	190	1
dry roasted	1 oz	187	1
dry roasted, salted	1 oz	187	1

FOOD	PORTION	CALORIES	IRON
halves, dried	1 cup	721	2
oil roasted	1 oz	195	1
oil roasted, salted	1 oz	195	1

PEPPER

black	1 tsp	5	1
cayenne	1 tsp	6	tr
red	1 tsp	6	tr
white	1 tsp	7	tr

PEPPERS

CANNED

Hot Banana Pepper Rings (Vlasic)	1 oz	4	tr
Jalapeno Mexican Hot (Vlasic)	1 oz	8	tr
Mild Cherry (Vlasic)	1 oz	8	tr
Mild Greek Pepperoncini Salad Peppers (Vlasic)	1 oz	4	tr
green chili, hot	1 (2.6 oz)	18	tr
green chili, hot, chopped	½ cup	17	tr
green halves	½ cup	13	1
jalapeno, chopped	½ cup	17	2
red chili, hot	1 (2.6 oz)	18	tr
red chili, hot, chopped	½ cup	17	tr
red halves	½ cup	13	1

DRIED

green	1 tbsp	1	tr
red	1 tbsp	1	tr

FRESH

green chili, hot, raw	1	18	1
green chili, hot, raw, chopped	½ cup	30	1

FOOD	PORTION	CALORIES	IRON
green, chopped, cooked	½ cup	19	tr
green, cooked	1 (2.6 oz)	20	tr
green, raw	1 (2.6 oz)	20	tr
green, raw, chopped	½ cup	13	tr
red chili, hot, raw	1 (1.6 oz)	18	1
red chili, raw, chopped	½ cup	30	1
red, chopped, cooked	½ cup	19	tr
red, cooked	1 (2.6 oz)	20	tr
red, raw	1 (2.6 oz)	20	tr
red, raw, chopped	½ cup	13	tr
FROZEN			
green, chopped, not prep	1 oz	6	tr
red, chopped	1 oz	6	tr

PERCH

FRESH			
atlantic, cooked	3 oz	103	1
atlantic fillet, cooked	1.8 oz	60	1
atlantic, raw	3 oz	80	1
cooked	3 oz	99	1
fillet, cooked	1.6 oz	54	1
raw	3 oz	77	1
red, raw	3.5 oz	114	1

PERSIMMONS

dried japanese	1	93	tr
fresh	1	32	1
fresh japanese	1	118	tr

FOOD	PORTION	CALORIES	IRON
PHEASANT			
FRESH			
breast w/o skin, raw	½ (6.4 oz)	243	1
leg w/o skin, raw	1 (3.6 oz)	143	2
w/ skin, raw	½ fowl (14 oz)	723	5
w/o skin, raw	½ fowl (12.4 oz)	470	4
PHYLLO DOUGH			
Ekizian	½ lb	865	9
phyllo dough	1 oz	85	1
sheet	1	57	1
PICKLES			
Hot & Spicy Garden Mix (Vlasic)	1 oz	4	tr
Kosher Baby Dills (Vlasic)	1 oz	4	tr
Kosher Crunchy Dills (Vlasic)	1 oz	4	tr
Kosher Dill Gherkins (Vlasic)	1 oz	4	tr
No Garlic Dill Spears (Vlasic)	1 oz	4	tr
dill	1 (2.3 oz)	12	tr
dill low sodium	1 (2.3 oz)	12	tr
dill low sodium, sliced	1 slice	1	tr
dill, sliced	1 slice	1	tr
gerkins	3.5 oz	21	2
kosher dill	1 (2.3 oz)	12	tr
piccalilli	1.4 oz	13	tr
polish dill	1 (2.3 oz)	12	tr
quick sour	1 (1.2 oz)	4	tr
quick sour low sodium	1 (1.2 oz)	4	tr
quick sour, sliced	1 slice	1	tr

FOOD	PORTION	CALORIES	IRON
sweet	1 (1.2 oz)	41	tr
sweet gerkin	1 sm (.5 oz)	20	tr
sweet low sodium	1 (1.2 oz)	41	tr
sweet, sliced	1 slice	7	tr

PIE

FOOD	PORTION	CALORIES	IRON
CANNED FILLING			
Mincemeat Old Fashioned (S&W)	½ cup	206	1
pumpkin pie mix	1 cup	282	1
FROZEN			
Apple (Banquet)	1 slice (3.3 oz)	250	1
Apple Homestyle (Sara Lee)	1 slice (4 oz)	280	1
Apple Homestyle High (Sara Lee)	1 slice (4.9 oz)	400	1
Apple Streusel Free & Light (Sara Lee)	1 slice (2.9 oz)	170	1
Blackberry (Banquet)	1 slice (3.3 oz)	270	1
Blueberry (Banquet)	1 slice (3.3 oz)	270	1
Blueberry Homestyle (Sara Lee)	1 slice (4 oz)	300	2
Cherry (Banquet)	1 slice (3.3 oz)	250	tr
Cherry Homestyle (Sara Lee)	1 slice (4 oz)	270	1
Cherry Streusel Free & Light (Sara Lee)	1 slice (3.6 oz)	160	1
Dutch Apple Homestyle (Sara Lee)	1 slice (4 oz)	300	1
Hyannis Boston Cream Pie (Pepperidge Farm)	1	230	2
Mince Homestyle (Sara Lee)	1 slice (4 oz)	300	2
Mincemeat (Banquet)	1 slice (3.3 oz)	260	1
Mississippi Mud (Pepperidge Farm)	1	310	3
Peach (Banquet)	1 slice (3.3 oz)	245	1
Peach Homestyle (Sara Lee)	1 slice (3.4 oz)	280	1

FOOD	PORTION	CALORIES	IRON
Pecan Homestyle (Sara Lee)	1 slice (3.4 oz)	400	1
Pumpkin (Banquet)	1 slice (3.3 oz)	200	1
Pumpkin Homestyle (Sara Lee)	1 slice (4 oz)	240	1
Raspberry Homestyle (Sara Lee)	1 slice (4 oz)	280	1
HOME RECIPE			
pecan	⅙ of 9" pie	575	5
MIX			
Boston Cream Classic Dessert (Betty Crocker)	⅛ pie	270	1
Chocolate Mousse (Jell-O)	⅛ pie	259	1
Coconut Cream (Jell-O)	⅛ pie	258	tr
Coconut Cream, as prep w/ whole milk (Jell-O)	⅙ of 8" pie	111	tr
Lemon (Jell-O)	⅙ of 8" pie	175	tr
Lemon Meringue No-Bake (Royal)	⅛ pie	210	tr
Pumpkin (Jell-O)	⅛ pie	253	1
READY-TO-USE			
apple	⅙ of 9" pie	405	2
blueberry	⅙ of 9" pie	380	2
cherry	⅙ of 9" pie	410	2
creme	⅙ of 9" pie	455	1
custard	⅙ of 9" pie	330	2
lemon meringue	⅙ of 9" pie	355	1
peach	⅙ of 9" pie	405	2
pumpkin	⅙ of 9" pie	320	1
SNACK			
Apple (Drake's)	1 (2 oz)	210	1
Blueberry (Drake's)	1 (2 oz)	210	tr
Cherry (Drake's)	1 (2 oz)	220	1
Dutch Apple (Little Debbie)	1 pkg (2.17 oz)	270	1

FOOD	PORTION	CALORIES	IRON
Lemon (Drake's)	1 (2 oz)	210	1
Marshmallow Banana (Little Debbie)	1 pkg (1.38 oz)	170	1
Marshmallow Chocolate (Little Debbie)	1 pkg (1.38 oz)	170	1
Oatmeal Creme (Little Debbie)	1 pkg (1.33 oz)	170	1
Pecan (Little Debbie)	1 pkg (1.83 oz)	200	1
Raisin Creme (Little Debbie)	1 pkg (1.17 oz)	170	tr
apple	1 (3 oz)	266	tr
cherry	1 (3 oz)	266	tr
lemon	1 (3 oz)	266	tr

PIE CRUST

FOOD	PORTION	CALORIES	IRON
FROZEN			
Pepperidge Farm Patty Shells	1	210	tr
Pepperidge Farm Puff Pastry Sheets	¼ sheet	260	1
puff pastry, baked	1 shell (1.4 oz)	223	1
HOME RECIPE			
9-inch crust	1	900	5
MIX			
Betty Crocker	¹⁄₁₆ pkg	120	tr
Betty Crocker Sticks	¹⁄₁₆ pkg	120	tr
Flako	⅙ of 9" pie	250	1
Pillsbury Stick	⅙ of 2-crust pie	270	1
Pillsbury Mix	⅙ of 2-crust pie	270	1
as prep	2 crusts	1485	9
READY-TO-USE			
Ready Crust Chocolate	1 (3" diam)	110	tr
Ready Crust Chocolate	⅛ of 9" pie	100	tr
Ready Crust Graham	1 (3" diam)	110	tr

FOOD	PORTION	CALORIES	IRON
Ready Crust Graham	⅛ of 9″ pie	100	tr
REFRIGERATED Pillsbury All Ready	⅛ of 2-crust pie	240	0

PIEROGI

TAKE-OUT pierogi	¾ cup (4.4 oz)	307	2

PIG'S EARS

ears, frzn, simmered	1 ear (3.7 oz)	183	2

PIGEON PEAS

DRIED catjang, cooked	1 cup	200	5
cooked	1 cup	204	2
cooked	½ cup	86	1

PIKE

FRESH northern, cooked	3 oz	96	1
northern fillet, cooked	½ (5.4 oz)	176	1
northern, raw	3 oz	75	tr
walleye, baked	3 oz	101	1
walleye fillet, baked	4.4 oz	147	2

PILLNUTS

canarytree, dried	1 oz	204	1

PIMIENTOS

canned	1 slice	0	tr
canned	1 tbsp	3	tr

FOOD	PORTION	CALORIES	IRON

PINE NUTS

FOOD	PORTION	CALORIES	IRON
pignolia, dried	1 oz	146	3
pignolia, dried	1 tbsp	51	1
pinyon, dried	1 oz	161	1

PINEAPPLE

FOOD	PORTION	CALORIES	IRON
CANNED			
All Cuts Juice Pack (Dole)	½ cup	70	tr
All Cuts Syrup Pack (Dole)	½ cup	90	tr
Hawaiian Slice Juice Pack (S&W)	½ cup	70	tr
chunks in heavy syrup	1 cup	199	1
chunks juice pack	1 cup	150	1
crushed in heavy syrup	1 cup	199	1
slices in heavy syrup	1 slice	45	tr
slices in light syrup	1 slice	30	tr
slices juice pack	1 slice	35	tr
slices water pack	1 slice	19	tr
tidbits in heavy syrup	1 cup	199	1
tidbits in juice	1 cup	150	1
tidbits in water	1 cup	79	1
FRESH			
diced	1 cup	77	1
sliced	1 slice	42	tr
FROZEN			
chunks sweetened	½ cup	104	tr
JUICE			
Dole	6 oz	100	tr
Dole New Breakfast Juice	6 oz	100	tr
Libby's Nectar	6 oz	110	tr

FOOD	PORTION	CALORIES	IRON
S&W Unsweetened	6 oz	100	tr
Tree Top	6 oz	100	tr
Veryfine 100%	8 oz	125	tr
canned	1 cup	139	1
frzn, as prep	1 cup	129	1
frzn, not prep	6 oz	387	2

PINK BEANS

CANNED Goya Spanish Style	7.5 oz	140	3
DRIED cooked	1 cup	252	4

PINTO BEANS

CANNED Gebhardt	4 oz	100	2
Goya Spanish Style	7.5 oz	140	4
Green Giant	½ cup	90	1
Green Giant Picante	½ cup	100	1
Trappey's	½ cup	90	1
Trappey's Hearty Texas	½ cup	110	2
Trappey's Jalapinto	½ cup	90	1
pinto	1 cup	186	4
DRIED cooked	1 cup	235	4
FROZEN cooked	3 oz	152	3

PISTACHIOS

California Natural (Dole)	1 oz	90	tr

FOOD	PORTION	CALORIES	IRON
Red Salted (Planters)	1 oz	170	1
Shelled & Roasted (Dole)	1 oz	163	2
dried	1 cup	739	9
dried	1 oz	164	2
dry roasted	1 oz	172	1
dry roasted, salted	1 cup	776	4
dry roasted, salted	1 oz	172	1

PITANGA

fresh	1	2	tr
fresh	1 cup	57	tr

PIZZA

FROZEN
Fox Deluxe
Golden Topping	½ pizza	240	2
Hamburger	½ pizza	260	2
Pepperoni	½ pizza	250	2
Sausage	½ pizza	260	2
Sausage & Pepperoni	½ pizza	260	2
Healthy Choice French Bread			
Cheese	1 (5.3 oz)	270	3
Deluxe	1 (6.25 oz)	330	3
Italian Turkey Sausage	1 (6.45 oz)	320	3
Pepperoni	1 (6.25 oz)	320	3
Jeno's 4-Pack			
Cheese	1 pizza	160	1
Combination	1 pizza	180	1
Hamburger	1 pizza	180	1
Pepperoni	1 pizza	170	1
Sausage	1 pizza	180	1

FOOD	PORTION	CALORIES	IRON
Jeno's Crisp 'n Tasty			
Canadian Bacon	½ pizza	250	2
Cheese	½ pizza	270	2
Hamburger	½ pizza	290	2
Pepperoni	½ pizza	280	2
Sausage	½ pizza	300	2
Sausage & Pepperoni	½ pizza	300	2
Jeno's Microwave Pizza Rolls			
Pepperoni & Cheese	6	240	3
Sausage & Cheese	6	250	3
Jeno's Pizza Rolls			
Cheese	6	240	2
Hamburger	6	240	3
Pepperoni & Cheese	6	230	3
Sausage & Pepperoni	6	230	3
Kid Cuisine Cheese	1 (6.85 oz)	380	3
Kid Cuisine Hamburger	6.85 oz	330	2
MicroMagic Deep Dish Combination	1 (6.5 oz)	605	3
MicroMagic Deep Dish Pepperoni	1 (6.5 oz)	615	3
MicroMagic Deep Dish Sausage	1 (6.5 oz)	590	3
Mr. P's Combination	½ pizza	260	2
Mr. P's Golden Topping	½ pizza	240	2
Mr. P's Hamburger	½ pizza	260	2
Mr. P's Pepperoni	½ pizza	250	2
Mr. P's Sausage	½ pizza	260	2
Pappalo's			
French Bread Cheese	1 pizza	360	2
French Bread Combination	1 pizza	430	2
French Bread Pepperoni	1 pizza	410	2
French Bread Sausage	1 pizza	410	2

FOOD	PORTION	CALORIES	IRON
Pappalo's *(cont.)*			
Pan Combination	⅙ pizza	340	2
Pan Hamburger	⅙ pizza	310	1
Pan Pepperoni	⅙ pizza	330	1
Pan Sausage	⅙ pizza	360	1
Thin Crust Combination	⅙ pizza	260	1
Thin Crust Hamburger	⅙ pizza	240	1
Thin Crust Pepperoni	⅙ pizza	270	1
Thin Crust Sausage	⅙ pizza	250	1
Pepperidge Farm			
Croissant Pastry Cheese	1	430	2
Croissant Pastry Deluxe	1	440	3
Croissant Pastry Pepperoni	1	420	2
Pillsbury Microwave			
Cheese	½ pizza	240	2
Combination	½ pizza	310	2
French Bread	1 pizza	370	2
French Bread Pepperoni	1 pizza	430	3
French Bread Sausage	1 pizza	410	5
French Bread Sausage & Pepperoni	1 pizza	450	3
Pepperoni	½ pizza	300	2
Sausage	½ pizza	280	2
Totino's			
Microwave Cheese	1 pizza	250	2
Microwave Pepperoni	1 pizza	280	2
Microwave Sausage	1 pizza	320	1
Microwave Sausage Pepperoni Combination	1 pizza	310	2
My Classic Deluxe Cheese	⅙ pizza	210	1
My Classic Deluxe Combination	⅙ pizza	270	2

FOOD	PORTION	CALORIES	IRON
My Classic Deluxe Pepperoni	⅙ pizza	260	1
Pan Pepperoni	⅙ pizza	330	1
Pan Sausage	⅙ pizza	320	2
Pan Sausage & Pepperoni Combination	⅙ pizza	340	2
Pan Three Cheese	⅙ pizza	290	1
Party Bacon	½ pizza	370	3
Party Canadian Bacon	½ pizza	310	2
Party Cheese	½ pizza	340	3
Party Combination	½ pizza	380	1
Party Hamburger	½ pizza	370	3
Party Mexican Style	½ pizza	380	3
Party Pepperoni	½ pizza	370	3
Party Sausage	½ pizza	390	3
Party Vegetable	½ pizza	300	3
Slices Cheese	1	170	1
Slices Combination	1	200	1
Slices Pepperoni	1	190	1
Slices Sausage	1	200	1
SAUCE			
Ragu Pizza Quick Sauce Garlic & Basil	1.7 oz	35	tr
Ragu Pizza Quick Sauce Mushrooms	1.7 oz	35	tr
Ragu Pizza Quick Sauce Traditional	1.7 oz	35	tr
Ragu Pizza Quick Sauce w/ Cheese	1.7 oz	35	tr
Ragu Pizza Quick Sauce w/ Pepperoni	1.7 oz	35	tr
Ragu Pizza Quick Sauce w/ Sausage	3 tbsp	35	tr

FOOD	PORTION	CALORIES	IRON
TAKE-OUT			
cheese	⅛ of 12″ pie	140	1
cheese	12″ pie	1121	5
cheese, meat & vegetables	⅛ of 12″ pie	184	2
cheese, meat & vegetables	12″ pie	1472	12
pepperoni	⅛ of 12″ pie	181	1
pepperoni	12″ pie	1445	7

PLANTAINS

FOOD	PORTION	CALORIES	IRON
All Natural Plantain Chips (Top Banana)	1 oz	150	1
FRESH			
sliced, cooked	½ cup	89	tr
uncooked	1	218	1
TAKE-OUT			
ripe, fried	2.8 oz	214	1

PLUMS

FOOD	PORTION	CALORIES	IRON
CANNED			
Halves Purple Fancy Unpeeled in Extra Heavy Syrup (S&W)	½ cup	135	1
Whole Purple Fancy Unpeeled in Extra Heavy Syrup (S&W)	½ cup	135	1
purple in heavy syrup	1 cup	320	2
purple in heavy syrup	3	119	1
purple in light syrup	1 cup	158	2
purple in light syrup	3	83	1
purple juice pack	1 cup	146	1
purple juice pack	3	55	tr
purple water pack	1 cup	102	tr
purple water pack	3	39	tr

FOOD	PORTION	CALORIES	IRON
FRESH			
plum	1	36	tr
sliced	1 cup	91	tr
JUICE			
Kern's Nectar	6 oz	110	1

POI

poi	½ cup	134	1

POKEBERRY SHOOTS

fresh, cooked	½ cup	16	1
fresh, raw	½ cup	18	1

POLLACK

atlantic, baked	3 oz	100	1
atlantic fillet, baked	5.3 oz	178	1
FROZEN			
Mrs. Paul's Light Fillets	1 (4.5 oz)	240	tr

POMEGRANATE

fresh	1	104	tr

POMPANO

florida, cooked	3 oz	179	1
florida, raw	3 oz	140	1

POPCORN

Newman's Own	3⅓ cups	80	1
Newman's Own, Microwave Butter	3 cups	140	1
Light Butter	3 cups	90	1
Light Natural	3 cups	90	1

FOOD	PORTION	CALORIES	IRON
Newman's Own, Microwave *(cont.)*			
Natural	3 cups	140	1
Natural No Salt	3 cups	140	1
Orville Redenbacher's			
Gourmet Hot Air	3 cups	40	tr
Gourmet Original	3 cups	80	tr
Gourmet White	3 cups	80	tr
Orville Redenbacher's, Microwave			
Gourmet	3 cups	100	tr
Gourmet Butter	3 cups	100	tr
Gourmet Butter Toffee	2½ cups	210	1
Gourmet Caramel	2½ cups	240	1
Gourmet Cheddar Cheese	3 cups	130	tr
Gourmet Frozen	3 cups	100	tr
Gourmet Frozen Butter	3 cups	100	tr
Gourmet Light	3 cups	70	tr
Gourmet Light Butter	3 cups	70	tr
Gourmet Salt Free	3 cups	100	tr
Gourmet Salt Free Butter	3 cups	100	tr
Gourmet Sour Cream 'n Onion	3 cups	160	1
Pillsbury Microwave Butter	3 cups	210	tr
Pillsbury Microwave Original	3 cups	210	tr
Pillsbury Microwave Salt Free	3 cups	170	1
Pop Secret			
Butter Flavor	3 cups	100	tr
Butter Flavor Singles	6 cups	250	1
Light Butter Flavor	3 cups	70	tr
Light Butter Flavor Singles	6 cups	140	1
Light Natural Flavor	3 cups	70	tr
Light Natural Flavor Singles	6 cups	150	1
Natural Flavor	3 cups	100	tr

FOOD	PORTION	CALORIES	IRON
Pop Qwiz Butter Flavor	3 cups	100	tr
Pop Qwiz Natural Flavor	3 cups	100	tr
Snyder's Butter	1 oz	140	1
Snyder's Cheese Gourmet White	1 oz	150	1
Ultra Slim-Fast Lite 'n Tasty	.5 oz	60	tr
air popped	1 cup	30	tr
popped w/ vegetable oil	1 cup	55	tr
sugar syrup coated	1 cup	135	1

POPPY SEEDS

poppy seeds	1 tsp	15	0

PORK

FRESH			
blade chop, roasted	1 (3.1 oz)	321	1
center loin chop, broiled	1 (3.1 oz)	275	1
center loin, roasted	3 oz	259	1
loin w/ fat, roasted	3 oz	271	1
shoulder, arm picnic, cured, lean only, roasted	3 oz	145	1
shoulder blade roll, cured, lean & fat	3 oz	304	1
shoulder whole, roasted	3 oz	277	1
spareribs, braised	3 oz	338	2
spleen, braised	3 oz	127	19
tenderloin, lean only, roasted	3 oz	141	1

POT PIE

FROZEN			
Beef (Swanson)	7 oz	370	3
Beef Hungry Man (Swanson)	16 oz	610	5

FOOD	PORTION	CALORIES	IRON
Chicken (Swanson)	7 oz	380	2
Chicken Homestyle (Swanson)	8 oz	410	2
Chicken Hungry Man (Swanson)	16 oz	630	4
Turkey (Swanson)	7 oz	380	2
Turkey Hungry Man (Swanson)	16 oz	650	4
Vegetable Pie w/ Beef (Banquet)	7 oz	510	2
Vegetable Pie w/ Beef (Morton)	7 oz	430	2
Vegetable Pie w/ Chicken (Banquet)	7 oz	550	2
Vegetable Pie w/ Chicken (Morton)	7 oz	420	2
Vegetable Pie w/ Turkey (Banquet)	7 oz	510	2
Vegetable Pie w/ Turkey (Morton)	7 oz	420	2
HOME RECIPE			
beef, baked	⅓ of 9" pie (7.4 oz)	515	4
chicken	⅓ of 9" pie (8.1 oz)	545	3

POTATO

CANNED			
Hunt's Whole New	4 oz	70	1
S&W New Extra Small	½ cup	45	tr
potatoes	½ cup	54	1
FRESH			
baked w/ skin	1 (6.5 oz)	220	3
baked w/o skin	1 (5 oz)	145	1
baked w/o skin	½ cup	57	tr
boiled	½ cup	68	tr
microwaved	1 (7 oz)	212	3
microwaved w/o skin	½ cup	78	tr

FOOD	PORTION	CALORIES	IRON
raw w/o skin	1 (3.9 oz)	88	1
skin only, baked	1 skin (2 oz)	115	4
FROZEN			
Baked Potato w/ Broccoli & Cheddar (Lean Cuisine)	10.38 oz	290	1
Baked Potato w/ Broccoli & Cheese Sauce (Healthy Choice)	10 oz	240	3
Cheddar Browns (Ore Ida)	3 oz	90	1
Cheddared Potatoes (Budget Gourmet)	1 pkg	260	1
Cheddared Potatoes w/ Broccoli (Budget Gourmet)	1 pkg	150	tr
Cottage Fries (Ore Ida)	3 oz	130	1
Crispers! (Ore Ida)	3 oz	220	1
Crispy Crowns! (Ore Ida)	3 oz	190	tr
Crispy Crunchers (Ore Ida)	3 oz	180	1
Deep Fries Crinkle Cuts (Ore Ida)	3 oz	160	tr
Deep Fries French Fries (Ore Ida)	3 oz	170	tr
Dinner Fries Country Style (Ore Ida)	3 oz	110	tr
French Fries (MicroMagic)	1 pkg (3 oz)	290	1
Golden Crinkles (Ore Ida)	3 oz	120	1
Golden Fries (Ore Ida)	3 oz	120	tr
Golden Twirls (Ore Ida)	3 oz	160	1
Hash Browns Shredded (Ore Ida)	3 oz	70	1
Lites Crinkle Cuts (Ore Ida)	3 oz	90	tr
Microwave Crinkle Cuts (Ore Ida)	3.5 oz	190	1
Microwave Hash Browns (Ore Ida)	2 oz	110	tr
Microwave Tater Tots (Ore Ida)	4 oz	210	1
Nacho Potatoes (Budget Gourmet)	1 pkg	200	tr
O'Brien Potatoes (Ore Ida)	3 oz	60	tr

FOOD	PORTION	CALORIES	IRON
One Serve Potatoes & Broccoli in Cheese Sauce (Green Giant)	1 pkg	130	tr
One Serve Potatoes au Gratin (Green Giant)	1 pkg	200	tr
Shoestrings (Ore Ida)	3 oz	150	tr
Skinny Fries (MicroMagic)	1 pkg (3 oz)	350	2
Stuffed Potatoes w/ Cheddar Cheese (Oh Boy!)	1 (6 oz)	150	tr
Stuffed Potatoes w/ Real Bacon (Oh Boy!)	1 (6 oz)	120	tr
Stuffed Potatoes w/ Sour Cream & Chives (Oh Boy!)	1 (6 oz)	110	1
Tater Tots (Ore Ida)	3 oz	160	1
Tater Tots w/ Bacon (Ore Ida)	3 oz	150	tr
Tater Tots w/ Onion (Ore Ida)	3 oz	150	1
Three-Cheese Potatoes (Budget Gourmet)	1 pkg	230	tr
Toaster Hash Browns (Ore Ida)	1 (1.75 oz)	100	tr
Topped Broccoli & Cheese (Ore Ida)	1 (5.63 oz)	160	1
Topped Vegetable Primavera (Ore Ida)	1 (6.13 oz)	160	1
Twice Baked Butter Flavor (Ore Ida)	1 (5 oz)	200	1
Twice Baked Cheddar Cheese (Ore Ida)	1 (5 oz)	210	1
Twice Baked Sour Cream & Chives (Ore Ida)	1 (5 oz)	190	1
Wedges Home Style (Ore Ida)	3 oz	110	1
Zesties! (Ore Ida)	3 oz	160	1
french fries	10 strips	111	1
french fries, thick cut	10 strips	109	1
hashed browns	½ cup	170	1
potato puffs	½ cup	138	1

FOOD	PORTION	CALORIES	IRON
potato puffs, as prep	1 puff	16	tr
HOME RECIPE			
au gratin	½ cup	160	1
hash browns	½ cup	163	1
mashed	½ cup	111	tr
o'brien	1 cup	157	1
potato pancakes	1 (2.7 oz)	495	1
scalloped	½ cup	105	1
MIX			
Au Gratin, as prep (Betty Crocker)	½ cup	140	tr
Cheddar & Bacon Casserole (French's)	½ cup	130	0
Cheesy Scalloped, as prep (Betty Crocker)	½ cup	140	tr
Creamy Italian Scalloped (French's)	½ cup	120	0
Creamy Stroganoff (French's)	½ cup	130	tr
Crispy Top Scalloped w/ Savory Onion (French's)	½ cup	140	tr
Hash Browns, as prep (Betty Crocker)	½ cup	160	tr
Hash Browns, as prep w/o salt (Betty Crocker)	½ cup	160	tr
Homestyle American Cheese, as prep (Betty Crocker)	½ cup	140	tr
Homestyle Broccoli Au gratin, as prep (Betty Crocker)	½ cup	130	tr
Homestyle Cheddar Cheese, as prep (Betty Crocker)	½ cup	140	tr
Homestyle Cheesy Scalloped, as prep (Betty Crocker)	½ cup	140	tr
Julienne, as prep (Betty Crocker)	½ cup	130	tr

FOOD	PORTION	CALORIES	IRON
Mashed Potato Flakes (Hungry Jack)	½ cup	40	0
Potatoes & Cheese Broccoli Au Gratin (Kraft)	½ cup	120	tr
Potatoes & Cheese Scalloped (Kraft)	½ cup	140	tr
Real Cheese Scalloped (French's)	½ cup	140	tr
Real Sour Cream & Chives (French's)	½ cup	150	tr
Scalloped & Ham, as prep (Betty Crocker)	½ cup	160	tr
Scalloped, as prep (Betty Crocker)	½ cup	140	tr
Smokey Cheddar, as prep (Betty Crocker)	½ cup	140	tr
Sour Cream 'n Chives, as prep (Betty Crocker)	½ cup	140	tr
Spuds Mashed (French's)	½ cup	140	tr
Tangy Au Gratin (French's)	½ cup	130	tr
Twice Baked Bacon & Cheddar, as prep (Betty Crocker)	½ cup	210	tr
Twice Baked Herbed Butter, as prep (Betty Crocker)	½ cup	220	1
Twice Baked Mild Cheddar w/ Onion, as prep (Betty Crocker)	½ cup	190	1
Twice Baked Sour Cream & Chives, as prep (Betty Crocker)	½ cup	200	tr
au gratin, as prep	4.5 oz	127	tr
instant mashed flakes, as prep w/ whole milk & butter	½ cup	118	tr
instant mashed flakes, not prep	½ cup	78	tr
instant mashed granules, as prep w/ whole milk & butter	½ cup	114	tr
instant mashed granules, not prep	½ cup	372	1

FOOD	PORTION	CALORIES	IRON
scalloped, as prep	4.5 oz	127	1
SHELF-STABLE Au Gratin Potatoes (Pantry Express)	½ cup	120	tr
TAKE-OUT au gratin w/ cheese	½ cup	178	1
baked, topped w/ cheese sauce	1	475	3
baked, topped w/ cheese sauce & bacon	1	451	3
baked, topped w/ cheese sauce & broccoli	1	402	3
baked, topped w/ cheese sauce & chili	1	481	409
baked, topped w/ sour cream & chives	1	394	3
curry	1 serv (6 oz)	292	2
french fried in beef tallow	1 lg	358	2
french fried in beef tallow	1 reg	237	1
french fried in vegetable oil	1 lg	355	2
french fried in vegetable oil	1 reg	235	1
hash browns	½ cup	151	tr
mashed w/ whole milk & margarine	⅓ cup	66	tr
mustard potato salad	3.5 oz	120	tr
potato salad	½ cup	179	1
potato salad	⅓ cup	108	tr
scalloped	½ cup	127	1

POTATO STARCH

FOOD	PORTION	CALORIES	IRON
potato starch	3.5 oz	335	2

FOOD	PORTION	CALORIES	IRON

POUT

FRESH
ocean, baked	3 oz	86	tr
ocean fillet, baked	4.8 oz	139	tr

PRETZELS

A & Eagle	1 oz	110	tr
A & Eagle Beer	1 oz	110	tr
Mister Salty Fat Free Sticks	1 oz	100	1
Mister Salty Fat Free Twists	1 oz	100	1
Mister Salty Twists	1 oz	110	1
Mister Salty Very Thin Sticks	1 oz	110	1
Mr. Phipps Chips	8	60	1
Mr. Phipps Chips Lightly Salted	8	60	1
Mr. Phipps Chips Sesame	8	60	1
Snyder's Logs	1 oz	310	tr
Snyder's Minis	1 oz	310	tr
Snyder's Minis Unsalted	1 oz	310	tr
Snyder's Nibblers	1 oz	310	tr
Snyder's Old Fashioned Hard	1 oz	100	tr
Snyder's Old Fashioned Hard Unsalted	1 oz	100	tr
Snyder's Old Tyme	1 oz	310	tr
Snyder's Old Tyme Unsalted	1 oz	110	tr
Snyder's Rods	1 oz	310	tr
Snyder's Stix	1 oz	310	tr
Snyder's Very Thins	1 oz	310	tr
Ultra Slim-Fast Lite 'n Tasty	1 oz	100	2
Wege Sourdough	1 oz	102	1
Wege Unsalted	1 oz	102	tr

FOOD	PORTION	CALORIES	IRON
Wege Whole Wheat	1 oz	109	1
sticks	10	10	tr
twist	1 (.5 oz)	65	tr
twists thin	10 (2 oz)	240	1

PRICKLY PEAR

fresh	1	42	tr

PRUNES

CANNED			
in heavy syrup	1 cup	245	1
in heavy syrup	5	90	tr
DRIED			
cooked w/ sugar	½ cup	147	1
cooked w/o sugar	½ cup	113	1
dried	1 cup	385	4
dried	10	201	2
JUICE			
S&W Unsweetened	6 oz	120	2
canned	1 cup	181	3

PUDDING

HOME RECIPE			
bread w/ raisins	½ cup	180	2
corn	⅔ cup	181	1
yorkshire, as prep w/ skim milk	3.5 oz	93	1
yorkshire, as prep w/ whole milk	3.5 oz	104	1
MIX WITH 2% MILK			
Banana Instant Sugar Free (Jell-O)	½ cup	84	tr
Chocolate Instant Sugar Free (Jell-O)	½ cup	92	tr

FOOD	PORTION	CALORIES	IRON
Chocolate Sugar Free (Jell-O)	½ cup	91	1
Pistachio Instant Sugar Free (Jell-O)	½ cup	94	tr
Vanilla Instant Sugar Free (Jell-O)	½ cup	82	tr
MIX WITH SKIM MILK Butterscotch (D-Zerta)	½ cup	68	tr
Chocolate (D-Zerta)	½ cup	65	tr
Vanilla (D-Zerta)	½ cup	69	tr
MIX WITH WHOLE MILK Banana Cream Instant (Jell-O)	½ cup	165	tr
Butter Pecan Instant (Jell-O)	½ cup	170	tr
Butterscotch (Jell-O)	½ cup	169	tr
Butterscotch Instant (Jell-O)	½ cup	164	tr
Chocolate Fudge Instant (Jell-O)	½ cup	175	1
Chocolate Instant (Jell-O)	½ cup	176	tr
Chocolate Tapioca Americana (Jell-O)	½ cup	169	1
Coconut Cream Instant (Jell-O)	½ cup	178	tr
French Vanilla (Jell-O)	½ cup	169	tr
French Vanilla Instant (Jell-O)	½ cup	165	tr
Lemon Instant (Jell-O)	½ cup	168	tr
Milk Chocolate Instant (Jell-O)	½ cup	179	tr
Pineapple Cream Instant (Jell-O)	½ cup	165	tr
Pistachio Instant (Jell-O)	½ cup	170	tr
Rice Americana (Jell-O)	½ cup	175	1
Vanilla (Jell-O)	½ cup	156	tr
Vanilla Instant (Jell-O)	½ cup	168	tr
Vanilla Tapioca Americana (Jell-O)	½ cup	160	tr
chocolate	½ cup	150	tr
chocolate instant	½ cup	155	tr

FOOD	PORTION	CALORIES	IRON
rice	½ cup	155	1
tapioca	½ cup	145	tr
vanilla	½ cup	145	tr
vanilla instant	½ cup	150	tr
READY-TO-USE			
Butterscotch (Ultra Slim-Fast)	4 oz	100	2
Chocolate (Jell-O)	1 (4 oz)	171	1
Chocolate (Snack Pack)	4.25 oz	170	tr
Chocolate (Swiss Miss)	4 oz	180	1
Chocolate (Ultra Slim-Fast)	4 oz	100	2
Chocolate Caramel Swirl (Jell-O)	1 (4 oz)	175	tr
Chocolate Light (Jell-O)	1 (4 oz)	104	tr
Chocolate Vanilla Light (Jell-O)	1 (4 oz)	104	tr
Chocolate Vanilla Swirl (Jell-O)	1 (5.5 oz)	240	1
Chocolate Vanilla Swirl (Jell-O)	1 (4 oz)	175	tr
Chocolate Fudge (Jell-O)	1 (4 oz)	171	1
Chocolate Fudge (Snack Pack)	4.25 oz	165	tr
Chocolate Fudge (Swiss Miss)	4 oz	220	1
Chocolate Fudge Light (Jell-O)	1 (4 oz)	101	tr
Chocolate Fudge Light (Swiss Miss)	4 oz	100	tr
Chocolate Fudge Milk Chocolate Swirl (Jell-O)	1 (4 oz)	171	1
Chocolate Light (Snack Pack)	4.25 oz	100	1
Chocolate Light (Swiss Miss)	4 oz	100	1
Chocolate Sundae (Swiss Miss)	4 oz	220	1
Lemon (Snack Pack)	4.25 oz	150	tr
Milk Chocolate (Jell-O)	1 (4 oz)	173	tr
Tapioca (Jell-O)	1 (5.5 oz)	229	tr
Tapioca (Jell-O)	1 (4 oz)	167	tr

FOOD	PORTION	CALORIES	IRON
Tapioca (Snack Pack)	4.25 oz	150	tr
Tapioca (Swiss Miss)	4 oz	160	tr
Vanilla (Jell-O)	1 (5.5 oz)	250	tr
Vanilla (Jell-O)	1 (4 oz)	182	tr
Vanilla (Ultra Slim-Fast)	4 oz	100	2
Vanilla Chocolate Parfait Light (Swiss Miss)	4 oz	100	tr
Vanilla Chocolate Swirl (Jell-O)	1 (4 oz)	178	tr
Vanilla Parfait (Swiss Miss)	4 oz	180	1
Vanilla Sundae (Swiss Miss)	4 oz	200	1
TAKE-OUT			
blancmange	1 serv (4.7 oz)	154	tr
bread	1 serv (6.7 oz)	564	3
queen of puddings	1 serv (4.4 oz)	266	1
rice	1 serv (3 oz)	110	tr
rice w/ raisins	½ cup	246	2
tapioca	½ cup	169	1

PUDDING POPS

FOOD	PORTION	CALORIES	IRON
Jell-O Chocolate	1	79	tr
Jell-O Chocolate Caramel Swirl	1	74	tr
Jell-O Chocolate Fudge	1	79	tr
Jell-O Chocolate Peanut Butter Swirl	1	78	tr
Jell-O Chocolate Swirl	1	80	tr
Jell-O Chocolate Vanilla Swirl	1	78	tr
Jell-O Milk Chocolate	1	80	tr
Jell-O Vanilla	1	77	tr
Jell-O Deluxe Chocolate Covered	1	201	1
Jell-O Deluxe Peanuts & Chocolate	1	185	tr

FOOD	PORTION	CALORIES	IRON

PUMMELO

FOOD	PORTION	CALORIES	IRON
fresh	1	228	1
sections	1 cup	71	tr

PUMPKIN

CANNED
FOOD	PORTION	CALORIES	IRON
pumpkin	½ cup	41	2

FRESH
FOOD	PORTION	CALORIES	IRON
cooked, mashed	½ cup	24	2
flowers, cooked	½ cup	10	1
flowers, raw	1	0	tr
leaves, cooked	½ cup	7	1
leaves, raw	½ cup	4	tr
raw, cubed	½ cup	15	tr

SEEDS
FOOD	PORTION	CALORIES	IRON
dried	1 oz	154	4
roasted	1 cup	1184	34
roasted	1 oz	148	4
salted & roasted	1 cup	1184	34
salted & roasted	1 oz	148	4
whole roasted	1 cup	285	2
whole roasted	1 oz	127	1
whole, salted, roasted	1 cup	285	2
whole, salted, roasted	1 oz	127	1

PURSLANE

FOOD	PORTION	CALORIES	IRON
cooked	1 cup	21	1
raw	1 cup	7	1

FOOD	PORTION	CALORIES	IRON

QUAIL

FRESH
breast w/o skin, raw	1 (2 oz)	69	1
w/ skin, raw	1 quail (3.8 oz)	210	4
w/o skin, raw	1 quail (3.2 oz)	123	4

QUICHE

HOME RECIPE
| lorraine | ⅛ of 8" pie | 600 | 1 |

TAKE-OUT
cheese	1 slice (3 oz)	283	1
lorraine	1 slice (3 oz)	352	1
mushroom	1 slice (3 oz)	256	1

QUINCE

| fresh | 1 | 53 | 1 |

QUINOA

| quinoa | ½ cup | 318 | 8 |

RABBIT

| domestic w/o bone, roasted | 3 oz | 167 | 2 |
| wild w/o bone, stewed | 3 oz | 147 | 4 |

RADISHES

DRIED
| chinese | ½ cup | 157 | 4 |
| daikon | ½ cup | 157 | 4 |

FRESH
| chinese, raw | 1 (12 oz) | 62 | 1 |
| chinese, raw, sliced | ½ cup | 8 | tr |

FOOD	PORTION	CALORIES	IRON
chinese, sliced, cooked	½ cup	13	tr
daikon, raw	1 (12 oz)	62	1
daikon, raw, sliced	½ cup	8	tr
daikon, sliced, cooked	½ cup	13	tr
red, raw	10	7	tr
red, sliced	½ cup	10	tr
white icicle, raw	1 (.5 oz)	2	tr
white icicle, raw, sliced	½ cup	7	tr
SPROUTS			
raw	½ cup	8	tr

RAISINS

Dole Golden	½ cup	260	2
Dole Seedless	½ cup	260	2
Sunbelt	1 bar (1 oz)	90	1
golden seedless	1 cup	437	3
seedless	1 cup	434	3
sultanas	1 oz	88	1

RASPBERRIES

CANNED			
in heavy syrup	½ cup	117	1
FRESH			
raspberries	1 cup	61	1
raspberries	1 pint	154	2
FROZEN			
Red (Big Valley)	3.5 oz	55	1
Whole in Lite Syrup (Birds Eye)	½ cup	100	tr
sweetened	1 cup	256	2
sweetened	1 pkg (10 oz)	291	2

FOOD	PORTION	CALORIES	IRON
JUICE			
Dole Pure & Light	6 oz	90	tr
Smucker's	8 oz	120	1
Smucker's Juice Sparkler	10 oz	130	1

RED BEANS

CANNED			
Green Giant	½ cup	90	1
Hunt's Small	4 oz	90	2
Van Camp's	1 cup	194	3

RELISH

Hot Dog (Vlasic)	1 oz	40	tr
cranberry orange	½ cup	246	tr
hamburger	1 tbsp	19	tr
hamburger	½ cup	158	1
hot dog	1 tbsp	14	tr
hot dog	½ cup	111	2
piccalilli	1.4 oz	13	tr
sweet	1 cup	159	1
sweet	1 tbsp	19	tr

RHUBARB

Big Valley, frzn	3.5 oz	16	tr
fresh	½ cup	13	tr
frzn	½ cup	60	tr
frzn, as prep w/ sugar	½ cup	139	tr

RICE

(*see also* BRAN, CEREAL, FLOUR, WILD RICE)

FOOD	PORTION	CALORIES	IRON
BROWN			
Minute Precooked, as prep	½ cup	121	tr
S&W Quick Natural Long Grain	3.5 oz	110	tr
S&W Quick Natural Long Grain, cooked	3.5 oz	119	1
long-grain, cooked	½ cup	109	tr
medium-grain, cooked	½ cup	109	tr
CANNED			
Van Camp's Spanish	1 cup	160	3
DRY MIX			
Knorr Risotto Milanese w/ Saffron	½ cup	130	1
Knorr Risotto Tomato	½ cup	110	1
Knorr Risotto w/ Mushrooms	½ cup	110	1
Knorr Risotto w/ Onion	½ cup	110	1
Knorr Risotto w/ Peas & Corn	½ cup	110	1
La Choy Chinese Fried Rice	¾ cup	190	3
Lipton Golden Saute			
Fried Rice Beef	½ cup	124	1
Fried Rice Chicken	½ cup	129	1
Fried Rice Oriental	½ cup	127	1
Lipton Rice & Sauce			
Beef	½ cup	119	1
Cajun	½ cup	123	2
Cheddar Broccoli	½ cup	125	3
Chicken	½ cup	124	1
Chicken Broccoli	½ cup	129	1
Creamy Chicken	½ cup	142	2
Herbs & Butter	½ cup	123	2
Long Grain & Wild Rice Original	½ cup	121	2
Mushroom	½ cup	123	2
Pilaf	½ cup	122	1

FOOD	PORTION	CALORIES	IRON
Lipton Rice & Sauce *(cont.)*			
Skillet Style Spanish	½ cup	104	1
Spanish	½ cup	118	1
Rice Asparagus w/ Hollandaise	½ cup	123	2
Minute Fried Rice w/ Vermicelli, as prep	½ cup	158	1
Minute Microwave Broccoli Almondine	½ cup	143	1
Minute Microwave Cheddar Cheese Broccoli	½ cup	164	1
Minute Microwave French Pilaf	½ cup	133	1
Minute Microwave Long Grain Brown & Wild	½ cup	140	1
Minute Microwave Rice w/ Savory Cheese Sauce, as prep	½ cup	162	1
Minute Rice Drumstick w/ Vermicelli, as prep	½ cup	153	1
Rice-A-Roni			
Beef	½ cup	140	1
Beef & Mushroom	½ cup	150	1
Chicken	½ cup	150	1
Chicken & Broccoli	½ cup	150	1
Chicken & Mushroom	½ cup	180	1
Chicken & Vegetables	½ cup	140	1
Fried Rice	½ cup	110	1
Herb & Butter	½ cup	130	tr
Long Grain & Wild, Chicken w/ Almonds	½ cup	140	1
Long Grain & Wild, Original	½ cup	130	1
Long Grain & Wild, Pilaf	½ cup	130	1
Pilaf	½ cup	150	1
Risotto	½ cup	200	1

FOOD	PORTION	CALORIES	IRON
Spanish	½ cup	150	1
Stroganoff	½ cup	200	1
Yellow Rice	½ cup	140	1
Ultra Slim-Fast Oriental Style	2.3 oz	240	5
Ultra Slim-Fast Rice & Chicken Sauce	2.3 oz	240	5
FROZEN			
Birds Eye French Style	½ cup	170	tr
Birds Eye Rice & Broccoli Au Gratin	½ pkg	150	tr
Budget Gourmet Oriental Rice w/ Vegetables	1 pkg	240	tr
Budget Gourmet Rice Mexicana	1 pkg	240	1
Budget Gourmet Rice Pilaf w/ Green Beans	1 pkg	240	tr
Green Giant Garden Gourmet Asparagus Pilaf	1 pkg	190	5
Green Giant Garden Gourmet Sherry Wild Rice	1 pkg	210	3
Green Giant One Serve Rice 'n Broccoli in Cheese Sauce	1 pkg	180	1
Green Giant One Serve Rice, Peas & Mushrooms w/ Sauce	1 pkg	130	1
Green Giant Rice Originals Italian Rice & Spinach in Cheese Sauce	½ cup	140	1
Green Giant Rice Originals Pilaf	½ cup	110	1
Green Giant Rice Originals Rice Medley	½ cup	100	1
Green Giant Rice Originals Rice 'n Broccoli in Cheese Sauce	½ cup	120	1
Green Giant Rice Originals White & Wild	½ cup	130	1

FOOD	PORTION	CALORIES	IRON
TAKE-OUT			
pilaf	½ cup	84	1
risotto	6.6 oz	426	1
spanish	¾ cup	363	2
WHITE			
Minute, as prep	⅔ cup	141	1
Minute Boil in Bag Long Grain, as prep	½ cup	94	1
Minute Long Grain, as prep	⅔ cup	150	1
Minute Long Grain & Wild, as prep	½ cup	149	2
Minute Rib Roast w/ Vermicelli, as prep	½ cup	151	1
S&W Long Grain, cooked	3.5 oz	106	1
Superfino Arborio Rice	½ cup	100	1
glutinous, cooked	½ cup	116	tr
long-grain, cooked	½ cup	131	1
long-grain instant, cooked	½ cup	80	tr
long-grain parboiled, cooked	½ cup	100	tr
medium-grain, cooked	½ cup	132	2
short-grain, cooked	½ cup	133	1

ROCKFISH

FRESH			
pacific, cooked	3 oz	103	tr
pacific fillet, cooked	5.2 oz	180	1
pacific, raw	3 oz	80	tr

ROLL
(*see also* BISCUIT, CROISSANT, ENGLISH MUFFIN, MUFFIN, SCONE)

FROZEN			
All Butter Cinnamon Roll w/ Icing (Sara Lee)	1	280	tr

FOOD	PORTION	CALORIES	IRON
All Butter Cinnamon Roll w/o Icing (Sara Lee)	1	230	tr
Cinnamon Roll (Pepperidge Farm)	1 (2.25 oz)	220	1
HOME RECIPE			
dinner, as prep w/ 2% milk	1 (2½")	111	1
dinner, as prep w/ whole milk	1 (2½")	112	1
raisin & nut	1 (2 oz)	196	1
MIX			
Hot Roll (Dromedary)	2	239	3
Hot Roll (Pillsbury)	2	240	2
READY-TO-EAT			
Bran'nola Buns (Arnold)	1	99	2
Brown 'n Serve Club (Pepperidge Farm)	1	100	1
Brown 'n Serve French (Pepperidge Farm)	½	180	2
Brown 'n Serve Hearth (Pepperidge Farm)	1	50	1
Buns (Wonder)	1	70	2
Deli Egg Old Country (Levy's)	1	146	2
Deli Kaiser Old Country (Levy's)	1	170	3
Deli Onion Old Country (Levy's)	1	153	3
Deli Sub Old Country (Levy's)	1	163	3
Dinner (Pepperidge Farm)	1	60	1
Dinner Country Style Classic (Pepperidge Farm)	1	50	1
Dinner Party (Arnold)	1	51	1
Dutch Egg Buns (Arnold)	1	123	1
Finger Poppy Seed (Pepperidge Farm)	1	50	tr
Finger Sesame Seed (Pepperidge Farm)	1	60	1

FOOD	PORTION	CALORIES	IRON
Frankfurter Dijon (Pepperidge Farm)	1	160	1
Frankfurter Side Sliced (Pepperidge Farm)	1	140	1
Frankfurter Top Sliced (Pepperidge Farm)	1	140	1
Frankfurter w/ Poppy Seeds (Pepperidge Farm)	1	130	1
French Francisco International (Arnold)	1	108	2
French Style (Pepperidge Farm)	1	100	1
Hamburger (Arnold)	1	115	1
Hamburger (Pepperidge Farm)	1	130	1
Hamburger Light (Wonder)	1	80	2
Heat & Serve Butter Crescent (Pepperidge Farm)	1	110	1
Heat & Serve Golden Twist (Pepperidge Farm)	1	110	1
Hoagie Soft (Pepperidge Farm)	1	210	1
Hot Dog (Arnold)	1	100	1
Hot Dog Light (Wonder)	1	80	2
Hot Dog New England Style (Arnold)	1	108	1
Kaiser Francisco (Arnold)	1	184	3
Old Fashioned (Pepperidge Farm)	1	50	tr
Parker House (Pepperidge Farm)	1	60	tr
Party (Pepperidge Farm)	1	30	tr
Potato Sandwich (Pepperidge Farm)	1	160	1
Salad Roll (Matthew's)	1	110	1
Sandwich (Matthew's)	1	110	1
Sandwich Onion w/ Poppy Seeds (Pepperidge Farm)	1	150	1

FOOD	PORTION	CALORIES	IRON
Sandwich Salad (Pepperidge Farm)	1	110	1
Sandwich Soft (Arnold)	1	110	1
Sandwich w/ Sesame Seeds (Pepperidge Farm)	1	140	1
Soft Family (Pepperidge Farm)	1	100	1
Sourdough French (Pepperidge Farm)	1	100	1
brown & serve	1 (1 oz)	85	1
cheese	1 (2.3 oz)	238	1
cinnamon raisin	1 (2¾")	223	1
dinner	1 (1 oz)	85	1
egg	1 (2½")	107	1
french	1 (1.3 oz)	105	1
hamburger	1 (1.5 oz)	123	1
hamburger multi-grain	1 (1.5 oz)	113	2
hamburger reduced calorie	1 (1.5 oz)	84	1
hard	1 (3½")	167	2
hot cross bun	1	202	1
hot dog	1 (1.5 oz)	123	1
hot dog multi-grain	1 (1.5 oz)	113	2
hot dog reduced calorie	1 (1.5 oz)	84	1
kaiser	1 (3½")	167	2
oat bran	1 (1.2 oz)	78	1
rye	1 (1 oz)	81	1
submarine	1 (4.7 oz)	155	1
wheat	1 (1 oz)	77	1
whole wheat	1 (1 oz)	75	1
REFRIGERATED Pillsbury Best Quick Cinnamon Rolls w/ Icing	1	110	tr

FOOD	PORTION	CALORIES	IRON
Pillsbury Butterflake	1	140	1
Pillsbury Crescent	1	100	tr
cinnamon w/ frosting	1	109	1
crescent	1 (1 oz)	98	1

ROSE APPLE

fresh	3.5 oz	32	1

ROSE HIP

fresh	3.5 oz	91	1

ROSELLE

fresh	1 cup	28	1

ROSEMARY

dried	1 tsp	4	tr

ROUGHY

orange, baked	3 oz	75	tr

RUTABAGA

FRESH			
cooked, mashed	½ cup	41	1
raw, cubed	½ cup	25	tr

SABLEFISH

baked	3 oz	213	1
fillet, baked	5.3 oz	378	2

SAFFRON

saffron	1 tsp	2	tr

FOOD	PORTION	CALORIES	IRON

SAGE

ground	1 tsp	2	tr

SALAD
(*see also* PASTA SALAD)

MIX

Suddenly Salad Caesar, as prep	½ cup	170	1
Suddenly Salad Ranch & Bacon, as prep	½ cup	210	1
Suddenly Salad Ranch & Bacon, as prep lowfat recipe	½ cup	160	1

TAKE-OUT

chef w/o dressing	1½ cups	386	3
tossed w/o dressing	1½ cups	32	1
tossed w/o dressing	¾ cup	16	tr
tossed w/o dressing w/ cheese & egg	1½ cups	102	tr
tossed w/o dressing w/ chicken	1½ cups	105	1
tossed w/o dressing w/ pasta & seafood	1½ cups	380	3
tossed w/o dressing w/ shrimp	1½ cups	107	tr
waldorf	½ cup	79	tr

SALAD DRESSING

HOME RECIPE

french	1 tbsp	88	0

MIX

Good Seasons Buttermilk Farm, as prep	1 tbsp	58	tr
Good Seasons Classic Dill	1 pkg	28	1
Good Seasons Ranch, as prep	1 tbsp	57	tr

FOOD	PORTION	CALORIES	IRON
READY-TO-USE			
Healthy Sensation			
Blue Cheese	1 tbsp	19	tr
French	1 tbsp	21	0
Honey Dijon	1 tbsp	26	tr
Italian	1 tbsp	7	tr
Ranch	1 tbsp	15	0
Thousand Island	1 tbsp	20	0
Ultra Slim-Fast French	1 tbsp	20	2
Ultra Slim-Fast Italian	1 tbsp	6	2
Wishbone			
Blue Cheese Chunky	1 tbsp	73	0
Blue Cheese Chunky Lite	1 tbsp	40	0
Caesar w/ Olive Oil Lite	1 tbsp	28	0
Dijon Vinaigrette Classic	1 tbsp	57	tr
Dijon Vinaigrette Classic Lite	1 tbsp	30	0
French Deluxe	1 tbsp	57	0
French Lite	1 tbsp	30	0
French Red	1 tbsp	64	0
French Red Lite	1 tbsp	17	0
French Sweet 'n Spicy	1 tbsp	61	tr
French Sweet 'n Spicy Lite	1 tbsp	17	0
Italian	1 tbsp	45	tr
Italian Creamy	1 tbsp	54	tr
Italian Creamy Lite	1 tbsp	26	0
Italian Lite	1 tbsp	6	0
Italian Robusto	1 tbsp	46	tr
Olive Oil Italian Classic	1 tbsp	33	tr
Olive Oil Italian Classic Lite	1 tbsp	20	0
Olive Oil Vinaigrette	1 tbsp	30	0
Olive Oil Vinaigrette Lite	1 tbsp	16	0

FOOD	PORTION	CALORIES	IRON
Ranch	1 tbsp	76	0
Ranch Lite	1 tbsp	42	0
Russian	1 tbsp	54	tr
Russian Lite	1 tbsp	21	0
Thousand Island	1 tbsp	66	tr
Thousand Island Lite	1 tbsp	22	0
blue cheese	1 tbsp	77	0
french	1 tbsp	67	tr
french reduced calorie	1 tbsp	22	tr
italian	1 tbsp	69	0
italian reduced calorie	1 tbsp	16	0
russian	1 tbsp	76	tr
russian reduced calorie	1 tbsp	23	tr
thousand island	1 tbsp	59	tr
thousand island reduced calorie	1 tbsp	24	tr

SALMON

CANNED

FOOD	PORTION	CALORIES	IRON
Bumble Bee Pink	2 oz	160	1
Bumble Bee Pink Skinless Boneless	3.25 oz	120	tr
Bumble Bee Red Sockeye	2 oz	180	1
Deming's Alaska Keta	½ cup	140	1
Deming's Alaska Pink	½ cup	140	1
Deming's Alaska Red Sockeye	½ cup	170	1
Double "Q" Alaska Pink	½ cup	140	1
Humpty Dumpty Alaska Chum	½ cup	140	1
S&W Red Fancy Sockeye Bluepack	½ cup	190	1
pink w/ bone	1 can (15.9 oz)	631	4
pink w/ bone	3 oz	118	1

FOOD	PORTION	CALORIES	IRON
sockeye w/ bone	1 can (12.9 oz)	566	4
sockeye w/ bone	3 oz	130	1
FRESH			
atlantic, baked	3 oz	155	1
chinook, baked	3 oz	196	1
chum, baked	3 oz	131	1
coho, cooked	3 oz	157	1
coho fillet, cooked	½ (5.4 oz)	286	1
coho, raw	3 oz	124	1
pink, baked	3 oz	127	1
sockeye, cooked	3 oz	183	1
sockeye fillet, cooked	½ (5.4 oz)	334	1
sockeye, raw	3 oz	143	tr
SMOKED			
chinook	1 oz	33	tr
chinook	3 oz	99	1
TAKE-OUT			
salmon cake	1 (3 oz)	241	1

SALSA

FOOD	PORTION	CALORIES	IRON
Casa Fiesta Chili Salsa	1 oz	9	tr
Rosarita Chunky Hot	3 tbsp	25	1
Rosarita Chunky Medium	3 tbsp	25	tr
Rosarita Chunky Mild	3 tbsp	25	tr
Rosarita Taco Salsa Chunky Medium	3 tbsp	25	1
Rosarita Taco Salsa Chunky Mild	3 tbsp	25	1

SALSIFY

FOOD	PORTION	CALORIES	IRON
FRESH			
cooked, sliced	½ cup	46	tr

FOOD	PORTION	CALORIES	IRON
raw, sliced	½ cup	55	tr

SALT/SEASONED SALT

salt	1 tsp	0	tr

SAPODILLA

fresh	1	140	1
fresh, cut up	1 cup	199	2

SAPOTES

fresh	1	301	2
CANNED			
Empress Skinless & Boneless in Olive Oil	1 can (3.8 oz)	420	1
Empress Skinless & Boneless in Soy Oil	1 can (4.4 oz)	500	1
S&W Norwegian Brisling	1.5 oz	130	1
atlantic w/ bone in oil	1 can (3.2 oz)	192	3
atlantic w/ bone in oil	2	50	1
pacific w/ bone in tomato sauce	1	68	1
pacific w/ bone in tomato sauce	1 can (13 oz)	658	9
FRESH			
raw	3.5 oz	135	2

SAUCE
(*see also* GRAVY, PIZZA, SPAGHETTI SAUCE, TOMATO)

DRY			
Etoufee Seasoning Mix (Cajun King)	3.5 oz	383	6
Jambalaya Seasoning Mix (Cajun King)	3.5 oz	375	4
Napoli, as prep (Knorr)	4 oz	100	1

FOOD	PORTION	CALORIES	IRON
cheese, as prep w/ milk	1 cup	307	tr
sour cream, as prep w/ milk	1 cup	509	1
stroganoff	1 cup	271	1
sweet & sour	1 cup	294	2
teriyaki	1 cup	131	3
white, as prep w/ milk	1 cup	241	tr
JARRED			
Bandito Diavalo Spicy (Newman's Own)	4 oz	70	1
Barbecue			
Country Style (Hunt's)	1 tbsp	20	tr
Hickory (Hunt's)	1 tbsp	20	tr
Homestyle (Hunt's)	1 tbsp	20	tr
Kansas City Style (Hunt's)	1 tbsp	20	tr
Kansas City Style (Kraft)	2 tbsp	50	1
New Orleans Style (Hunt's)	1 tbsp	20	tr
Original (Hunt's)	1 tbsp	20	tr
Southern Style (Hunt's)	1 tbsp	20	tr
Texas Style (Hunt's)	1 tbsp	25	tr
Thick 'n Spicy Chunky (Kraft)	2 tbsp	60	tr
Thick 'n Spicy Hickory Smoke (Kraft)	2 tbsp	50	tr
Thick 'n Spicy Kansas City Style (Kraft)	2 tbsp	60	tr
Thick 'n Spicy Mesquite Smoke (Kraft)	2 tbsp	50	tr
Thick 'n Spicy Original (Kraft)	2 tbsp	50	tr
Thick 'n Spicy w/ Honey (Kraft)	2 tbsp	60	tr
Western Style (Hunt's)	1 tbsp	20	tr
Chili 7 Spice Tabasco (McIlhenny)	4 oz	56	4
Enchilada Sauce (Gebhardt)	3 tbsp	25	1

FOOD	PORTION	CALORIES	IRON
Ginger Teriyaki Marinade (Golden Dipt)	1 oz	120	1
Hot Dog (Just Rite)	2 oz	60	1
Hot Dog (Wolf Brand)	1.25 oz	44	1
Hot Dog Chili (Gebhardt)	2 tbsp	30	tr
Manwich Mexican	2.5 oz	35	2
Sloppy Joe (Manwich)	2.5 oz	40	1
Tabasco (McIlhenny)	¼ tsp	tr	tr
Worcestershire (Heinz)	1 tbsp	6	tr
barbecue	1 cup	188	2
teriyaki	1 oz	30	1
teriyaki	1 tbsp	15	tr

SAUERKRAUT

CANNED			
SnowFloss Kraut	4 oz	28	tr
SnowFloss Kraut Bavarian Style	4 oz	64	tr
Vlasic Old Fashioned	1 oz	4	tr
canned	½ cup	22	2
JUICE			
S&W	4 oz	14	1

SAUSAGE
(*see also* HOT DOG)

FROZEN			
Louis Rich Breakfast Links	1	46	1
Louis Rich Polska Kielbasa	1 oz	40	tr
Louis Rich Smoked Sausage, cooked	1 (1 oz)	43	tr
Louis Rich Smoked Sausage w/ Cheese, cooked	1 oz	47	tr

FOOD	PORTION	CALORIES	IRON
Oscar Mayer Little Friers Pork, cooked	1 (.75 oz)	82	tr
Oscar Mayer Smokies Beef	1 (1.5 oz)	124	1
Oscar Mayer Smokies Cheese	1 (1.5 oz)	126	tr
Oscar Mayer Smokies Links	1 (1.5 oz)	126	1
Oscar Mayer Smokies Little	1 (.33 oz)	27	tr
blutwurst, uncooked	3.5 oz	424	6
bratwurst pork	1 oz	92	tr
bratwurst pork, cooked	1 link (3 oz)	256	1
bratwurst pork & beef	1 link (2.5 oz)	226	1
country-style pork, cooked	1 link (.5 oz)	48	tr
country-style pork, cooked	1 patty (1 oz)	100	tr
italian pork, cooked	1 (2.4 oz)	216	1
italian pork, cooked	1 (3 oz)	268	1
kielbasa pork	1 oz	88	tr
knockwurst pork & beef	1 (2.4 oz)	209	1
knockwurst pork & beef	1 oz	87	tr
mettwurst, uncooked	3.5 oz	483	2
polish pork	1 (8 oz)	739	3
polish pork	1 oz	92	tr
pork & beef, cooked	1 link (.5 oz)	52	tr
pork & beef, cooked	1 patty (1 oz)	107	tr
pork, cooked	1 link (.5 oz)	48	tr
pork, cooked	1 patty (1 oz)	100	tr
smoked pork	1 link (2.4 oz)	265	1
smoked pork	1 sm link (.5 oz)	62	tr
smoked pork & beef	1 link (2.4 oz)	229	tr
smoked pork & beef	1 sm link (.5 oz)	54	tr
vienna, canned	1 (.5 oz)	45	tr

FOOD	PORTION	CALORIES	IRON
vienna, canned	7 (4 oz)	315	1
TAKE-OUT			
pork	1 link (.5 oz)	48	tr
pork	1 patty (1 oz)	100	tr

SAUSAGE DISHES

sausage roll	1 (2.3 oz)	311	1

SAVORY

ground	1 tsp	4	1

SCALLOP

FRESH			
raw	3 oz	75	tr
HOME RECIPE			
breaded & fried	2 lg	67	tr
TAKE-OUT			
breaded & fried	6 (5 oz)	386	2

SCONE

HOME RECIPE			
apricot scone	1	232	2
TAKE-OUT			
cheese	1 (1.75 oz)	182	1
fruit	1 (1.75 oz)	158	1
plain	1 (1.75 oz)	181	1

SCROD

FROZEN			
Microwave Entree Baked (Gorton's)	1 pkg	320	tr

FOOD	PORTION	CALORIES	IRON

SCUP

fresh, baked	3 oz	115	1

SEA BASS
(*see* BASS)

SEA TROUT
(*see* TROUT)

SEAWEED

DRIED			
agar	1 oz	87	6
FRESH			
agar	1 oz	tr	1
irish moss	1 oz	14	3
kelp	1 oz	12	1
kombu	1 oz	12	1
laver	1 oz	10	1
nori	1 oz	10	1
tangle	1 oz	12	1
wakame	1 oz	13	1

SEMOLINA

dry	½ cup	303	4

SESAME

Sesame Butter (Erewhon)	2 tbsp	190	2
Sesame Tahini (Erewhon)	2 tbsp	200	2
seeds	1 tsp	16	tr
seeds, dried	1 cup	825	21
seeds, dried	1 tbsp	52	1

FOOD	PORTION	CALORIES	IRON
seeds, roasted & toasted	1 oz	161	4
sesame butter	1 tbsp	95	3
tahini from roasted & toasted kernels	1 tbsp	89	1
tahini from stone-ground kernels	1 tbsp	86	tr
tahini from unroasted kernels	1 tbsp	85	1

SESBANIA

flower	1	1	tr
flowers	1 cup	5	tr
flowers, cooked	1 cup	23	1

SHAD

american, baked	3 oz	214	1

SHALLOTS

dried	1 tbsp	3	tr
raw, chopped	1 tbsp	7	tr

SHARK

FRESH
batter dipped & fried	3 oz	194	1
raw	3 oz	111	1

SHEEPSHEAD (FISH)

cooked	3 oz	107	1
fillet, cooked	6.5 oz	234	1
raw	3 oz	92	tr

SHELLFISH
    (*see individual names*, SHELLFISH SUBSTITUTES)

FOOD	PORTION	CALORIES	IRON
SHELLFISH SUBSTITUTES			
Louis Kemp Crab Delights & Cocktail Sauce	4.5 oz	119	1
Louis Kemp Crab Delights Chunk Style	2 oz	54	tr
Louis Kemp Crab Delights Flake Style	2 oz	54	tr
Louis Kemp Crab Delights Leg Style	2 oz	56	tr
Louis Kemp Lobster Delights & Margarine	4.5 oz	393	tr
Louis Kemp Lobster Delights Chunk Style	2 oz	57	tr
crab, imitation	3 oz	87	tr
scallop, imitation	3 oz	84	tr
shrimp, imitation	3 oz	86	1
surimi	1 oz	28	tr
surimi	3 oz	84	tr
SHELLIE BEANS			
canned shellie beans	½ cup	37	1
SHERBET			
(*see also* ICES AND ICE POPS)			
orange	1 cup	270	tr
orange	½ gal	2158	2
SHRIMP			
CANNED			
Deveined Medium Whole Shrimp (S&W)	2 oz	65	1
shrimp	1 cup	154	4

FOOD	PORTION	CALORIES	IRON
shrimp	3 oz	102	2
FRESH			
cooked	3 oz	84	3
cooked	4 large	22	1
raw	3 oz	90	2
raw	4 large	30	1
FROZEN			
Butterfly Shrimp (Gorton's)	4 oz	160	2
Light Seafood Entrees Shrimp & Clams w/ Linguini (Mrs. Paul's)	10 oz	240	3
Microwave Crunchy Shrimp (Gorton's)	5 oz	380	1
Microwave Entree Shrimp Scampi (Gorton's)	1 pkg	390	tr
Shrimp Crisps (Gorton's)	4 oz	280	1
TAKE-OUT			
breaded & fried	3 oz	206	1
breaded & fried	4 large	73	tr
breaded & fried	6–8 (6 oz)	454	3
jambalaya	¾ cup	188	3

SMELT

rainbow, cooked	3 oz	106	1
rainbow, raw	3 oz	83	1

SNACKS

(*see also* CHIPS; FRUIT SNACKS; NUTS, MIXED; POPCORN; PRETZELS)

Bugles	1 oz	150	1
Bugles Nacho Cheese	1 oz	160	1
Bugles Ranch	1 oz	150	1
Chex Snack Mix Barbeque	⅔ cup	130	2

FOOD	PORTION	CALORIES	IRON
Chex Snack Mix Cool Sour Cream & Onion	⅔ cup	130	4
Chex Snack Mix Golden Cheddar	⅔ cup	130	4
Chex Snack Mix Traditional	⅔ cup	120	5
Cornnuts Barbecue	1 oz	120	tr
Cornnuts Nacho Cheese	1 oz	120	tr
Cornnuts Original	1 oz	120	tr
Cornnuts Picante	1 oz	120	tr
Cornnuts Ranch	1 oz	120	tr
Doo Dads	1 oz	140	1
Health Valley Cheddar Lites	.25 oz	40	tr
Snyder's Onion Toasters	1 oz	150	1
Snyder's Snack Mix	1 oz	130	1
Snyder's Sopaipillas Apple & Cinnamon	1 oz	150	tr
Ultra Slim-Fast Lite 'n Tasty Cheese Curls	1 oz	110	tr

SNAIL

fresh, cooked	3 oz	233	9
fresh, raw	3 oz	117	4

SNAP BEANS

CANNED			
green	½ cup	13	1
green low sodium	½ cup	13	1
italian	½ cup	13	1
italian low sodium	½ cup	13	1
yellow	½ cup	13	1
yellow low sodium	½ cup	13	1

FOOD	PORTION	CALORIES	IRON
FRESH			
green, cooked	½ cup	22	1
green, raw	½ cup	17	1
yellow, cooked	½ cup	22	1
yellow, raw	½ cup	17	1
FROZEN			
green, cooked	½ cup	18	1
italian, cooked	½ cup	18	1
yellow, cooked	½ cup	18	1

SNAPPER

FRESH			
cooked	3 oz	109	tr
fillet, cooked	6 oz	217	tr
raw	3 oz	85	tr

SODA
(see also DRINK MIXERS)

FOOD	PORTION	CALORIES	IRON
Lucozade	7 oz	136	tr
Orangina	9 oz	150	tr
cola	12 oz	151	tr
cream	12 oz	191	tr
diet cola	12 oz	2	tr
diet cola w/ Nutrasweet	12 oz	2	tr
diet cola w/ saccharin	12 oz	2	tr
ginger ale	12-oz can	124	tr
grape	12 oz	161	tr
lemon line	12 oz	149	tr
orange	12 oz	177	tr
root beer	12 oz	152	tr

FOOD	PORTION	CALORIES	IRON

SOLE

FRESH

| raw | 3.5 oz | 90 | 1 |

FROZEN

Fishmarket Fresh (Gorton's)	5 oz	110	tr
Light Fillets (Mrs. Paul's)	1 fillet	240	1
Microwave Entree in Lemon Butter (Gorton's)	1 pkg	380	tr
Microwave Entree in Wine Sauce (Gorton's)	1 pkg	180	tr

SORBET
(*see* ICES AND ICE POPS, SHERBET)

SORGHUM

| sorghum | ½ cup | 325 | 4 |

SOUFFLE

HOME RECIPE

cheese	3.5 oz	253	1
grand marnier	1 cup	109	1
lemon, chilled	1 cup	176	tr
raspberry, chilled	1 cup	173	1
spinach souffle	1 cup	218	1

SOUP

CANNED

Bean & Ham (Healthy Choice)	½ can (7.5 oz)	220	2
Bean & Ham Home Cookin' (Campbell)	10.75 oz	210	3
Bean Homestyle, as prep (Campbell)	8 oz	130	1

FOOD	PORTION	CALORIES	IRON
Bean w/ Bacon, as prep (Campbell)	8 oz	140	2
Bean w/ Bacon Healthy Request, as prep (Campbell)	8 oz	140	2
Beef, as prep (Campbell)	8 oz	80	1
Beef Broth (Health Valley)	7.5 oz	10	tr
Beef Broth No Salt Added (Health Valley)	7.5 oz	10	tr
Beef Chunky Ready-to-Serve (Campbell)	10.75 oz	200	2
Beef Noodle, as prep (Campbell)	8 oz	70	1
Beef Noodle Homestyle, as prep (Campbell)	8 oz	80	1
Beef Stroganoff Chunky Ready-to-Serve (Campbell)	10.75 oz	320	3
Beef w/ Vegetables & Pasta Home Cookin' (Campbell)	10.75 oz	140	2
Beefy Mushroom, as prep (Campbell)	8 oz	60	tr
Black Bean (Goya)	7.5 oz	160	4
Black Bean (Health Valley)	7.5 oz	150	5
Black Bean No Salt Added (Health Valley)	7.5 oz	150	5
Borscht (Gold's)	8 oz	100	4
Borscht Lo-Cal (Gold's)	8 oz	20	1
Borscht Low Calorie (Manischewitz)	8 oz	20	1
Borscht w/ Beets (Manischewitz)	8 oz	80	1
Cheddar Cheese, as prep (Campbell)	8 oz	110	tr
Chicken Alphabet, as prep (Campbell)	8 oz	80	1
Chicken 'n Dumplings, as prep (Campbell)	8 oz	80	tr

FOOD	PORTION	CALORIES	IRON
Chicken & Stars, as prep (Campbell)	8 oz	60	tr
Chicken Barley, as prep (Campbell)	8 oz	70	tr
Chicken Broth (Health Valley)	7.5 oz	35	tr
Chicken Broth Low Sodium Ready-to-Serve (Campbell)	10.5 oz	30	1
Chicken Broth No Salt Added (Health Valley)	7.5 oz	35	tr
Chicken Corn Chowder Chunky Ready-to-Serve (Campbell)	10.75 oz	340	1
Chicken Gumbo w/ Sausage Home Cookin' (Campbell)	10.75 oz	140	2
Chicken Minestrone Home Cookin' (Campbell)	10.75 oz	180	2
Chicken Mushroom Creamy, as prep (Campbell)	8 oz	120	tr
Chicken Noodle, as prep (Campbell)	8 oz	60	tr
Chicken Noodle Chunky Ready-to-Serve (Campbell)	10.75 oz	200	2
Chicken Noodle Healthy Request, as prep (Campbell)	8 oz	60	1
Chicken Noodle Homestyle, as prep (Campbell)	8 oz	70	1
Chicken Noodle-O's, as prep (Campbell)	8 oz	70	tr
Chicken Nuggets w/ Vegetables & Noodles Chunky (Campbell)	10.75 oz	190	1
Chicken Rice Home Cookin' (Campbell)	10.75 oz	150	1
Chicken Vegetable, as prep (Campbell)	8 oz	70	1
Chicken Vegetable Beef Low Sodium Ready-to-Serve (Campbell)	10.75 oz	180	2

FOOD	PORTION	CALORIES	IRON
Chicken Vegetable Chunky Ready-to-Serve (Campbell)	9.5 oz	170	1
Chicken w/ Noodles Home Cookin' (Campbell)	10.75 oz	140	1
Chicken w/ Noodles Low Sodium Ready-to-Serve (Campbell)	10.75 oz	170	2
Chicken w/ Rice (Healthy Choice)	½ can (7.5 oz)	140	tr
Chicken w/ Rice Chunky Ready-to-Serve (Campbell)	9.5 oz	140	1
Chicken w/ Rice Healthy Request, as prep (Campbell)	8 oz	60	tr
Chili Beef, as prep (Campbell)	8 oz	140	1
Chili Beef Chunky Ready-to-Serve (Campbell)	11 oz	290	5
Chunky Beef Vegetable (Healthy Choice)	½ can (7.5 oz)	110	1
Chunky Chicken Noodle & Vegetable (Healthy Choice)	½ can (7.5 oz)	160	1
Chunky Chicken Vegetable (Health Valley)	7.5 oz	125	1
Chunky Five Bean Vegetable (Health Valley)	7.5 oz	110	2
Chunky Five Bean Vegetable No Salt Added (Health Valley)	7.5 oz	110	2
Chunky Vegetable Chicken No Salt Added (Health Valley)	7.5 oz	125	1
Clam Chowder Manhattan Style, as prep (Campbell)	8 oz	70	tr
Clam Chowder Manhattan Style Chunky Ready-to-Serve (Campbell)	10.75 oz	160	2
Clam Chowder New England, as prep (Campbell)	8 oz	80	1
Clam Chowder New England, as prep w/ whole milk (Campbell)	8 oz	150	1

FOOD	PORTION	CALORIES	IRON
Clam Chowder New England Chunky Ready-to-Serve (Campbell)	10.75 oz	290	2
Consomme, as prep (Campbell)	8 oz	25	tr
Country Vegetable (Healthy Choice)	½ can (7.5 oz)	120	1
Country Vegetable Home Cookin' (Campbell)	10.75 oz	120	1
Cream of Asparagus, as prep (Campbell)	8 oz	80	tr
Cream of Broccoli, as prep (Campbell)	8 oz	80	tr
Cream of Broccoli, as prep w/ 2% milk (Campbell)	8 oz	140	tr
Cream of Chicken Healthy Request (Campbell)	8 oz	70	tr
Cream of Mushroom Healthy Request (Campbell)	8 oz	60	tr
Cream of Mushroom Low Sodium Ready-to-Serve (Campbell)	10.5 oz	210	1
Cream of Onion, as prep w/ whole milk & water (Campbell)	8 oz	140	tr
Cream of Potato, as prep w/ whole milk & water (Campbell)	8 oz	120	tr
Cream of Shrimp, as prep w/ whole milk (Campbell)	8 oz	160	tr
Cream of Tomato Homestyle, as prep (Campbell)	8 oz	110	tr
Cream of Tomato Homestyle, as prep w/ whole milk (Campbell)	8 oz	180	tr
Creamy Chicken Mushroom Chunky Ready-to-Serve (Campbell)	10.5 oz	270	1
Creole Style Chunky Ready-to-Serve (Campbell)	10.75 oz	240	2
Curly Noodle w/ Chicken, as prep (Campbell)	8 oz	80	1

FOOD	PORTION	CALORIES	IRON
French Onion, as prep (Campbell)	8 oz	60	tr
Green Pea, as prep (Campbell)	8 oz	160	1
Green Split Pea (Health Valley)	7.5 oz	180	2
Green Split Pea No Salt Added (Health Valley)	7.5 oz	180	2
Ham 'n Butter Bean Chunky Ready-to-Serve (Campbell)	10.75 oz	280	2
Hearty Beef (Healthy Choice)	½ can (7.5 oz)	120	1
Hearty Chicken (Healthy Choice)	½ can (7.5 oz)	150	1
Hearty Chicken Noodle Healthy Request Ready-to-Serve (Campbell)	8 oz	80	1
Hearty Chicken Rice Healthy Request Ready-to-Serve (Campbell)	80 oz	110	tr
Hearty Chicken Vegetable Healthy Request (Campbell)	8 oz	120	tr
Hearty Lentil Home Cookin' (Campbell)	10.75 oz	170	4
Hearty Minestrone Healthy Request Ready-to-Serve (Campbell)	8 oz	90	1
Hearty Vegetable Beef Healthy Request Ready-to-Serve (Campbell)	8 oz	120	1
Hearty Vegetable Healthy Request Ready-to-Serve (Campbell)	8 oz	110	1
Lentil (Health Valley)	7.5 oz	220	5
Lentil No Salt Added (Health Valley)	7.5 oz	220	5
Manhattan Clam Chowder (Health Valley)	7.5 oz	110	4
Manhattan Clam Chowder No Salt Added (Health Valley)	7.5 oz	110	4
Mediterranean Vegetable Chunky Ready-to-Serve (Campbell)	9.5 oz	170	1

FOOD	PORTION	CALORIES	IRON
Minestrone (Health Valley)	7.5 oz	130	2
Minestrone (Healthy Choice)	½ can (7.5 oz)	160	1
Minestrone, as prep (Campbell)	8 oz	80	1
Minestrone Chunky Ready-to-Serve (Campbell)	9.5 oz	160	2
Minestrone Home Cookin' (Campbell)	10.75 oz	140	1
Minestrone No Salt Added (Health Valley)	7.5 oz	130	2
Mushroom Barley (Health Valley)	7.5 oz	100	9
Mushroom Barley No Salt Added (Health Valley)	7.5 oz	100	9
Mushroom Golden, as prep (Campbell)	8 oz	70	tr
Nacho Cheese, as prep w/ milk (Campbell)	8 oz	180	tr
New England Clam Chowder, as prep w/ whole milk (Gorton's)	¼ can	140	1
Noodles & Ground Beef, as prep (Campbell)	8 oz	90	1
Old Fashioned Bean w/ Ham Chunky Ready-to-Serve (Campbell)	11 oz	290	3
Old Fashioned Chicken Chunky Ready-to-Serve (Campbell)	10.75 oz	180	1
Old Fashioned Chicken Noodle (Healthy Choice)	½ can (7.5 oz)	90	tr
Old Fashioned Vegetable Beef Chunky Ready-to-Serve (Campbell)	10.75 oz	190	2
Oyster Stew, as prep (Campbell)	8 oz	70	1
Oyster Stew, as prep w/ whole milk (Campbell)	8 oz	140	1
Pepper Pot, as prep (Campbell)	8 oz	90	1
Pepper Steak Chunky Ready-to-Serve (Campbell)	10.75 oz	180	2

FOOD	PORTION	CALORIES	IRON
Potato Leek (Health Valley)	7.5 oz	130	2
Potato Leek No Salt Added (Health Valley)	7.5 oz	130	2
Schav (Gold's)	8 oz	25	4
Scotch Broth, as prep (Campbell)	8 oz	80	tr
Sirloin Burger Chunky Ready-to-Serve (Campbell)	10.75 oz	220	3
Split Pea & Ham (Healthy Choice)	½ can (7.5 oz)	170	1
Split Pea Low Sodium Ready-to-Serve (Campbell)	10.75 oz	230	2
Split Pea w/ Bacon, as prep (Campbell)	8 oz	160	2
Split Pea w/ Ham Chunky Ready-to-Serve (Campbell)	10.75 oz	230	2
Split Pea w/ Ham Home Cookin' (Campbell)	10.75 oz	230	3
Steak & Potato Chunky Ready-to-Serve (Campbell)	10.75 oz	200	2
Teddy Bear, as prep (Campbell)	8 oz	70	1
Tomato (Health Valley)	7.5 oz	130	1
Tomato, as prep (Campbell)	8 oz	90	tr
Tomato, as prep w/ 2% milk (Campbell)	8 oz	150	1
Tomato Bisque, as prep (Campbell)	8 oz	120	tr
Tomato Garden (Healthy Choice)	½ can (7.5 oz)	130	1
Tomato Garden Home Cookin' (Campbell)	10.75 oz	150	2
Tomato Healthy Request, as prep (Campbell)	8 oz	90	tr
Tomato Healthy Request, as prep w/ skim milk (Campbell)	8 oz	130	1
Tomato No Salt Added (Health Valley)	7.5 oz	130	2

FOOD	PORTION	CALORIES	IRON
Tomato Rice Old Fashioned, as prep (Campbell)	8 oz	110	tr
Tomato w/ Tomato Pieces Low Sodium Ready-to-Serve (Campbell)	10.5 oz	190	1
Tomato Zesty, as prep (Campbell)	8 oz	100	1
Turkey Noodle, as prep (Campbell)	8 oz	70	tr
Turkey Vegetable, as prep (Campbell)	8 oz	70	tr
Turkey Vegetable Chunky Ready-to-Serve (Campbell)	9.5 oz	150	1
Vegetable (Health Valley)	7.5 oz	110	2
Vegetable, as prep (Campbell)	8 oz	90	tr
Vegetable Beef (Healthy Choice)	½ can (7.5 oz)	130	1
Vegetable Beef, as prep (Campbell)	8 oz	70	1
Vegetable Beef Healthy Request, as prep (Campbell)	8 oz	70	1
Vegetable Beef Home Cookin' (Campbell)	10.75 oz	140	2
Vegetable Chunky Ready-to-Serve (Campbell)	10.75 oz	160	2
Vegetable Healthy Request, as prep (Campbell)	8 oz	90	1
Vegetable Homestyle, as prep (Campbell)	8 oz	60	tr
Vegetable No Salt Added (Health Valley)	7.5 oz	110	2
Vegetable Old Fashioned, as prep (Campbell)	8 oz	60	tr
Vegetarian Vegetable, as prep (Campbell)	8 oz	80	tr
Won Ton, as prep (Campbell)	8 oz	40	tr
asparagus, cream of, as prep w/ milk	1 cup	161	1

FOOD	PORTION	CALORIES	IRON
asparagus, cream of, as prep w/ water	1 cup	87	1
beef broth ready-to-serve	1 can (14 oz)	27	1
beef broth ready-to-serve	1 cup	16	tr
beef noodle, as prep w/ water	1 cup	84	1
black bean, as prep w/ water	1 cup	116	2
black bean turtle soup	1 cup	218	5
celery, cream of, as prep w/ milk	1 cup	165	1
celery, cream of, as prep w/ water	1 cup	90	1
celery, cream of, not prep	1 can (10.75 oz)	219	2
cheese, as prep w/ milk	1 cup	230	1
cheese, as prep w/ water	1 cup	155	1
cheese, not prep	1 can (11 oz)	377	2
chicken broth, as prep w/ water	1 cup	39	1
chicken, cream of, as prep w/ milk	1 cup	191	1
chicken, cream of, as prep w/ water	1 cup	116	1
chicken gumbo, as prep w/ water	1 cup	56	1
chicken noodle, as prep w/ water	1 cup	75	1
chicken rice, as prep w/ water	1 cup	251	1
clam chowder, manhattan, as prep w/ water	1 cup	77	2
clam chowder, new england, as prep w/ milk	1 cup	163	1
clam chowder, new england, as prep w/ water	1 cup	95	1
consomme w/ gelatin, as prep w/ water	1 cup	29	1
consomme w/ gelatin, not prep	1 can (10.5 oz)	71	1
escarole ready-to-serve	1 cup	27	1
french onion, as prep w/ water	1 cup	57	1

FOOD	PORTION	CALORIES	IRON
gazpacho ready-to-serve	1 cup	57	1
minestrone, as prep w/ water	1 cup	83	1
mushroom, cream of, as prep w/ milk	1 cup	203	1
mushroom, cream of, as prep w/ water	1 cup	129	1
oyster stew, as prep w/ milk	1 cup	134	1
oyster stew, as prep w/ water	1 cup	59	1
pepperpot, as prep w/ water	1 cup	103	1
potato, cream of, as prep w/ water	1 cup	73	tr
potato, cream of, as prep w/ milk	1 cup	148	1
scotch broth, as prep w/ water	1 cup	80	1
split pea w/ ham, as prep w/ water	1 cup	189	2
tomato, as prep w/ milk	1 cup	160	2
tomato, as prep w/ water	1 cup	86	2
vegetarian vegetable, as prep w/ water	1 cup	72	1
vichyssoise	1 cup	148	1
DRY			
Asparagus, as prep (Knorr)	8 oz	80	tr
Bean w/ Bacon 'n Ham Microwave (Campbell)	7.5 oz	230	2
Beef, as prep (Ramen Noodle)	8 oz	190	1
Beef Instant Oriental Noodle (Lipton)	8 oz	177	2
Beef Low Fat, as prep (Ramen Noodle)	8 oz	160	2
Beef Mushroom (Lipton)	8 oz	38	tr
Beef Noodle (Campbell's Cup)	1 (1.35 oz)	130	1
Beef Noodle (Ultra Slim-Fast)	6 oz	45	2
Beef w/ Vegetables, as prep (Cup-A-Ramen)	8 oz	270	2

FOOD	PORTION	CALORIES	IRON
Beef w/ Vegetables Low Fat, as prep (Cup-A-Ramen)	8 oz	220	2
Beefy Onion (Lipton)	8 oz	27	tr
Cauliflower, as prep (Knorr)	8 oz	100	1
Chicken, as prep (Ramen Noodle)	8 oz	190	2
Chicken 'N Pasta, as prep (Knorr)	8 oz	90	1
Chicken Broth (Cup-A-Soup)	6 oz	19	0
Chicken Instant Oriental Noodle (Lipton)	8 oz	180	2
Chicken Leek (Ultra Slim-Fast)	6 oz	50	2
Chicken Low Fat, as prep (Ramen Noodle)	8 oz	160	2
Chicken Noodle (Campbell's Cup)	1 (1.35 oz)	140	1
Chicken Noodle (Lipton)	8 oz	82	1
Chicken Noodle (Ultra Slim-Fast)	6 oz	45	2
Chicken Noodle, as prep (Campbell)	8 oz	100	1
Chicken Noodle, as prep (Knorr)	8 oz	100	tr
Chicken Noodle Hearty (Lipton)	8 oz	81	1
Chicken Noodle Microwave (Campbell)	7.5 oz	100	1
Chicken Noodle w/ White Meat, as prep (Campbell's Cup)	6 oz	90	1
Chicken Vegetable (Cup-A-Soup)	6 oz	47	tr
Chicken w/ Rice Microwave (Campbell)	7.5 oz	100	4
Chicken w/ Vegetables, as prep (Cup-A-Ramen)	8 oz	270	2
Chicken w/ Vegetables Low Fat, as prep (Cup-A-Ramen)	8 oz	220	2
Chili Beef Microwave (Campbell)	7.5 oz	190	2
Country Barley, as prep (Knorr)	8 oz	120	2

FOOD	PORTION	CALORIES	IRON
Country Vegetable (Lipton)	8 oz	80	1
Creamy Broccoli (Ultra Slim-Fast)	6 oz	75	2
Creamy Broccoli & Cheese (Cup-A-Soup)	6 oz	70	tr
Creamy Tomato (Ultra Slim-Fast)	6 oz	60	2
Fine Herb, as prep (Knorr)	8 oz	130	1
French Onion, as prep (Knorr)	8 oz	50	tr
Giggle Noodle (Lipton)	8 oz	72	1
Green Pea (Cup-A-Soup)	6 oz	113	1
Hearty Chicken & Noodles (Cup-A-Soup)	6 oz	110	1
Hearty Creamy Chicken Lots-A-Noodles (Cup-A-Soup)	7 oz	179	2
Hearty Minestrone, as prep (Knorr)	10 oz	130	1
Hearty Noodle, as prep (Campbell)	8 oz	90	1
Hearty Noodles w/ Vegetables (Campbell's Cup)	1 (1.7 oz)	180	2
Hearty Noodles w/ Vegetables (Lipton)	8 oz	75	1
Hearty Vegetable (Ultra Slim-Fast)	6 oz	50	2
Leek, as prep (Knorr)	8 oz	110	1
Manhattan Clam Chowder (Golden Dipt)	¼ pkg	80	tr
Minestrone, as prep (Manischewitz)	6 oz	50	1
Mushroom, as prep (Knorr)	8 oz	100	tr
Noodle (4C)	8 oz	50	tr
Noodle, as prep (Campbell)	8 oz	110	1
Noodle w/ Chicken Broth, as prep (Campbell's Cup)	6 oz	90	1
Onion (Cup-A-Soup)	6 oz	27	0

FOOD	PORTION	CALORIES	IRON
Onion (Lipton)	8 oz	20	tr
Onion (Ultra Slim-Fast)	6 oz	45	2
Onion Golden (Lipton)	8 oz	62	tr
Onion Mushroom (Lipton)	8 oz	41	tr
Oriental, as prep (Ramen Noodle)	8 oz	190	2
Oriental Hot & Sour, as prep (Knorr)	8 oz	80	1
Oriental Low Fat, as prep (Ramen Noodle)	8 oz	150	2
Oriental w/ Vegetables, as prep (Cup-A-Ramen)	8 oz	270	3
Oriental w/ Vegetables Low Fat, as prep (Cup-A-Ramen)	8 oz	220	2
Oxtail Hearty Beef, as prep (Knorr)	8 oz	70	1
Pork, as prep (Ramen Noodle)	8 oz	200	1
Pork Low Fat, as prep (Ramen Noodle)	8 oz	150	3
Potato Leek (Ultra Slim-Fast)	6 oz	80	2
Ring-O-Noodle (Lipton)	8 oz	67	tr
Shrimp w/ Vegetables, as prep (Cup-A-Ramen)	8 oz	280	2
Shrimp w/ Vegetables Low Fat, as prep (Cup-A-Ramen)	8 oz	230	3
Split Pea Soup Mix, as prep (Manischewitz)	6 oz	45	1
Tomato (Cup-A-Soup)	6 oz	103	tr
Tomato Basil, as prep (Knorr)	8 oz	90	1
Vegetable (Lipton)	8 oz	37	1
Vegetable, as prep (Knorr)	8 oz	35	tr
Vegetable Beef Microwave (Campbell)	7.5 oz	100	1
Vegetable Soup Mix, as prep (Manischewitz)	6 oz	50	1

FOOD	PORTION	CALORIES	IRON
beef broth cube	3.6 g	6	tr
beef broth cube, as prep w/ water	1 cup	8	tr
chicken broth	1 pkg (.2 oz)	16	tr
chicken broth, as prep w/ water	1 cup	21	tr
chicken broth cube	4.8 g	9	tr
chicken broth cube, as prep w/ water	1 cup	13	tr
chicken noodle, as prep w/ water	1 cup	53	1
french onion, not prep	1 pkg (1.4 oz)	115	1
onion, as prep w/ water	1 cup	28	tr
tomato, as prep w/ water	1 cup	102	tr
FROZEN			
Kettle Ready			
Black Bean w/ Ham	6 oz	154	2
Boston Clam Chowder	6 oz	131	tr
Chicken Gumbo	6 oz	94	1
Chicken Noodle	6 oz	94	1
Chili	6 oz	161	1
Corn & Broccoli Chowder	6 oz	102	tr
Cream of Asparagus	6 oz	62	tr
Cream of Broccoli	6 oz	94	tr
Cream of Cauliflower	6 oz	93	tr
Cream of Cheddar Broccoli	6 oz	137	tr
Cream of Chicken	6 oz	98	tr
Cream of Mushroom	6 oz	85	tr
Cream of Potato	6 oz	121	tr
Creamy Cheddar	6 oz	158	tr
French Onion	6 oz	42	tr
Garden Vegetable	6 oz	85	1
Hearty Beef Vegetable	6 oz	85	tr

FOOD	PORTION	CALORIES	IRON
Hearty Minestrone	6 oz	104	tr
Manhattan Clam Chowder	6 oz	69	1
New England Clam Chowder	6 oz	116	tr
Savory Bean w/ Ham	6 oz	113	2
Split Pea w/ Ham	6 oz	155	2
Tomato Florentine	6 oz	106	tr
Tortellini in Tomato	6 oz	122	3
HOME RECIPE			
black bean turtle soup	1 cup	241	5
corn & cheese chowder	¾ cup	215	1
greek	¾ cup	63	1
SHELF-STABLE			
Chunky Beef Vegetable (Healthy Choice)	7.5-oz cup	110	1
Chunky Chicken Noodle & Vegetable (Healthy Choice)	7.5-oz cup	160	1
TAKE-OUT			
gazpacho	1 cup	46	tr
oxtail	5 oz	64	2

SOUR CREAM

sour cream	1 cup	493	tr
sour cream	1 tbsp	26	tr

SOURSOP

fresh	1	416	4
fresh, cut up	1 cup	150	1

SOY
(*see also* TOFU)

Soo Moo Beverage (Health Valley)	1 cup	120	1

FOOD	PORTION	CALORIES	IRON
milk	1 cup	79	1
soy sauce	1 tbsp	7	tr
soy sauce shoyu	1 tbsp	9	tr
soy sauce tamari	1 tbsp	11	tr
soya cheese	1.4 oz	128	tr
soybean sprouts, raw	½ cup	43	1
soybean sprouts, steamed	½ cup	38	1
soybean sprouts, stir fried	1 cup	125	tr
soybeans, cooked	1 cup	298	9
soybeans, dry roasted	½ cup	387	3
soybeans, roasted	½ cup	405	3
soybeans, roasted & toasted	1 cup	490	5
soybeans, roasted & toasted	1 oz	129	1
soybeans, salted, roasted & toasted	1 cup	490	5
soybeans salted, roasted & toasted	1 oz	129	1

SPAGHETTI
(*see* PASTA, PASTA DISHES, PASTA SALAD, SPAGHETTI SAUCE)

SPAGHETTI SAUCE
(*see also* PIZZA, TOMATO)

JARRED
Hunt's Chunky	4 oz	50	1
Hunt's Homestyle	4 oz	60	2
Hunt's Homestyle w/ Meat	4 oz	60	2
Hunt's Homestyle w/ Mushrooms	4 oz	50	2
Hunt's Traditional	4 oz	70	2
Hunt's w/ Meat	4 oz	70	2
Hunt's w/ Mushrooms	4 oz	70	2
Newman's Own	4 oz	70	1

FOOD	PORTION	CALORIES	IRON
Newman's Own Sockarooni	4 oz	70	1
Newman's Own w/ Mushrooms	4 oz	70	1
Prego Chunky Sausage & Green Peppers	4 oz	160	1
Prego Extra Chunky Garden Combination	4 oz	80	1
Prego Extra Chunky Mushroom & Green Pepper	4 oz	100	1
Prego Extra Chunky Mushroom & Onion	4 oz	100	1
Prego Extra Chunky Mushroom & Tomato	4 oz	110	1
Prego Extra Chunky Mushroom w/ Extra Spice	4 oz	100	1
Prego Extra Chunky Tomato & Onion	4 oz	110	1
Prego Marinara	4 oz	100	1
Prego Meat Flavored	4 oz	140	1
Prego Mushroom	4 oz	130	1
Prego Onion & Garlic	4 oz	110	1
Prego Regular	4 oz	130	1
Prego Three Cheese	4 oz	100	1
Prego Tomato & Basil	4 oz	100	1
Ragu Chunky Gardenstyle Extra Tomatoes, Garlic & Onions	4 oz	70	1
Ragu Chunky Gardenstyle Green & Red Peppers	4 oz	70	1
Ragu Chunky Gardenstyle Italian Garden Combination	4 oz	70	1
Ragu Chunky Gardenstyle Mushrooms & Onions	4 oz	70	1
Ragu Homestyle w/ Meat	4 oz	110	1
Ragu Homestyle w/ Mushrooms	4 oz	110	1

FOOD	PORTION	CALORIES	IRON
Ragu Homestyle w/ Tomato & Herbs	4 oz	110	1
Ragu Italian Cooking Sauce	4 oz	70	1
Ragu Joe	3.5 oz	50	1
Ragu Old World Style Marinara	4 oz	80	1
Ragu Old World Style Plain	4 oz	80	1
Ragu Old World Style w/ Mushrooms	4 oz	80	1
Ragu Old World Style w/ Meat	4 oz	80	1
Ragu Thick & Hearty Plain	4 oz	100	1
Ragu Thick & Hearty w/ Meat	4 oz	120	2
Ragu Thick & Hearty w/ Mushrooms	4 oz	100	1
marinara sauce	1 cup	171	2
spaghetti sauce	1 cup	272	2
TAKE-OUT bolognese	5 oz	195	2

SPANISH FOOD

CANNED			
Enchilada Sauce Mild (Rosarita)	2.5 oz	25	1
Enchiladas (Gebhardt)	2	310	2
Picante Chunky Hot (Rosarita)	3 tbsp	18	1
Picante Chunky Medium (Rosarita)	3 tbsp	16	tr
Picante Chunky Mild (Rosarita)	3 tbsp	25	tr
Picante Mild (Casa Fiesta)	1 oz	9	tr
Taco Sauce Mild (Casa Fiesta)	1 oz	9	tr
Tamales (Derby)	2	160	2
Tamales (Gebhardt)	2	290	2
Tamales (Wolf Brand)	7.5 oz	328	2
Tamales Jumbo (Gebhardt)	2	400	3

FOOD	PORTION	CALORIES	IRON
Tamales w/ Sauce (Van Camp's)	1 cup	293	3
FROZEN			
Banquet Beef Enchilada & Tamale w/ Chili Gravy	10 oz	300	3
Budget Gourmet Beef Mexicana	1 pkg	520	4
Budget Gourmet Chicken Enchilada Suiza	1 pkg	290	1
Budget Gourmet Chicken Mexicana	1 pkg	560	5
Budget Gourmet Sirloin Enchilada Ranchero	1 pkg	280	1
Healthy Choice Enchiladas Beef	12.75 oz	350	2
Healthy Choice Enchiladas Chicken	12.75 oz	330	2
Healthy Choice Enchiladas Chicken	9.5 oz	280	1
Healthy Choice Fajitas Beef	7 oz	210	3
Healthy Choice Fajitas Chicken	7 oz	200	3
Le Menu Entree LightStyle Enchiladas Chicken	8 oz	280	2
Lean Cuisine Enchanadas Beef & Bean	9.25 oz	240	2
Lean Cuisine Enchanadas Chicken	9.88 oz	290	3
Patio Britos Beef & Bean	1 (3 oz)	210	1
Patio Britos Nacho Beef	1 (3 oz)	220	1
Patio Britos Nacho Cheese	1 (3.63 oz)	250	1
Patio Britos Spicy Chicken & Cheese	1 (3 oz)	210	1
Patio Burritos Hot Beef & Bean Red Chili	1 (5 oz)	340	3
Patio Burritos Medium Beef & Bean	1 (5 oz)	370	3
Patio Burritos Mild Beef & Bean Green Chili	1 (5 oz)	330	4
Patio Enchilada Beef Dinner	13.25 oz	520	4
Patio Enchilada Cheese Dinner	12 oz	370	3

FOOD	PORTION	CALORIES	IRON
Patio Fiesta Dinner	12 oz	460	4
Patio Mexican Dinner	13.25 oz	540	4
Patio Tamale Dinner	13 oz	470	4
Swanson Enchiladas Beef	13.75 oz	480	3
Swanson Mexican Style Combination	14.25 oz	490	3
Swanson Mexican Style Hungry Man	20.25 oz	820	5
MIX			
Masa Harina De Maiz (Quaker)	2 tortillas	137	2
Masa Trigo (Quaker)	2 tortillas	149	2
Menudo Mix (Gebhardt)	1 tsp	5	tr
Taco Meat Seasoning Mix Mild (Ortega)	1 filled taco	90	2
READY-TO-USE			
Taco Shells (Casa Fiesta)	3.5 oz	480	4
Taco Shells (Gebhardt)	1	50	1
Taco Shells (Rosarita)	1	50	1
Tortilla Wheat Flour (Mariachi)	1	112	2
Tostada Shells (Rosarita)	1	60	1
taco shell, baked	1 med	61	tr
taco shell, baked w/o salt	1 med	61	tr
tortilla corn	1 (6" diam)	56	tr
tortilla corn w/o salt	1 (6" diam)	56	tr
tortilla flour w/o salt	1 (8" diam)	114	1
TAKE-OUT			
burrito w/ apple	1 lg (5.4 oz)	484	2
burrito w/ apple	1 sm (2.6 oz)	231	1
burrito w/ beans	2 (7.6 oz)	448	5
burrito w/ beans & cheese	2 (6.5 oz)	377	2

FOOD	PORTION	CALORIES	IRON
burrito w/ beans & chili peppers	2 (7.2 oz)	413	5
burrito w/ beans & meat	2 (8.1 oz)	508	5
burrito w/ beans, cheese & beef	2 (7.1 oz)	331	4
burrito w/ beans, cheese & chili peppers	2 (11.8 oz)	663	8
burrito w/ beef	2 (7.7 oz)	523	6
burrito w/ beef & chili peppers	2 (7.1 oz)	426	4
burrito w/ beef, cheese & chili peppers	2 (10.7 oz)	634	8
burrito w/ cherry	1 lg (5.4 oz)	484	2
burrito w/ cherry	1 sm (2.6 oz)	231	1
chimichanga w/ beef	1 (6.1 oz)	425	5
chimichanga w/ beef & cheese	1 (6.4 oz)	443	4
chimichanga w/ beef & red chili peppers	1 (6.7 oz)	424	4
chimichanga w/ beef, cheese & red chili peppers	1 (6.3 oz)	364	3
enchilada w/ cheese	1 (5.7 oz)	320	1
enchilada w/ cheese & beef	1 (6.7 oz)	324	3
enchirito w/ cheese, beef & beans	1 (6.8 oz)	344	2
frijoles w/ cheese	1 cup (5.9 oz)	226	2
nachos w/ cheese	6–8 (4 oz)	345	1
nachos w/ cheese & jalapeno peppers	6–8 (7.2 oz)	607	2
nachos w/ cheese, beans, ground beef & peppers	6–8 (8.9 oz)	568	3
nachos w/ cinnamon & sugar	6–8 (3.8 oz)	592	3
taco	1 sm (6 oz)	370	2
taco salad	1½ cups	279	2
taco salad w/ chili con carne	1½ cups	288	3
tostada w/ beans & cheese	1 (5.1 oz)	223	2

FOOD	PORTION	CALORIES	IRON
tostada w/ beans, beef & cheese	1 (7.9 oz)	334	2
tostada w/ beef & cheese	1 (5.7 oz)	315	3
tostada w/ guacamole	2 (9.2 oz)	360	2

SPARE RIBS
(*see* PORK)

SPICES
(*see* HERBS/SPICES, *individual spice names*)

SPINACH

CANNED
S&W Northwest Premium	½ cup	25	2
spinach	½ cup	25	2

FRESH
cooked	½ cup	21	3
mustard, chopped, cooked	½ cup	14	1
mustard, raw, chopped	½ cup	17	1
new zealand, chopped, cooked	½ cup	11	1
new zealand, raw	½ cup	4	tr
raw, chopped	1 pkg (10 oz)	46	6
raw, chopped	½ cup	6	1

FROZEN
Birds Eye Chopped	½ cup	20	2
Birds Eye Creamed	½ cup	90	1
Birds Eye Leaf	½ cup	20	2
Budget Gourmet Au Gratin	1 pkg	160	1
Green Giant	½ cup	25	2
Green Giant Creamed	½ cup	70	1
Green Giant Cut Leaf in Butter Sauce	½ cup	40	2

FOOD	PORTION	CALORIES	IRON
Green Giant Harvest Fresh	½ cup	25	1
cooked	½ cup	27	1

SPOT

fresh, baked	3 oz	134	tr

SQUASH
   (*see also* ZUCCHINI)

CANNED			
crookneck, sliced	½ cup	14	1
FRESH			
acorn, cooked & mashed	½ cup	41	1
acorn, cubed & baked	½ cup	57	1
butternut, baked	½ cup	41	1
crookneck, raw, sliced	½ cup	12	tr
crookneck, sliced & cooked	½ cup	18	tr
hubbard, baked	½ cup	51	tr
hubbard, cooked & mashed	½ cup	35	tr
scallop, raw, sliced	½ cup	12	tr
scallop, sliced & cooked	½ cup	14	tr
spaghetti, cooked	½ cup	23	tr
FROZEN			
Winter Cooked (Birds Eye)	½ cup	45	1
butternut, cooked & mashed	½ cup	47	1
crookneck, sliced & cooked	½ cup	24	tr
SEEDS			
dried	1 cup	747	21
dried	1 oz	154	4
roasted	1 cup	1184	34
roasted	1 oz	148	4

FOOD	PORTION	CALORIES	IRON
salted & roasted	1 cup	1184	34
salted & roasted	1 oz	148	4
whole, roasted	1 cup	285	2
whole, roasted	1 oz	127	1
whole, salted & roasted	1 cup	285	2
whole, salted & roasted	1 oz	127	1

SQUID

fresh, fried	3 oz	149	1
fresh, raw	3 oz	78	1

SQUIRREL

roasted	3 oz	147	6

STRAWBERRIES

CANNED			
in heavy syrup	½ cup	117	1
FRESH			
strawberries	1 cup	45	1
strawberries	1 pint	97	1
FROZEN			
Big Valley	3.5 oz	35	tr
Halved in Delicious Syrup (Birds Eye)	½ cup	120	1
Halved in Lite Syrup (Birds Eye)	½ cup	90	tr
sweetened, sliced	1 cup	245	1
sweetened, sliced	1 pkg (10 oz)	273	2
unsweetened	1 cup	52	1
whole, sweetened	1 cup	200	1
whole, sweetened	1 pkg (10 oz)	223	1

FOOD	PORTION	CALORIES	IRON
JUICE			
Kool-Aid Koolers	1 (8.45 oz)	136	tr
Smucker's	8 oz	130	1

STUFFING/DRESSING

FOOD	PORTION	CALORIES	IRON
HOME RECIPE			
bread, as prep w/ water & fat	½ cup	251	1
bread, as prep w/ water, egg & fat	½ cup	107	1
plain, as prep	½ cup	195	2
sausage	½ cup	292	1
MIX			
Arnold All Purpose Seasoned	.5 oz	51	1
Arnold Corn	.5 oz	50	tr
Betty Crocker Chicken	½ cup	180	1
Betty Crocker Traditional Herb	½ cup	180	1
Brownberry Corn	1 oz	103	1
Brownberry Herb	1 oz	100	1
Brownberry Sage & Onion	1 oz	97	2
Golden Grain Bread Stuffing Chicken	½ cup	180	1
Golden Grain Bread Stuffing Corn Bread	½ cup	180	1
Golden Grain Bread Stuffing Herb & Butter	½ cup	180	1
Golden Grain Bread Stuffing w/ Wild Rice	½ cup	180	1
Pepperidge Farm Corn Bread	1 oz	110	1
Pepperidge Farm Country Style	1 oz	100	1
Pepperidge Farm Cube	1 oz	110	1
Pepperidge Farm Distinctive Apple Raisin	1 oz	110	2

FOOD	PORTION	CALORIES	IRON
Pepperidge Farm Distinctive Classic Chicken	1 oz	110	1
Pepperidge Farm Distinctive Country Garden Herb	1 oz	120	2
Pepperidge Farm Distinctive Vegetable & Almond	1 oz	110	3
Pepperidge Farm Distinctive Wild Rice & Mushroom	1 oz	130	1
Pepperidge Farm Herb Seasoned	1 oz	110	1
Stove Top Beef, as prep	½ cup	178	1
Stove Top Chicken, as prep	½ cup	176	1
Stove Top Chicken w/ Rice, as prep	½ cup	182	1
Stove Top Cornbread, as prep	½ cup	175	1
Stove Top Flex Serve Chicken, as prep	½ cup	173	1
Stove Top Flex Serve Cornbread, as prep	½ cup	181	1
Stove Top Flex Serve Homestyle Herb, as prep	½ cup	173	1
Stove Top Long Grain & Wild Rice, as prep	½ cup	182	1
bread, dry, as prep	½ cup	178	1
cornbread, as prep	½ cup	179	1

SUCKER

white, baked	3 oz	101	1

SUGAR
(*see also* SUGAR SUBSTITUTES, SYRUP)

brown	1 cup	820	5
powdered, sifted	1 cup	385	tr
white	1 cup	770	tr

FOOD	PORTION	CALORIES	IRON
white	1 packet (6 g)	25	tr
white	1 tbsp	45	tr

SUGAR APPLE

fresh	1	146	1
fresh, cut up	1 cup	236	2

SUGAR SUBSTITUTES

S&W Liquid Table Sweetener	⅛ tsp	0	0
Sprinkle Sweet	1 tsp	2	0
Sweet*10	⅛ tsp	0	0

SUNDAE TOPPINGS
(see ICE CREAM TOPPINGS)

SUNFISH

pumpkinseed, baked	3 oz	97	1

SUNFLOWER SEEDS

Sunflower Butter (Erewhon)	2 tbsp	200	1
Sunflower Nuts Dry Roasted Unsalted (Planters)	1 oz	170	1
Sunflower Seeds (Planters)	1 oz	160	1
dried	1 cup	821	10
dried	1 oz	162	2
dry roasted	1 cup	745	5
dry roasted	1 oz	165	1
dry roasted, salted	1 cup	745	5
dry roasted, salted	1 oz	165	1
oil roasted	1 cup	830	9
oil roasted, salted	1 cup	830	9

FOOD	PORTION	CALORIES	IRON
oil roasted, salted	1 oz	175	2
sunflower butter	1 tbsp	93	1
sunflower butter w/o salt	1 tbsp	93	1
toasted	1 cup	826	9
toasted	1 oz	176	2
toasted, salted	1 cup	826	9
toasted, salted	1 oz	176	2

SWAMP CABBAGE

FRESH
chopped, cooked	½ cup	10	1
raw, chopped	1 cup	11	1

SWEET POTATO
(*see also* YAM)

CANNED
in syrup	½ cup	106	1
pieces	1 cup	183	2

FRESH
baked w/ skin	1 (3.5 oz)	118	1
leaves, cooked	½ cup	11	tr
mashed	½ cup	172	1

FROZEN
Candied Sweet Potatoes (Mrs. Paul's)	4 oz	170	1
Candied Sweets 'n Apples (Mrs. Paul's)	4 oz	160	1
cooked	½ cup	88	tr

HOME RECIPE
candied	3.5 oz	144	1

FOOD	PORTION	CALORIES	IRON

SWEETBREADS

beef, braised	3 oz	230	2
lamb, braised	3 oz	199	2
veal, braised	3 oz	218	2

SWISS CHARD

FRESH			
cooked	½ cup	18	2
raw, chopped	½ cup	3	tr

SWORDFISH

cooked	3 oz	132	1
raw	3 oz	103	1

SYRUP
(*see also* ICE CREAM TOPPINGS, PANCAKE/WAFFLE SYRUP)

Blueberry (Whistling Wings)	1 oz	45	tr
Raspberry (Whistling Wings)	1 oz	60	tr
corn	2 tbsp	122	tr
raspberry	3.5 oz	267	2

TAHINI
(*see* SESAME)

TAMARIND

fresh	1	5	tr
fresh, cut up	1 cup	287	3

TANGERINE

CANNED			
in light syrup	½ cup	76	tr

FOOD	PORTION	CALORIES	IRON
juice pack	½ cup	46	tr
FRESH			
sections	1 cup	86	tr
tangerine	1	37	tr
JUICE			
Dole Pure & Light	6 oz	100	tr
canned, sweetened	1 cup	125	1
fresh	1 cup	106	tr
frzn, sweetened, as prep	1 cup	110	tr
frzn, sweetened, not prep	6 oz	344	1

TAPIOCA

pearl, dry	⅓ cup	174	tr
starch	3.5 oz	344	1

TARO

chips	½ cup	57	tr
chips	10	110	tr
leaves, cooked	½ cup	18	1
raw, sliced	½ cup	56	tr
shoots, sliced & cooked	½ cup	10	tr
sliced, cooked	½ cup	94	tr
tahitian, sliced & cooked	½ cup	30	1

TARRAGON

ground	1 tsp	5	1

TEA/HERBAL TEA

REGULAR			
Lipton Iced Tea Lemon w/ Vitamin C	6 oz	58	0

FOOD	PORTION	CALORIES	IRON
Lipton Iced Tea Mix Lemon	6 oz	55	0
Lipton Iced Tea Sugar Free	8 oz	1	0
Lipton Iced Tea Sugar Free Peach	8 oz	5	0
Lipton Iced Tea Sugar Free Raspberry	8 oz	5	0
Lipton Iced Tea w/ Nutrasweet	8 oz	3	0
Lipton Iced Tea w/ Nutrasweet Decaffeinated	8 oz	3	0
Lipton Instant	6 oz	0	0
Lipton Instant Decaffeinated	6 oz	0	0
Lipton Instant Lemon	8 oz	3	0
Lipton Instant Raspberry	8 oz	3	0
brewed tea	6 oz	2	tr
instant artificially sweetened lemon flavor, as prep w/ water	8 oz	5	tr
instant sweetened lemon flavor, as prep w/ water	9 oz	87	tr
instant unsweetened, as prep w/ water	8 oz	2	tr
instant unsweetened lemon flavor, as prep w/ water	8 oz	4	tr

TEMPEH

tempeh	½ cup	165	2

THYME

ground	1 tsp	4	2

TILEFISH

FRESH
cooked	3 oz	125	tr
fillet, cooked	½ (5.3 oz)	220	tr
raw	3 oz	81	tr

FOOD	PORTION	CALORIES	IRON

TOFU

FOOD	PORTION	CALORIES	IRON
Azumaya Blue Label	3.5 oz	46	tr
Azumaya Green Label	3.5 oz	68	1
Azumaya Name Age Fried	3.5 oz	144	1
Azumaya Red Label	3.5 oz	68	1
Mori-Nu Silken Extra Firm	½ box (5.25 oz)	90	2
Mori-Nu Silken Firm	½ box (5.25 oz)	90	2
Mori-Nu Silken Soft	½ box (5.25 oz)	80	1
Spring Creek Great Balls of Tofu!	2 (3 oz)	107	2
Spring Creek Nigari Firm	4 oz	140	2
firm	½ cup	183	13
firm	¼ block (3 oz)	118	8
fresh, fried	1 piece (.5 oz)	35	1
fuyu, salted & fermented	1 block (.33 oz)	13	tr
koyadofu, dried & frozen	1 piece (.5 oz)	82	2
okara	½ cup	47	1
regular	½ cup	94	7
regular	¼ block (4 oz)	88	6
YOGURT			
Stir Fruity Black Cherry	6 oz	141	2
Stir Fruity Blueberry	6 oz	140	1
Stir Fruity Lemon Chiffon	6 oz	152	1
Stir Fruity Mixed Berry	6 oz	149	1
Stir Fruity Orange	6 oz	143	1
Stir Fruity Peach	6 oz	160	2
Stir Fruity Pina Colada	6 oz	162	1
Stir Fruity Raspberry	6 oz	155	1

FOOD	PORTION	CALORIES	IRON
Stir Fruity Spiced Apple	6 oz	167	2
Stir Fruity Strawberry	6 oz	140	1
Stir Fruity Tropical Fruit	6 oz	170	2

TOFUTTI
(*see* ICE CREAM AND FROZEN DESSERTS)

TOMATO
(*see also* PIZZA, SPAGHETTI SAUCE)

CANNED

FOOD	PORTION	CALORIES	IRON
Health Valley Sauce	1 cup	70	2
Health Valley Sauce Low Sodium	1 cup	70	2
Hunt's Crushed Angela Mia	4 oz	35	1
Hunt's Crushed Italian	4 oz	40	1
Hunt's Italian Pear Shaped	4 oz	20	tr
Hunt's Paste	2 oz	45	1
Hunt's Paste Italian Style	2 oz	50	1
Hunt's Paste No Salt Added	2 oz	45	2
Hunt's Paste w/ Garlic	2 oz	50	1
Hunt's Peeled Choice-Cut	4 oz	20	1
Hunt's Puree	4 oz	45	1
Hunt's Sauce	4 oz	30	1
Hunt's Sauce Herb	4 oz	70	1
Hunt's Sauce Italian	4 oz	60	1
Hunt's Sauce Meatloaf Fixin's	4 oz	20	tr
Hunt's Sauce No Salt Added	4 oz	35	1
Hunt's Sauce Special	4 oz	35	1
Hunt's Sauce w/ Bits	4 oz	30	tr
Hunt's Sauce w/ Garlic	4 oz	70	3
Hunt's Sauce w/ Mushrooms	4 oz	25	1
Hunt's Stewed	4 oz	35	1

FOOD	PORTION	CALORIES	IRON
Hunt's Stewed Italian	4 oz	40	1
Hunt's Stewed No Salt Added	4 oz	35	1
Hunt's Whole	4 oz	20	tr
Hunt's Whole Italian	4 oz	25	tr
Hunt's Whole No Salt Added	4 oz	20	1
S&W Aspic Supreme	½ cup	60	1
S&W Diced in Rich Puree	½ cup	35	tr
S&W Italian Stewed Sliced	½ cup	35	tr
S&W Italian Style w/ Basil	½ cup	25	tr
S&W Mexican Style Stewed	½ cup	40	tr
S&W Paste	6 oz	150	2
S&W Peeled Ready Cut	½ cup	25	tr
S&W Puree	½ cup	60	1
S&W Sauce	½ cup	40	1
S&W Sauce Chunky	½ cup	45	1
S&W Stewed Sliced	½ cup	35	tr
S&W Stewed 50% Salt Reduced	½ cup	35	1
S&W Whole Diet	½ cup	25	tr
S&W Whole Peeled	½ cup	25	tr
paste	½ cup	110	4
puree	1 cup	102	2
puree w/o salt	1 cup	102	2
red, whole	½ cup	24	1
sauce	½ cup	37	1
sauce spanish style	½ cup	40	4
sauce w/ green chilis	½ cup	18	tr
sauce w/ mushrooms	½ cup	42	1
sauce w/ onions	½ cup	52	1
stewed	½ cup	34	1
wedges in tomato juice	½ cup	34	1

FOOD	PORTION	CALORIES	IRON
FRESH			
cooked	½ cup	32	1
green	1	30	1
red	1 (4.5 oz)	26	1
red, chopped	1 cup	35	1
JUICE			
Campbell	6 oz	40	1
Hunt's	6 oz	30	1
Hunt's No Salt Added	6 oz	35	1
Libby's	6 oz	35	1
S&W California	6 oz	35	1
S&W Diet	½ cup	35	1
beef broth & tomato	5.5 oz	61	1
clam & tomato	1 can (5.5 oz)	77	1
tomato juice	½ cup	21	1
tomato juice	6 oz	32	1
TAKE-OUT			
stewed	1 cup	80	1

TOPPINGS
(*see* ICE CREAM TOPPINGS)

TORTILLA CHIPS
(*see* CHIPS)

TRITICALE
(*see also* FLOUR)

dry	½ cup	323	2

TONGUE

beef, simmered	3 oz	241	3

FOOD	PORTION	CALORIES	IRON
lamb, braised	3 oz	234	2
pork, braised	3 oz	230	4

TREE FERN

chopped, cooked	½ cup	28	tr

TROUT

FRESH

baked	3 oz	162	2
rainbow, cooked	3 oz	129	2
sea trout, baked	3 oz	113	tr

TRUFFLES

fresh	3.5 oz	25	4

TUNA

(*see also* TUNA DISHES)

CANNED

Bumble Bee Chunk Light in Oil	2 oz	160	1
Bumble Bee Chunk Light in Water	2 oz	60	1
Bumble Bee Solid White in Oil	2 oz	130	tr
Bumble Bee Solid White in Water	2 oz	70	tr
Empress Chunk Light	2 oz	60	tr
Empress Chunk Light Tongol	2 oz	50	1
S&W Chunk Light Fancy in Oil	2 oz	140	1
S&W Chunk Light Fancy in Water	2 oz	60	1
light in oil	1 can (6 oz)	399	2
light in oil	3 oz	169	1
light in water	1 can (5.8 oz)	192	3
light in water	3 oz	99	1

FOOD	PORTION	CALORIES	IRON
white in oil	1 can (6.2 oz)	331	1
white in oil	3 oz	158	1
white in water	1 can (6 oz)	234	1
white in water	3 oz	116	1
FRESH			
bluefin, cooked	3 oz	157	1
bluefin, raw	3 oz	122	1
skipjack, baked	3 oz	112	1
yellowfin, baked	3 oz	118	1

TUNA DISHES

FOOD	PORTION	CALORIES	IRON
FROZEN			
Microwave Tuna Sandwich (Mrs. Paul's)	1	200	2
MIX			
Tuna Helper Au Gratin, as prep	⅕ pkg (6 oz)	280	1
Tuna Helper Buttery Rice, as prep	⅕ pkg (6 oz)	280	1
Tuna Helper Cheesy Noodles, as prep	⅕ pkg (7.75 oz)	240	1
Tuna Helper Creamy Mushroom, as prep	⅕ pkg (7 oz)	220	1
Tuna Helper Creamy Noodles, as prep	⅕ pkg (8 oz)	300	1
Tuna Helper Fettucine Alfredo, as prep	⅕ pkg (7 oz)	300	1
Tuna Helper Romanoff, as prep	⅕ pkg (8 oz)	290	1
Tuna Helper Tetrazzini, as prep	⅕ pkg (6 oz)	240	1
Tuna Helper Tuna Pot Pie, as prep	⅙ pkg (5.1 oz)	420	2
Tuna Helper Tuna Salad, as prep	⅕ pkg (5.5 oz)	420	2
TAKE-OUT			
tuna salad	1 cup	383	2

FOOD	PORTION	CALORIES	IRON
tuna salad	3 oz	159	1
tuna salad submarine sandwich w/ lettuce & oil	1	584	3

TURKEY
(*see also* DINNERS, HOT DOG, TURKEY DISHES)

CANNED

FOOD	PORTION	CALORIES	IRON
White (Swanson)	2.5 oz	80	tr
w/ broth	1 can (5 oz)	231	3
w/ broth	½ can (2.5 oz)	116	1

FRESH

FOOD	PORTION	CALORIES	IRON
Breast Hen w/o Wing, cooked (Louis Rich)	1 oz	50	tr
Breast Roast, cooked (Louis Rich)	1 oz	41	tr
Breast Slices, cooked (Louis Rich)	1 oz	39	tr
Breast Steaks, cooked (Louis Rich)	1 oz	39	tr
Breast Tenderloins, cooked (Louis Rich)	1 oz	39	tr
Drumsticks, cooked (Louis Rich)	1 oz	56	1
Ground, cooked (Louis Rich)	1 oz	60	1
Ground, cooked (Louis Rich)	3.5 oz	216	2
Ground Lean 90% Fat Free, cooked (Louis Rich)	3.5 oz	186	1
Thighs, cooked (Louis Rich)	1 oz	64	1
Whole, cooked (Louis Rich)	1 oz	52	tr
Whole, cooked (Louis Rich)	3.5 oz	186	1
Wing Drumettes, cooked (Louis Rich)	1 oz	51	tr
Wings, cooked (Louis Rich)	1 oz	54	tr
back w/ skin, roasted	½ back (9 oz)	637	6
breast w/ skin, roasted	4 oz	212	2

FOOD	PORTION	CALORIES	IRON
dark meat w/ skin, roasted	3.6 oz	230	2
dark meat w/o skin, roasted	1 cup (5 oz)	262	3
dark meat w/o skin, roasted	3 oz	170	2
ground, cooked	3 oz	188	2
leg w/ skin, roasted	1 (1.2 lbs)	1133	13
leg w/ skin, roasted	2.5 oz	147	2
light meat w/ skin, roasted	4.7 oz	268	2
light meat w/ skin, roasted	from ½ turkey (2.3 lbs)	2069	15
light meat w/o skin, roasted	4 oz	183	2
neck, simmered	1 (5.3 oz)	274	3
skin, roasted	1 oz	141	1
skin, roasted	from ½ turkey (9 oz)	1096	4
wing w/ skin, roasted	1 (6.5 oz)	426	3
w/ skin, neck & giblets, roasted	½ turkey (8.8 lbs)	4123	40
w/ skin, roasted	½ turkey (4 lbs)	3857	33
w/ skin, roasted	8.4 oz	498	4
w/o skin, roasted	1 cup (5 oz)	238	2
w/o skin, roasted	7.3 oz	354	4
FROZEN roast boneless seasoned light & dark meat, roasted	1 pkg (1.7 lbs)	1213	13
READ-TO-USE Carl Buddig	1 oz	50	tr
Carl Buddig Turkey Ham	1 oz	40	tr
Louis Rich Barbecued Breast Skinless	1 oz	29	tr
Louis Rich Bologna	1 slice (28 g)	61	tr
Louis Rich Bologna Mild	1 slice (28 g)	59	tr

FOOD	PORTION	CALORIES	IRON
Louis Rich Breaded Nuggets	1 (.75 oz)	62	tr
Louis Rich Breaded Patties	1 (2.8 oz)	209	1
Louis Rich Breaded Sticks	1 (1 oz)	81	tr
Louis Rich Chopped Ham	1 slice (28 g)	46	tr
Louis Rich Cotto Salami	1 slice (28 g)	53	tr
Louis Rich Ham Round	1 slice (28 g)	34	tr
Louis Rich Ham Thin Sliced	1 slice	12	tr
Louis Rich Hickory Smoked Breast Skinless	1 oz	28	tr
Louis Rich Honey Cured Ham	1 slice	25	tr
Louis Rich Honey Roasted Breast	1 slice (1 oz)	32	tr
Louis Rich Honey Roasted Breast Skinless	1 oz	31	tr
Louis Rich Luncheon Loaf	1 slice (28 g)	45	tr
Louis Rich Oven Roasted Breast	1 slice (1 oz)	31	tr
Louis Rich Oven Roasted Breast Skinless	1 oz	26	tr
Louis Rich Oven Roasted Thin Sliced Breast	1 slice	12	tr
Louis Rich Pastrami	1 slice (1 oz)	32	tr
Louis Rich Pastrami Thin Sliced	1 slice	11	tr
Louis Rich Salami	1 slice (28 g)	54	tr
Louis Rich Smoked	1 slice (28 g)	32	tr
Louis Rich Smoked Breast	1 slice	21	tr
Louis Rich Smoked Breast Chunk	1 oz	33	tr
Louis Rich Smoked Breast Thin Sliced	1 slice	11	tr
Louis Rich Summer Sausage	1 slice (28 g)	55	1
Oscar Mayer Breast Roast Thin Sliced	1 slice (.4 oz)	12	tr
Oscar Mayer Oven Roasted Breast	1 slice (.75 oz)	23	tr
Oscar Mayer Smoked Breast	1 slice (.75 oz)	20	tr

FOOD	PORTION	CALORIES	IRON
bologna	1 oz	57	tr
breast	1 slice (.75 oz)	23	tr
diced light & dark, seasoned	1 oz	39	1
diced light & dark, seasoned	½ lb	313	4
ham thigh meat	1 pkg (8 oz)	291	6
ham thigh meat	2 oz	73	2
pastrami	1 pkg (8 oz)	320	4
pastrami	2 oz	80	1
patties, battered & fried	1 (2.3 oz)	181	1
patties, battered & fried	1 (3.3 oz)	266	2
poultry salad sandwich spread	1 oz	238	tr
poultry salad sandwich spread	1 tbsp	109	tr
prebasted breast w/ skin, roasted	3.8 lbs	2175	11
prebasted breast w/ skin, roasted	½ breast (1.9 lbs)	1087	6
prebasted thigh w/ skin, roasted	11 oz	495	5
roll, light & dark meat	1 oz	42	tr
roll, light meat	1 oz	42	tr
salami, cooked	1 pkg (8 oz)	446	4
salami, cooked	2 oz	111	1
turkey loaf breast meat	1 pkg (6 oz)	187	1
turkey loaf breast meat	2 slices (1.5 oz)	47	tr
turkey sticks, battered & fried	1 (2.3 oz)	178	1
turkey sticks, breaded & fried	1 (2.3 oz)	178	1

TURKEY DISHES

FROZEN

gravy & turkey	1 cup (8.4 oz)	160	2
gravy & turkey	1 pkg (5 oz)	95	1

FOOD	PORTION	CALORIES	IRON

TURMERIC

ground	1 tsp	8	1

TURNIPS

CANNED

greens	½ cup	17	2

FRESH

cooked, mashed	½ cup	21	tr
greens, chopped & cooked	½ cup	15	1
greens, raw, chopped	½ cup	7	tr
raw, cubed	½ cup	18	tr

FROZEN

greens, cooked	½ cup	24	2

TURTLE

raw	3.5 oz	85	2

VEAL

(*see also* BEEF, DINNERS, VEAL DISHES)

FRESH

cutlet, lean only, braised	3 oz	172	1
cutlet, lean only, fried	3 oz	156	1
ground, broiled	3 oz	146	1
loin chop w/ bone, lean & fat, braised	1 chop (2.8 oz)	227	1
loin chop w/ bone, lean only, braised	1 chop (2.4 oz)	155	1
shoulder w/ bone, lean only, braised	3 oz	169	1
sirloin w/ bone, lean & fat, roasted	3 oz	171	1
sirloin w/ bone, lean only, roasted	3 oz	143	1

FOOD	PORTION	CALORIES	IRON

VEAL DISHES

TAKE-OUT
| parmigiana | 4.2 oz | 279 | 3 |

VEGETABLES, MIXED
(see also individual vegetables)

CANNED
Chop Suey Vegetables (La Choy)	½ cup	10	tr
Garden Medley (Green Giant)	½ cup	40	tr
Garden Salad Marinated (S&W)	½ cup	60	1
Mixed Vegetables Old Fashion Harvest Time (S&W)	½ cup	35	tr
Peas & Carrots Water Pack (S&W)	½ cup	35	1
Succotash Country Style (S&W)	½ cup	80	1
Sweet Peas & Diced Carrots (S&W)	½ cup	50	1
Sweet Peas w/ Tiny Pearl Onions (S&W)	½ cup	60	1
mixed vegetables	½ cup	39	1
peas & carrots	½ cup	48	1
peas & carrots low sodium	½ cup	48	1
peas & onions	½ cup	30	1
succotash	½ cup	102	1

FROZEN
American Mixtures California (Green Giant)	½ cup	25	0
American Mixtures Heartland (Green Giant)	½ cup	25	tr
American Mixtures New England (Green Giant)	½ cup	70	1

FOOD	PORTION	CALORIES	IRON
American Mixtures San Francisco (Green Giant)	½ cup	25	tr
American Mixtures Sante Fe (Green Giant)	½ cup	70	tr
American Mixtures Seattle (Green Giant)	½ cup	25	tr
Breaded Medley (Ore Ida)	3 oz	160	1
Broccoli, Cauliflower & Carrots in Butter Sauce (Green Giant)	½ cup	30	tr
Broccoli, Cauliflower & Carrots in Cheese Sauce (Birds Eye)	½ pkg	80	tr
Broccoli, Cauliflower & Carrots in Cheese Sauce (Green Giant)	½ cp	60	tr
California Florentine Blend (Big Valley)	3.5 oz	25	tr
Farm Fresh Broccoli & Cauliflower (Birds Eye)	¾ cup	30	1
Farm Fresh Broccoli, Carrots & Water Chestnuts (Birds Eye)	¾ cup	40	1
Farm Fresh Broccoli, Cauliflower & Carrots (Birds Eye)	¾ cup	35	1
Farm Fresh Broccoli, Cauliflower & Red Peppers (Birds Eye)	¾ cup	30	1
Farm Fresh Broccoli, Corn & Red Peppers (Birds Eye)	⅔ cup	60	1
Farm Fresh Broccoli, Green Beans, Pearl Onions & Red Peppers (Birds Eye)	¾ cup	35	1
Farm Fresh Broccoli, Red Peppers, Onions & Mushrooms (Birds Eye)	¾ cup	30	1
Farm Fresh Brussels Sprouts, Cauliflower & Carrots (Birds Eye)	¾ cup	40	1
Farm Fresh Cauliflower, Carrots & Snow Peas (Birds Eye)	⅔ cup	35	1
Harvest Fresh Mixed Vegetables (Green Giant)	½ cup	40	tr

FOOD	PORTION	CALORIES	IRON
In Butter Sauce Broccoli, Cauliflower & Carrots (Birds Eye)	½ cup	40	tr
In Sauce Peas & Pearl Onions w/ Seasonings (Birds Eye)	½ cup	70	1
Internationals Austrian (Birds Eye)	3.3 oz	70	tr
Internationals Bavarian (Birds Eye)	3.3 oz	90	1
Internationals California (Birds Eye)	3.3 oz	90	1
Internationals French Country (Birds Eye)	3.3 oz	70	1
Internationals Italian (Birds Eye)	3.3 oz	80	1
Internationals Japanese (Birds Eye)	3.3 oz	60	1
Internationals New England (Birds Eye)	3.3 oz	100	tr
Mandarin Vegetables (Budget Gourmet)	1 pkg	160	1
Mixed (Birds Eye)	½ cup	60	1
Mixed (Green Giant)	½ cup	40	1
Mixed in Butter Sauce (Green Giant)	½ cup	60	1
Mixed Fancy (La Choy)	½ cup	12	tr
New England Recipe Vegetables (Budget Gourmet)	1 pkg	230	tr
One Serve Broccoli, Carrots & Rotini in Cheese Sauce (Green Giant)	1 pkg	120	1
One Serve Broccoli, Cauliflower & Carrots (Green Giant)	1 pkg	25	tr
Peas & Cauliflower in Cream Sauce (Budget Gourmet)	1 pkg	150	tr
Peas & Potatoes w/ Cream Sauce (Birds Eye)	½ cup	100	1
Peas & Water Chestnuts Oriental (Budget Gourmet)	1 pkg	110	tr

FOOD	PORTION	CALORIES	IRON
Polybag (Birds Eye)	½ cup	60	1
Spring Vegetables in Cheese Sauce (Budget Gourmet)	1 pkg	150	1
Valley Combinations Broccoli & Cauliflower (Green Giant)	½ cup	60	0
mixed vegetables, cooked	½ cup	54	1
peas & carrots, cooked	½ cup	38	1
peas & onions, cooked	½ cup	40	1
succotash, cooked	½ cup	79	1
HOME RECIPE succotash	½ cup	111	1
JUICE Smucker's Vegetable Juice Hearty	8 oz	58	tr
Smucker's Vegetable Juice Hot & Spicy	8 oz	58	tr
V8	6 oz	35	1
V8 No Salt Added	6 oz	35	1
V8 Spicy Hot	6 oz	35	1
vegetable juice cocktail	½ cup	22	1
vegetable juice cocktail	6 oz	34	1
SHELF-STABLE Corn, Green Beans, Carrots, Pasta in Tomato Sauce (Pantry Express)	½ cup	80	1
Green Beans, Potatoes & Mushrooms in Seasoned Sauce (Pantry Express)	½ cup	50	tr
TAKE-OUT curry	1 serv (7.7 oz)	398	2
pakoras	1 (2 oz)	108	2
ratatouille	8.8 oz	190	1
samosa	2 (4 oz)	519	1

FOOD	PORTION	CALORIES	IRON

VENISON

roasted	3 oz	134	4

VINEGAR

cider	1 tbsp	tr	tr

WAFFLES

FROZEN

FOOD	PORTION	CALORIES	IRON
Apple Cinnamon (Aunt Jemima)	2.5 oz	176	4
Apple Cinnamon (Eggo)	1	130	2
Belgian Waffles & Sausage (Great Starts)	2.85 oz	280	1
Belgian Waffles Strawberries & Sausage (Great Starts)	3.5 oz	210	1
Blueberry (Aunt Jemima)	2.5 oz	175	4
Blueberry (Eggo)	1	130	2
Blueberry Batter, as prep (Aunt Jemima)	3.6 oz	204	2
Buttermilk (Aunt Jemima)	2.5 oz	179	4
Buttermilk (Eggo)	1	130	2
Homestyle (Eggo)	1	130	2
Minis (Eggo)	4	90	2
Multi Bran (Nutri-Grain)	1	120	2
Nut & Honey (Eggo)	1	130	2
Oat Bran (Common Sense)	1	110	2
Oat Bran w/ Fruit & Nuts (Common Sense)	1	120	2
Original (Aunt Jemima)	2.5 oz	173	4
Plain (Nutri-Grain)	1	120	2
Raisin & Bran (Nutri-Grain)	1	120	2
Special K (Kellogg's)	1	80	2

FOOD	PORTION	CALORIES	IRON
Strawberry (Eggo)	1	130	2
Waffle w/ Bacon (Great Starts)	2.2 oz	230	1
Whole-Grain Wheat/Oat Bran (Aunt Jemima)	2.5 oz	154	6
buttermilk	1 (4" sq)	88	1
plain	1 (4" sq)	88	1
HOME RECIPE plain	1 (7" diam)	218	2
MIX plain, as prep	1 (7" diam)	218	1

WALNUTS

FOOD	PORTION	CALORIES	IRON
Black (Planters)	1 oz	180	1
English Halves (Planters)	1 oz	190	1
black, dried	1 oz	172	1
black, dried & chopped	1 cup	759	4
english, dried	1 oz	182	1
english, dried & chopped	1 cup	770	3

WATER CHESTNUTS

FOOD	PORTION	CALORIES	IRON
CANNED La Choy Sliced	¼ cup	18	tr
La Choy Whole	4	14	tr
chinese, sliced	½ cup	35	1
FRESH sliced	½ cup	66	tr

WATERCRESS
(see also CRESS)

FOOD	PORTION	CALORIES	IRON
raw, chopped	½ cup	2	tr

FOOD	PORTION	CALORIES	IRON

WATERMELON

FOOD	PORTION	CALORIES	IRON
cut up	1 cup	50	tr
wedge	1/16	152	1
seeds dried	1 cup	602	2
dried	1 oz	158	2

WAX BEANS

FOOD	PORTION	CALORIES	IRON
CANNED			
Golden Cut Premium (S&W)	1/2 cup	20	1

WHALE

FOOD	PORTION	CALORIES	IRON
raw	3.5 oz	134	4

WHEAT
(see also BRAN, BULGUR, COUSCOUS, CEREAL, FLOUR, WHEAT GERM)

FOOD	PORTION	CALORIES	IRON
sprouted	1/3 cup	71	tr
starch	3.5 oz	348	0
WHEAT GERM			
Kretschmer	1/4 cup	103	2
Kretschmer Honey Crunch	1/4 cup	105	2
plain, toasted	1 cup	431	10
plain, toasted	1/4 cup	108	3
plain, untoasted	1/4 cup	104	2
w/ brown sugar & honey, toasted	1 cup	426	8
w/ brown sugar & honey, toasted	1 oz	107	2

WHIPPED TOPPINGS
(see also CREAM)

FOOD	PORTION	CALORIES	IRON
cream, pressurized	1 cup	154	tr
cream, pressurized	1 tbsp	8	tr
nondairy powdered, as prep w/ whole milk	1 cup	151	tr

FOOD	PORTION	CALORIES	IRON
nondairy powdered, as prep w/ whole milk	1 tbsp	8	tr
nondairy, pressurized	1 cup	184	tr
nondairy, pressurized	1 tbsp	11	tr
nondairy, frzn	1 tbsp	13	tr

WHITE BEANS

CANNED			
Goya Spanish Style	7.5 oz	130	4
white beans	1 cup	306	8
DRIED			
regular, cooked	1 cup	249	7
small, cooked	1 cup	253	5

WHITEFISH

FRESH			
baked	3 oz	146	tr
SMOKED			
whitefish	1 oz	39	tr
whitefish	3 oz	92	tr

WHITING

fresh, cooked	3 oz	98	tr
fresh, raw	3 oz	77	tr

WILD RICE

cooked	½ cup	83	tr

WINE

red	3.5 oz	74	tr
rose	3.5 oz	73	tr

FOOD	PORTION	CALORIES	IRON
sweet dessert	2 oz	90	tr
white	3.5 oz	70	tr

WINGED BEANS

dried, cooked	1 cup	252	7

WOLFFISH

fresh atlantic, baked	3 oz	105	tr

YAM

(*see also* SWEET POTATO)

FOOD	PORTION	CALORIES	IRON
CANNED			
Bruce Cut	½ cup	139	tr
Bruce Mashed	½ cup	130	1
Bruce Vacuum Pack	½ cup	122	tr
Bruce Whole	½ cup	139	tr
S&W Candied	½ cup	180	tr
S&W Southern Whole in Extra Heavy Syrup	½ cup	139	1
FRESH			
hawaiian mountain yam, cooked	½ cup	59	tr
yam, cubed & cooked	½ cup	79	tr

YAM BEAN

cooked	¾ cup	38	1
dried, cooked	1 cup	202	5

YEAST

baker's compressed	1 cake (0.6 oz)	18	1
baker's, dry	1 pkg (.25 oz)	21	1
baker's, dry	1 tbsp	35	2
brewer's, dry	1 tbsp	25	1

FOOD	PORTION	CALORIES	IRON
YELLOW BEANS			
dried, cooked	1 cup	254	4
YELLOWTAIL			
fresh, baked	3 oz	159	1
YOGURT			
Apple Crisp Lowfat (New Country)	6 oz	150	tr
Apples 'n Spice Nonfat Lite (Colombo)	8 oz	190	1
Banana Fruit on Bottom (Dannon)	8 oz	240	0
Banana Strawberry Classic (Colombo)	8 oz	250	1
Banana Strawberry Nonfat Lite (Colombo)	8 oz	190	1
Banana Strawberry Nonfat Lite Swiss Style (Colombo)	4.4 oz	100	tr
Black Cherry Classic (Colombo)	8 oz	230	1
Blueberry (Dannon)	8 oz	200	0
Blueberry Classic (Colombo)	8 oz	230	1
Blueberry Fruit on Bottom (Dannon)	4.4 oz	130	0
Blueberry Fruit on Bottom (Dannon)	8 oz	240	0
Blueberry Nonfat (Dannon)	6 oz	140	0
Blueberry Nonfat Light (Dannon)	4.4 oz	60	0
Blueberry Nonfat Light (Dannon)	8 oz	100	0
Blueberry Nonfat Lite (Colombo)	8 oz	190	1
Blueberry Nonfat Lite Swiss Style (Colombo)	4.4 oz	100	tr
Blueberry Supreme Lowfat (New Country)	6 oz	150	tr

FOOD	PORTION	CALORIES	IRON
Boysenberry Fruit on Bottom (Dannon)	8 oz	240	0
Cherry Fruit on Bottom (Dannon)	4.4 oz	130	0
Cherry Fruit on Bottom (Dannon)	8 oz	240	0
Cherry Nonfat Lite (Colombo)	8 oz	190	1
Cherry Supreme Lowfat (New Country)	6 oz	150	tr
Cherry Vanilla Nonfat Light (Dannon)	8 oz	100	0
Coffee Lowfat (Dannon)	8 oz	200	0
Coffee Nonfat Lite (Colombo)	8 oz	190	1
Dutch Apple Fruit on Bottom (Dannon)	8 oz	240	0
Exotic Fruit Fruit on Bottom (Dannon)	8 oz	240	0
French Vanilla Classic (Colombo)	8 oz	215	1
French Vanilla Lowfat (New Country)	6 oz	150	tr
Fruit Cocktail Nonfat Lite (Colombo)	8 oz	190	1
Fruit Crunch Lowfat (New Country)	6 oz	150	tr
Hawaiian Salad Lowfat (New Country)	6 oz	150	tr
Lemon Lowfat (Dannon)	8 oz	200	0
Lemon Nonfat Lite (Colombo)	8 oz	190	1
Lemon Supreme Lowfat (New Country)	6 oz	150	tr
Mixed Berries Fruit on Bottom (Dannon)	4.4 oz	130	0
Mixed Berries Fruit on Bottom (Dannon)	8 oz	240	0
Mixed Berries Lowfat (Dannon)	8 oz	240	0

FOOD	PORTION	CALORIES	IRON
Mixed Berries Lowfat (New Country)	6 oz	150	tr
Orange Supreme Lowfat (New Country)	6 oz	150	tr
Peach Fruit Mousette (Colombo)	3.5 oz	80	tr
Peach Fruit on Bottom (Dannon)	8 oz	240	0
Peach Lowfat Blended w/ Fruit (Dannon)	4.4 oz	130	0
Peach Melba Classic (Colombo)	8 oz	230	1
Peach Nonfat (Dannon)	6 oz	140	0
Peach Nonfat Light (Dannon)	8 oz	100	0
Peach Nonfat Lite (Colombo)	8 oz	190	1
Peach Nonfat Lite Swiss Style (Colombo)	4.4 oz	100	tr
Peaches 'n Cream Lowfat (New Country)	6 oz	150	tr
Pina Colada Fruit on Bottom (Dannon)	8 oz	240	0
Plain Classic (Colombo)	8 oz	150	1
Plain Extra Mild Sweetened (Colombo)	8 oz	200	1
Plain Lowfat (Dannon)	8 oz	140	0
Plain Nonfat (Colombo)	8 oz	110	1
Plain Nonfat (Dannon)	8 oz	110	0
Raspberry Classic (Colombo)	8 oz	230	1
Raspberry Fruit Mousette (Colombo)	3.5 oz	80	tr
Raspberry Fruit on Bottom (Dannon)	4.4 oz	120	0
Raspberry Fruit on Bottom (Dannon)	8 oz	240	0
Raspberry Lowfat Blended w/ Fruit (Dannon)	4.4 oz	130	0

FOOD	PORTION	CALORIES	IRON
Raspberry Nonfat (Dannon)	6 oz	140	0
Raspberry Nonfat (Dannon)	8 oz	200	0
Raspberry Nonfat Light (Dannon)	8 oz	100	0
Raspberry Nonfat Lite (Colombo)	8 oz	190	1
Raspberry Nonfat Lite Swiss Style (Colombo)	4.4 oz	100	tr
Raspberry Supreme Lowfat (New Country)	6 oz	150	tr
Strawberry Banana Fruit on Bottom (Dannon)	4.4 oz	130	0
Strawberry Banana Lowfat (New Country)	6 oz	150	tr
Strawberry Banana Lowfat Blended w/ Fruit (Dannon)	4.4 oz	130	0
Strawberry Banana Nonfat Light (Dannon)	8 oz	100	0
Strawberry Classic (Colombo)	8 oz	230	1
Strawberry Fruit Cup Lowfat (New Country)	6 oz	150	tr
Strawberry Fruit Cup Nonfat Light (Dannon)	8 oz	100	0
Strawberry Fruit Mousette (Colombo)	3.5 oz	80	tr
Strawberry Fruit on Bottom (Dannon)	4.4 oz	130	0
Strawberry Fruit on Bottom (Dannon)	8 oz	240	0
Strawberry Lowfat (Dannon)	8 oz	200	0
Strawberry Lowfat Blended w/ Fruit (Dannon)	4.4 oz	130	0
Strawberry Nonfat (Dannon)	6 oz	140	0
Strawberry Nonfat Light (Dannon)	4.4 oz	60	0
Strawberry Nonfat Light (Dannon)	8 oz	100	0

FOOD	PORTION	CALORIES	IRON
Strawberry Nonfat Lite (Colombo)	8 oz	190	1
Strawberry Nonfat Lite Swiss Style (Colombo)	4.4 oz	100	tr
Strawberry Supreme Lowfat (New Country)	6 oz	150	tr
Vanilla Lowfat (Dannon)	8 oz	200	0
Vanilla Nonfat Light (Dannon)	8 oz	100	0
Vanilla Nonfat Lite (Colombo)	8 oz	160	1
coffee lowfat	8 oz	194	tr
fruit lowfat	4 oz	113	tr
fruit lowfat	8 oz	225	tr
plain	8 oz	139	tr
plain lowfat	8 oz	144	tr
plain nonfat	8 oz	127	tr
vanilla lowfat	8 oz	194	tr

YOGURT, FROZEN
(see also TOFU)

Chocolate (Haagen-Dazs)	3 oz	130	1
Strawberry (Borden)	½ cup	100	0
Strawberry (Meadow Gold)	½ cup	100	0
Strawberry Nonfat (Dannon)	6 oz	140	0

ZUCCHINI

CANNED

Italian Style (S&W)	½ cup	45	1
italian style	½ cup	33	1

FRESH

raw, sliced	½ cup	9	tr
sliced, cooked	½ cup	14	tr

FOOD	PORTION	CALORIES	IRON
FROZEN			
Big Valley	3.5 oz	12	tr
Breaded Zucchini (Ore Ida)	3 oz	150	2
cooked	½ cup	19	1

PART II
Restaurant, Take-Out and Fast-Food Chains

FOOD	PORTION	CALORIES	IRON

ARBY'S

FOOD	PORTION	CALORIES	IRON
Hot Chocolate	8 oz	110	tr
BREAKFAST SELECTIONS			
Biscuit, Bacon	1	318	3
Biscuit, Ham	1	323	3
Biscuit, Plain	1	280	3
Biscuit, Sausage	1	460	4
Cinnamon Nut Danish	1	340	3
Croissant, Bacon/Egg	1	389	4
Croissant, Ham/Cheese	1	345	3
Croissant, Mushroom/Cheese	1	493	3
Croissant, Plain	1	260	3
Croissant, Sausage/Egg	1	519	4
Muffin, Blueberry	1	200	1
Platter, Bacon	1	860	2
Platter, Egg	1	460	4
Platter, Ham	1	518	2
Platter, Sausage	1	640	4
Toastix	1 serv	420	3
DESSERTS			
Cheese Cake	1 serv	306	1
Chocolate Chip Cookie	1	130	tr
Chocolate Shake	12 oz	451	1
Polar Swirl Butterfinger	1	457	tr
Polar Swirl Oreo	1	482	1
Turnover, Apple	1	303	1
Turnover, Blueberry	1	320	1
Turnover, Cherry	1	280	1

FOOD	PORTION	CALORIES	IRON
MAIN MENU SELECTIONS			
Arby's Sauce	.5 oz	15	tr
Bac 'N Cheddar Deluxe Sandwich	1	532	5
Baked Potato, Broccoli 'N Cheddar	1	417	3
Baked Potato, Deluxe	1	621	3
Baked Potato, Mushroom & Cheese	1	515	3
Baked Potato, Plain	1	240	3
Baked Potato w/ Butter or Margarine & Sour Cream	1	463	3
Beef 'N Cheddar Sandwich	1	451	4
Cheddar Fries	1 serv (5 oz)	399	1
Chicken Breast Sandwich	1	489	4
Chicken Cordon Bleu Sandwich	1	658	4
Curly Fries	1 serv (3.5 oz)	337	1
Fish Fillet Sandwich	1	537	4
French Dip	1	345	3
French Dip 'N Swiss	1	425	3
French Fries	1 serv	246	1
Grilled Chicken Barbeque Sandwich	1	378	4
Grilled Chicken Deluxe Sandwich	1	426	4
Ham 'N Cheese Sandwich	1	330	3
Philly Beef 'N Swiss Sandwich	1	498	4
Potato Cakes	1 serv	204	1
Roast Beef Sandwich, Giant	1	530	6
Roast Beef Sandwich, Junior	1	218	2
Roast Beef Sandwich, Regular	1	353	4
Roast Beef Sandwich, Super	1	529	5
Roast Chicken Club	1	513	4
Roast Chicken Deluxe Sandwich	1	373	4

FOOD	PORTION	CALORIES	IRON
Sub Deluxe	1	482	4
Turkey Deluxe Sandwich	1	399	3
SALADS AND DRESSINGS			
Blue Cheese Dressing	2 oz	295	tr
Cashew Chicken Salad	1	590	3
Chef Salad	1	210	1
Croutons	.5 oz	59	tr
Garden Salad	1	149	1
Honey French Dressing	2 oz	322	2
Thousand Island Dressing	2 oz	298	1
SOUPS			
Beef w/ Vegetables & Barley	8 oz	96	1
Boston Clam Chowder	8 oz	207	2
Cream of Broccoli	8 oz	180	1
French Onion	8 oz	67	1
Lumberjack Mixed Vegetable	8 oz	89	1
Old Fashioned Chicken Noodle	8 oz	99	1
Pilgrim's Corn Chowder	5 oz	193	1
Split Pea w/ Ham	8 oz	200	2
Tomato Florentine	8 oz	244	1
Wisconsin Cheese	8 oz	287	1

AU BON PAIN

FOOD	PORTION	CALORIES	IRON
BREAD AND ROLLS			
Alpine Roll	1	220	1
Baguette Loaf	1	810	8
Cheese Loaf	1	1670	12
Four Grain Loaf	1	1420	11
French Roll	1	320	3
Hearth Roll	1	250	2

FOOD	PORTION	CALORIES	IRON
Hearth Sandwich Roll	1	370	3
Onion Herb Loaf	1	1430	12
Parisienne Loaf	1	1490	14
Petit Pain Roll	1	220	2
Sandwich Croissant	1	300	2
Soft Roll	1	310	2
COOKIES			
Chocolate Chip	1	280	2
Chocolate Chunk Pecan	1	290	1
Oatmeal Raisin	1	250	1
Peanut Butter	1	290	1
White Chocolate Chunk Pecan	1	300	1
CROISSANTS			
Almond	1	420	2
Apple	1	250	1
Blueberry Cheese	1	380	2
Chocolate	1	400	2
Chocolate Hazelnut	1	480	2
Cinnamon Raisin	1	390	3
Coconut Pecan	1	440	2
Ham & Cheese	1	370	2
Plain	1	220	1
Raspberry Cheese	1	400	2
Spinach & Cheese	1	290	2
Strawberry Cheese	1	400	2
Sweet Cheese	1	420	2
Turkey & Cheddar	1	410	2
Turkey & Harvati	1	410	2

FOOD	PORTION	CALORIES	IRON
MUFFINS			
Blueberry	1	390	1
Bran	1	390	1
Carrot	1	450	2
Corn	1	460	2
Cranberry Walnut	1	350	1
Oat Bran Apple	1	400	3
Pumpkin	1	410	2
Whole Grain	1	440	1
SALADS			
Chicken, Cracked Pepper	1	100	2
Chicken, Grilled	1	110	2
Garden, Large	1	40	2
Garden, Small	1	20	1
Shrimp	1	102	3
SANDWICH FILLINGS			
Boursin	1 serv	290	1
Chicken, Grilled	1 serv	130	1
Roast Beef	1 serv	180	3
SOUPS			
Beef Barley	1 bowl	125	1
Beef Barley	1 cup	80	1
Chicken Noodle	1 bowl	125	2
Chicken Noodle	1 cup	80	1
Clam Chowder	1 bowl	390	1
Clam Chowder	1 cup	270	1
Cream of Broccoli	1 bowl	380	3
Cream of Broccoli	1 cup	250	2
Garden Vegetarian	1 bowl	70	3

FOOD	PORTION	CALORIES	IRON
Garden Vegetarian	1 cup	50	2
Minestrone	1 bowl	190	3
Minestrone	1 cup	120	2
Split Pea	1 bowl	380	3
Split Pea	1 cup	250	2
Tomato Florentine	1 bowl	120	3
Tomato Florentine	1 cup	90	2
Vegetarian Chili	1 bowl	280	3
Vegetarian Chili	1 cup	180	1

BURGER KING

BEVERAGES			
Shake, Chocolate	1 med	284	1
BREAKFAST SELECTIONS			
Blueberry Muffin	1	292	1
Breakfast Buddy w/ Sausage, Egg & Cheese	1	255	2
Croissan'wich w/ Bacon, Egg & Cheese	1	353	2
Croissan'wich w/ Ham, Egg & Cheese	1	351	2
Croissan'wich w/ Sausage, Egg & Cheese	1	534	3
French Toast Sticks	1 serv	440	3
Hash Browns	1	213	tr
DESSERTS			
Apple Pie	1	320	1
Cherry Pie	1	360	1
Lemon Pie	1	290	tr
Snickers Ice Cream Bar	1	220	tr

FOOD	PORTION	CALORIES	IRON
MAIN MENU SELECTIONS			
Bacon Double Cheeseburger	1	470	4
Bacon Double Cheeseburger Deluxe	1	530	4
BK Broiler	1	280	2
Cheeseburger	1	300	3
Chicken Sandwich	1	620	4
Chicken Tenders	6 pieces	236	1
Double Cheeseburger	1	450	4
Double Whopper	1	800	7
French Fries, Salted	1 med	372	1
Hamburger	1	260	3
Ocean Catch Fish Fillet Sandwich	1	450	2
Onion Rings	1 serv	339	1
Whopper	1	570	5
Whopper, Double w/ Cheese	1	890	7
Whopper Jr.	1	300	3
Whopper Jr. w/ Cheese	1	350	3
Whopper w/ Cheese	1	660	5
SALADS AND DRESSINGS			
Chef Salad	1	178	1
Chunky Chicken Salad	1	142	1
Garden Salad	1	95	1
Side Salad	1	25	1

CARL'S JR.

BAKERY SELECTIONS			
Chocolate Chip Cookies	2.5 oz	330	2
Cinnamon Roll	1	460	2
Danish	1	520	2

FOOD	PORTION	CALORIES	IRON
Fudge Brownie	1	430	2
Fudge Moussecake	1 slice	400	1
Muffin, Blueberry	1	340	4
Muffin, Bran	1	310	2
Raspberry Cheesecake	1 slice	310	1
BEVERAGES			
Orange Juice	1 sm	90	tr
Shake	1 reg	330	2
BREAKFAST SELECTIONS			
Breakfast Burrito	1	430	5
English Muffin w/ Margarine	1	190	1
French Toast Dips w/o Syrup	1 serv	490	3
Hash Brown Nuggets	1 serv	270	1
Hot Cakes w/ Margarine w/o Syrup	1 serv	510	2
Sausage	1 patty	190	1
Scrambled Eggs	1 serv	120	2
Sunrise Sandwich	1	300	2
MAIN MENU SELECTIONS			
All Star Chili Dog	1	720	4
All Star Hot Dog	1	540	3
Carl's Catch Fish Sandwich	1	560	4
Cheeseburger, Double Western w/ Bacon	1	1030	6
Cheeseburger, Western w/ Bacon	1	730	5
Chicken Club Charbroiler	1	570	4
Chicken Charbroiler BBQ Sandwich	1	310	2
Chicken Sante Fe Sandwich	1	540	4
Country Fried Steak Sandwich	1	720	4
CrissCut Fries	1 serv	330	2

FOOD	PORTION	CALORIES	IRON
French Fries	1 reg	420	1
Hamburger	1	220	3
Hamburger, Famous Star	1	610	4
Hamburger, Old Time Star	1	460	2
Hamburger, Super Star	1	820	6
Jr. Crisp Burrito	1	140	1
Onion Rings	1 serv	520	4
Potato, Bacon & Cheese	1	730	4
Potato, Broccoli & Cheese	1	590	5
Potato, Fiesta	1	720	5
Potato, Lite	1	250	3
Potato, Sour Cream & Chives	1	470	3
Potato w/ Cheese	1	690	2
Roast Beef Club	1	620	5
Roast Beef Deluxe Sandwich	1	540	4
Zucchini	1 serv	390	2
SALADS AND DRESSINGS			
1000 Island Dressing	1 oz	110	tr
Salad-to-Go Chicken	1	200	2
Salad-to-Go Garden	1 sm	50	tr

CARVEL

Lo-Yo Vanilla Frozen Yogurt	1 oz	34	tr

CHICK-FIL-A

BEVERAGES			
Iced Tea, Unsweetened	1 reg (9 oz)	3	tr
Lemonade	1 sm (10 oz)	138	tr
Lemonade, Diet	1 sm (10 oz)	32	tr

FOOD	PORTION	CALORIES	IRON
DESSERTS			
Cheesecake	1 slice	299	tr
Cheesecake w/ Blueberry Topping	1 slice	350	1
Cheesecake w/ Strawberry Topping	1 slice	343	tr
Fudge Brownie w/ Nuts	1	369	3
Lemon Pie	1 slice	329	1
MAIN MENU SELECTIONS			
Carrot & Raisin Salad	1 serv	116	1
Chargrilled Chicken Garden Salad	1 serv (10.4 oz)	126	3
Chargrilled Chicken Deluxe Sandwich	1	266	4
Chargrilled Chicken Sandwich	1	258	3
Chargrilled Chicken w/o Bun	3.6 oz	128	2
Chicken Sandwich	1	360	5
Chicken Deluxe Sandwich	1	368	5
Chicken Salad Plate	1 serv (12.6 oz)	291	5
Chicken Salad Sandwich on Whole Wheat	1	365	3
Chicken w/o Bun	1 piece (3.6 oz)	219	3
Chick-n-Q Sandwich	1	409	2
Cole Slaw	1 serv	175	1
Grilled 'n Lites	2 skewers	97	2
Hearty Breast of Chicken Soup	1 cup (8.5 oz)	152	2
Nuggets	8 pack	287	1
Potato Salad	1 serv	198	1
Tossed Salad	1 serv (4.5 oz)	21	1
Tossed Salad w/ Blue Cheese Dressing	1 serv (6 oz)	243	1
Tossed Salad w/ Honey French Dressing	1 serv (6 oz)	277	2

FOOD	PORTION	CALORIES	IRON
Tossed Salad w/ Lite Italian Dressing	1 serv (6 oz)	43	1
Tossed Salad w/ Lite Ranch Dressing	1 serv (6 oz)	171	1
Tossed Salad w/ Ranch Dressing	1 serv (6 oz)	298	1
Tossed Salad w/ Thousand Island Dressing	1 serv (6 oz)	250	1
Waffle Potato Fries	1 sm	270	1

DAIRY QUEEN/BRAZIER

FOOD SELECTION

FOOD	PORTION	CALORIES	IRON
¼ lb. Super Dog	1	590	3
BBQ Beef Sandwich	1	225	2
Baked Chicken Fillet Sandwich w/ Cheese	1	480	2
Breaded Chicken Fillet Sandwich	1	430	2
Double Hamburger	1	460	5
Double Hamburger w/ Cheese	1	570	5
DQ Homestyle Ultimate Burger	1	700	7
Fish Fillet Sandwich	1	370	2
Fish Fillet Sandwich w/ Cheese	1	420	2
French Fries	1 lg	390	1
French Fries	1 reg	300	1
French Fries	1 sm	210	1
Garden Salad	1	200	2
Grilled Chicken Fillet Sandwich	1	300	2
Hot Dog	1	280	1
Hot Dog w/ Cheese	1	330	1
Hot Dog w/ Chili	1	320	1
Onion Rings	1 reg	240	1
Side Salad	1	25	1

FOOD	PORTION	CALORIES	IRON
Single Hamburger	1	310	2
Single Hamburger w/ Cheese	1	365	2
ICE CREAM			
Banana Split	1	510	4
Blizzard, Strawberry	1 reg	740	2
Blizzard, Strawberry	1 sm	500	1
Breeze, Strawberry	1 reg	590	2
Breeze, Strawberry	1 sm	400	1
Buster Bar	1	450	1
Cone, Chocolate	1 lg	350	1
Cone, Chocolate	1 reg	230	1
Cone, Dipped Chocolate	1 reg	330	1
Cone, Vanilla	1 lg	340	1
Cone, Vanilla	1 reg	230	1
Cone, Vanilla	1 sm	140	tr
Cone, Yogurt	1 lg	260	1
Cone, Yogurt	1 reg	180	1
Cup, Yogurt	1 lg	230	1
Cup, Yogurt	1 reg	170	1
Dilly Bar	1	210	1
DQ Frozen Cake Slice, Undecorated	1	380	1
DQ Sandwich	1	140	1
Heath Blizzard	1 reg	820	2
Heath Blizzard	1 sm	560	1
Heath Breeze	1 reg	680	2
Heath Breeze	1 sm	450	1
Hot Fudge Brownie Delight	1	710	5
Malt, Vanilla	1 reg	610	1
Nutty Double Fudge	1	580	4

FOOD	PORTION	CALORIES	IRON
Peanut Buster Parfait	1	710	4
QC Big Scoop, Chocolate	1	310	1
Shake, Chocolate	1 reg	540	1
Shake, Vanilla	1 lg	600	1
Shake, Vanilla	1 reg	520	1
Sundae, Chocolate	1 reg	300	1
Waffle Cone Sundae, Strawberry	1	350	1
Yogurt Sundae, Strawberry	1 reg	200	1

EL POLLO LOCO

Beans	3.5 oz	110	1
Chicken	2 pieces	310	3
Coleslaw	2.8 oz	80	1
Combo Meal	1	720	9
Corn	3.3 oz	110	1
Potato Salad	4.3 oz	140	1
Rice	2.5 oz	100	1
Salsa	1.8 oz	10	1
Tortillas, Corn	3.3 oz	210	4
Tortillas, Flour	3.3 oz	280	4

GODFATHER'S PIZZA

Golden Crust Cheese	1/10 lg	261	2
Golden Crust Cheese	1/6 sm	213	2
Golden Crust Cheese	1/8 med	229	2
Golden Crust Combo	1/10 lg	322	3
Golden Crust Combo	1/6 sm	273	3
Golden Crust Combo	1/8 med	283	3
Original Crust Cheese	1/10 lg	271	2

FOOD	PORTION	CALORIES	IRON
Original Crust Cheese	¼ mini	138	1
Original Crust Cheese	⅙ sm	239	2
Original Crust Cheese	⅛ med	242	2
Original Crust Combo	⅒ lg	332	3
Original Crust Combo	¼ mini	164	1
Original Crust Combo	⅙ sm	299	3
Original Crust Combo	⅛ med	318	3

HAAGEN-DAZS

FOOD	PORTION	CALORIES	IRON
Blueberry Sorbet & Cream	4 oz	190	1
Butter Pecan	4 oz	390	tr
Caramel Almond Crunch Bar	1	240	tr
Caramel Nut Sundae	4 oz	310	tr
Chocolate	4 oz	270	tr
Chocolate Chocolate Chip	4 oz	290	2
Chocolate Chocolate Mint	4 oz	300	1
Chocolate Dark Chocolate Bar	1	390	1
Chocolate Frozen Yogurt	3 oz	130	1
Chocolate Nonfat Soft Yogurt	1 oz	30	tr
Coffee	4 oz	270	tr
Deep Chocolate	4 oz	290	1
Deep Chocolate Fudge	4 oz	290	1
Fudge Pop Bar	1	210	1
Keylime Sorbet & Cream	4 oz	190	1
Macadamia Brittle	4 oz	280	tr
Orange & Cream Pop	1	130	1
Orange Sorbet & Cream	4 oz	190	1
Peanut Butter Crunch Bar	1	270	1
Raspberry Sorbet & Cream	4 oz	180	1

FOOD	PORTION	CALORIES	IRON
Rum Raisin	4 oz	250	tr
Strawberry	4 oz	250	1
Vanilla Crunch Bar	1	220	tr
Vanilla Fudge	4 oz	270	tr
Vanilla Milk Chocolate Almond Bar	1	370	1
Vanilla Milk Chocolate Bar	1	360	1
Vanilla Milk Chocolate Brittle Bar	1	370	1
Vanilla Peanut Butter Swirl	4 oz	280	tr
Vanilla Swiss Almond	4 oz	290	tr

HARDEE'S

BEVERAGES			
Shake, Chocolate	12 oz	460	1
Shake, Strawberry	12 oz	440	tr
Shake, Vanilla	12 oz	400	tr

BREAKFAST SELECTIONS			
Bacon & Egg Biscuit	1	410	3
Bacon Biscuit	1	360	2
Bacon, Egg & Cheese Biscuit	1	460	3
Big Country Breakfast, Bacon	1	660	5
Big Country Breakfast, Country Ham	1	670	6
Big Country Breakfast, Ham	1	620	5
Big Country Breakfast, Sausage	1	850	6
Biscuit 'N' Gravy	1	440	2
Canadian Rise 'N' Shine Biscuit	1	470	4
Chicken Biscuit	1	430	2
Cinnamon 'N' Raisin	1	320	2
Country Ham Biscuit	1	350	3

FOOD	PORTION	CALORIES	IRON
Country Ham & Egg Biscuit	1	400	4
Ham & Egg Biscuit	1	370	3
Ham Biscuit	1	320	2
Ham, Egg & Cheese Biscuit	1	420	3
Hash Rounds	1 serv	230	1
Margarine/Butter Blend	1 tsp	35	tr
Rise 'N' Shine Biscuit	1	320	2
Sausage & Egg Biscuit	1	490	4
Sausage Biscuit	1	440	3
Steak & Egg Biscuit	1	550	5
Steak Biscuit	1	500	4
Syrup	1.5 oz	120	1
Three Pancakes	1 serv	280	3
Three Pancakes w/ 1 Sausage Pattie	1 serv	430	4
Three Pancakes w/ 2 Bacon Strips	1 serv	350	4
DESSERTS			
Apple Turnover	1	270	tr
Big Cookie	1	250	tr
Cool Twist Cone, Chocolate	1	200	2
Cool Twist Cone, Vanilla/Chocolate	1	190	2
Cool Twist Sundae, Caramel	1	330	tr
Cool Twist Sundae, Hot Fudge	1	320	1
Cool Twist Sundae, Strawberry	1	260	tr
MAIN MENU SELECTIONS			
Bacon Cheeseburger	1	610	6
Big Deluxe Burger	1	500	5
Big Fry	1 serv	500	2
Big Roast Beef	1	300	5
Big Twin	1	450	4

FOOD	PORTION	CALORIES	IRON
Cheeseburger	1	320	3
Chef Salad	1	240	2
Chicken Fillet	1	370	3
Chicken 'N' Pasta Salad	1	414	9
Chicken Stix	6 pieces	210	1
Chicken Stix	9 pieces	310	1
Crispy Curls	1 serv	300	1
Fisherman's Fillet	1	500	3
French Fries	1 lg	360	1
French Fries	1 reg	230	1
Garden Salad	1	210	1
Grilled Chicken Sandwich	1	310	3
Hamburger	1	270	3
Hot Dog, All Beef	1	300	3
Hot Ham 'N' Cheese	1	330	3
Mushroom 'N' Swiss Burger	1	490	5
Quarter-Pound Cheeseburger	1	500	5
Regular Roast Beef	1	260	4
Side Salad	1	20	tr
Turkey Club	1	390	3

JACK IN THE BOX

BEVERAGES			
Milk Shake, Chocolate	11 oz	330	1
Milk Shake, Strawberry	11 oz	320	tr
Orange Juice	6 oz	80	tr
BREAKFAST SELECTIONS			
Breakfast Jack	1	307	3
Hash Browns	1	156	tr
Pancake Platter	1	612	2

FOOD	PORTION	CALORIES	IRON
Sausage Crescent	1	584	3
Scrambled Egg Platter	1	559	5
Scrambled Egg Pocket	1	431	4
Sourdough Breakfast Sandwich	1	381	4
Supreme Crescent	1	547	3
DESSERTS			
Cheesecake	1	309	1
Double Fudge Cake	1 slice	288	2
Hot Apple Turnover	1	354	2
MAIN MENU SELECTIONS			
Bacon Bacon Cheeseburger	1	705	5
Cheeseburger	1	315	3
Chicken & Mushroom Sandwich	1	438	3
Chicken Fajita Pita	1	292	3
Chicken Strips	4 pieces	285	1
Chicken Strips	6 pieces	451	1
Chicken Supreme	1	641	3
Double Cheeseburger	1	467	3
Egg Rolls	3 pieces	437	4
Egg Rolls	5 pieces	753	6
Fish Supreme	1	510	3
French Fries	1 jumbo	396	1
French Fries	1 reg	351	1
French Fries	1 sm	219	1
Grilled Chicken Fillet	1	431	6
Grilled Sourdough Burger	1	712	4
Ham & Turkey Melt	1	592	2
Hamburger	1	267	2
Jumbo Jack	1	584	3
Jumbo Jack w/ Cheese	1	677	4

FOOD	PORTION	CALORIES	IRON
Old Fashioned Patty Melt	1	713	4
Onion Rings	1 serv	380	2
Pastrami Melt	1	556	4
Seasoned Curly French Fries	1 serv	358	2
Super Taco	1	281	2
Taco	1	187	1
Taquitos	7 pieces	511	4
Ultimate Cheeseburger	1	942	6
SALADS AND DRESSINGS			
Chef Salad	1	325	1
Taco Salad	1	503	4

KENTUCKY FRIED CHICKEN

FOOD	PORTION	CALORIES	IRON
CHICKEN DISHES			
Chicken Littles Sandwich	1	169	2
Colonel's Chicken Sandwich	1	482	1
Extra Crispy Center Breast	1	342	1
Extra Crispy Drumstick	1	204	1
Extra Crispy Thigh	1	406	1
Extra Crispy Wing	1	254	1
Kentucky Nuggets	1	46	tr
Original Center Breast	1	283	1
Original Drumstick	1	146	1
Original Side Breast	1	267	1
Original Wing	1	178	1
SIDE DISHES			
Buttermilk Biscuit	1	235	2
Cole Slaw	1 serv	119	tr
Corn-on-the-Cob	1 ear	176	1
French Fries	1 reg	244	1

FOOD	PORTION	CALORIES	IRON
Mashed Potatoes & Gravy	1 serv	71	tr
Sauce, Barbecue	1 oz	35	tr
Sauce, Honey	.5 oz	49	tr
Sauce, Mustard	1 oz	36	tr
Sauce, Sweet & Sour	1 oz	58	tr

LONG JOHN SILVER'S

FOOD	PORTION	CALORIES	IRON
CHILDREN'S MENU SELECTIONS			
Chicken Planks, 2 Pieces & Fryes	7.8 oz	510	4
Fish & Fryes, 1 Piece	6.9 oz	450	4
Fish, Chicken & Fryes	8.9 oz	580	4
DESSERTS			
Apple Pie	1 slice	320	1
Cherry Pie	1 slice	360	1
Chocolate Chip Cookie	1	230	tr
Lemon Pie	1 slice	340	1
Oatmeal Raisin Cookie	1	160	1
Walnut Brownie	1	440	2
MAIN MENU SELECTIONS			
Batter Dipped Fish, 1 Piece	3.1 oz	210	1
Batter Dipped Fish, 2 Pieces	6.2 oz	410	2
Chicken	17.3 oz	620	5
Chicken Plank, 1 Piece	2 oz	130	1
Chicken Planks, 2 Pieces	4 oz	270	1
Chicken Planks, 2 Pieces & Fryes	6.9 oz	440	3
Chicken Planks, 3 Pieces	5.9 oz	400	2
Chicken Planks, 3 Pieces w/ Fryes & Slaw	14.1 oz	860	5
Chicken Planks, 4 Pieces w/ Fryes & Slaw	16 oz	990	6

FOOD	PORTION	CALORIES	IRON
Clams w/ Fryes & Slaw	12.7 oz	910	5
Coleslaw	3.4 oz	140	1
Corn Cobbette	1 piece	140	tr
Fish & Chicken w/ Fryes & Slaw	15.2 oz	930	5
Fish & Fryes, 2 Pieces	9.2 oz	580	4
Fish & Fryes, 3 Pieces	14 oz	930	5
Fish & More, 2 Pieces	14 oz	860	5
Fish & More, 3 Pieces w/ Fryes & Slaw	17.5 oz	1070	6
Fish Light Portion w/ Lemon Crumb, 2 Pieces	10.3 oz	320	2
Fish Light Portion w/ Paprika, 2 Pieces	10 oz	300	2
Fish w/ Lemon Crumb, 3 Pieces	18.4 oz	640	5
Fish w/ Paprika, 3 Pieces	18.2 oz	610	5
Fish w/ Scampi Sauce, 3 Pieces	18.6 oz	660	5
Fryes	1 reg	170	2
Green Beans	4 oz	113	1
Hush Puppies	1	70	1
Long John's Homestyle Fish, 3 Pieces w/ Fryes & Slaw	13.1 oz	830	5
Ocean Chef Salad	8.2 oz	234	4
Rice Pilaf	5 oz	142	1
Sandwich, Baked Chicken	6.4 oz	310	2
Sandwich, Batter Dipped Chicken, 2 Pieces	6.5 oz	440	5
Sandwich, Batter Dipped Fish, 1 Piece	5.6 oz	380	5
Seafood Chowder w/ Cod	7 oz	140	2
Seafood Gumbo w/ Cod	7 oz	120	2
Seafood Salad	9.8 oz	230	5

FOOD	PORTION	CALORIES	IRON
Shrimp Scampi	10.6 oz	610	5
SALAD DRESSINGS AND SAUCES			
Seafood Sauce	.88 oz	35	tr

McDONALD'S

FOOD	PORTION	CALORIES	IRON
BEVERAGES			
Apple Juice	6 oz	90	1
BREAKFAST SELECTIONS			
Biscuit w/ Bacon, Egg & Cheese	1	440	3
Biscuit w/ Sausage	1	420	2
Biscuit w/ Sausage & Egg	1	505	4
Biscuit w/ Spread	1	260	1
Breakfast Burrito	1	280	1
Cheerios	¾ cup	80	5
Egg McMuffin	1	280	3
English Muffin w/ Spread	1	170	1
Fat-Free Apple Bran Muffin	1	180	1
Fat-Free Blueberry Muffin	1	170	1
Hotcakes w/ Margarine & Syrup	1 portion	440	2
Sausage	1	160	1
Sausage McMuffin	1	345	3
Sausage McMuffin w/ Egg	1	430	4
Scrambled Eggs	1 portion	140	2
Wheaties	¾ cup	90	4
DESSERTS			
Apple Pie	1 (3 oz)	260	1
Cookies, Chocolaty Chip	1 pkg (2 oz)	330	2
Cookies, McDonaldland	1 pkg (2 oz)	290	2
Danish, Apple	1	390	1

FOOD	PORTION	CALORIES	IRON
Danish, Cinnamon Raisin	1	440	2
Danish, Iced Cheese	1	390	1
Danish, Raspberry	1	410	1
Sundae, Lowfat Frozen Yogurt Hot Fudge	1 (6 oz)	240	tr

MAIN MENU SELECTIONS

Big Mac	1	500	4
Cheeseburger	1	305	3
Chicken Fajita	1	185	tr
Chicken McNuggets	6	270	1
Fillet-O-Fish	1	370	2
French Fries	1 lg	400	1
French Fries	1 med	320	1
French Fries	1 sm	220	tr
Hamburger	1	255	3
McChicken	1	415	3
McLean Deluxe	1	320	4
McLean Deluxe w/ Cheese	1	370	4
Quarter Pounder	1	410	4
Quarter Pounder w/ Cheese	1	510	4

SALADS, DRESSINGS AND SAUCES

Chef Salad	1 serv	170	1
Chunky Chicken Salad	1 serv	150	1
Garden Salad	1	50	1
McNuggets Sauce, Barbeque	1.12 oz	50	tr
Side Salad	1 serv	30	1

NATHAN'S

French Fries	1 (7 oz)	550	3
Hot Dog & Roll	1	290	2

FOOD	PORTION	CALORIES	IRON

PIZZA HUT

FOOD	PORTION	CALORIES	IRON
HAND-TOSSED MEDIUM			
Cheese	2 slices	518	5
Pepperoni	2 slices	500	5
Super Supreme	2 slices	556	7
Supreme	2 slices	540	8
PAN PIZZA MEDIUM			
Cheese	2 slices	492	5
Pepperoni	2 slices	540	6
Super Supreme	2 slices	563	7
Supreme	2 slices	589	5
PERSONAL PAN PIZZA			
Pepperoni	1 pie	675	6
Supreme	1 pie	647	7
THIN 'N CRISPY MEDIUM			
Cheese	2 slices	398	3
Pepperoni	2 slices	413	3
Super Supreme	2 slices	463	5
Supreme	2 slices	459	6

RED LOBSTER

FOOD	PORTION	CALORIES	IRON
Calamari, breaded & fried	1 lunch serv	360	1
Filet Mignon	8 oz	350	5
Hamburger	5 oz	410	3
Langostino	1 lunch serv	120	1
Maine Lobster	18 oz	240	1
Rib Eye Steak	12 oz	980	5
Sirloin Steak	8 oz	350	5
Snow Crab Legs	1 lb	150	tr

FOOD	PORTION	CALORIES	IRON
Strip Steak	9 oz	560	4
Tilefish	1 lunch serv	100	tr
Yellowfin Tuna	1 lunch serv	180	1

TACO BELL

FOOD	PORTION	CALORIES	IRON
Burrito, Bean	1	447	4
Burrito, Beef	1	493	4
Burrito, Chicken	1	334	8
Burrito, Combo	1	407	3
Burrito, Fiesta Bean	1	226	3
Burrito, Supreme	1	503	4
Chilito	1	383	3
Cinnamon Twists	1 order	171	tr
Enchirito	1	382	3
Guacamole	.66 oz	34	tr
Jalapeno Peppers	3.5 oz	20	tr
MexiMelt, Beef	1	266	2
MexiMelt, Chicken	1	257	4
Mexican Pizza	1	575	4
Nacho Cheese Sauce	2 oz	105	tr
Nachos	1	346	1
Nachos Bellgrande	1	649	3
Nachos Supreme	1	367	tr
Pico de Gallo	1	8	tr
Pintos 'N Cheese	1	190	1
Ranch Dressing	2.5 oz	236	1
Salsa	.33 oz	18	1
Taco	1	183	1
Taco Bellgrande	1	335	2
Taco, Fiesta	1	127	1

FOOD	PORTION	CALORIES	IRON
Taco Salad	1	905	6
Taco Salad w/o Shell	1	484	4
Taco Sauce, Hot	1 pkg	3	tr
Taco, Soft	1	225	2
Taco, Soft, Chicken	1	213	6
Taco, Soft, Fiesta	1	147	1
Taco, Soft, Steak	1	218	3
Taco, Soft, Supreme	1	272	2
Taco Supreme	1	230	1
Tostada	1	243	2
Tostada, Fiesta	1	167	1

TACO JOHN'S

FOOD	PORTION	CALORIES	IRON
Bean Burrito	1	197	2
Beef Burrito	1	303	3
Chicken Burrito w/ Green Chili	1	344	3
Chicken Super Taco Salad w/ Dressing	1	507	4
Chicken Super Taco Salad w/o Dressing	1	377	4
Chimichanga	1	464	4
Chimichanga w/ Chicken	1 serv	441	4
Combo Burrito	1	250	3
Mexican Rice	1 serv	340	3
Nachos	1 serv	468	1
Smothered Burrito w/ Green Chili	1	367	3
Smothered Burrito w/ Texas Chili	1	455	5
Soft Shell	1	140	3
Soft Shell w/ Chicken	1	180	2
Super Burrito	1	389	4

FOOD	PORTION	CALORIES	IRON
Super Burrito w/ Chicken	1	366	4
Super Nachos	1 serv	669	3
Super Taco Salad w/ 2 oz Dressing	1	558	5
Super Taco Salad w/o Dressing	1	428	5
Taco	1	178	1
Taco Bravo	1	319	3
Taco Burger	1	281	3
Taco Salad w/ 2 oz Dressing	1	359	3
Taco Salad w/o Dressing	1	228	3

T.J. CINNAMON'S

Doughnuts, Cake	2	454	2
Doughnuts, Raised	2	352	2
Mini-Cinn Plain	1	75	tr
Mini-Cinn w/ Icing	1	80	tr
Original Gourmet Cinnamon Roll, Plain	1	630	2
Original Gourmet Cinnamon Roll w/ Icing	1	686	2
Petite Cinnamon Roll, Plain	1	185	1
Petite Cinnamon Roll w/ Icing	1	202	1
Sticky Bun, Cinnamon Pecan	1	607	2
Sticky Bun Petite, Cinnamon Pecan	1	255	1
Triple Chocolate Classic Roll, Plain	1	412	2
Triple Chocolate Classic Roll w/ Icing	1	462	2

WENDY'S

BEVERAGES

Chocolate Milk	8 oz	160	1

FOOD	PORTION	CALORIES	IRON
Hot Chocolate	6 oz	110	tr
Lemonade	8 oz	90	tr
CHILDREN'S MENU SELECTIONS			
Kid's Meal Cheeseburger	1	300	4
Kid's Meal Hamburger	1	260	4
DESSERTS			
Chocolate Chip Cookie	1	275	1
Frosty Dairy Dessert	1 sm	340	1
MAIN MENU SELECTIONS			
¼ lb. Hamburger Patty, no bun	1	180	4
Big Classic	1	570	6
Chicken Breast Fillet	1	220	13
Chicken Sandwich	1	440	14
Chili	1 reg	220	6
Country Fried Steak Sandwich	1	440	4
Crispy Chicken Nuggets	6 pieces	280	1
Fish Fillet Sandwich	1	460	3
French Fries	1 sm order	240	1
Grilled Chicken Fillet	1	100	1
Grilled Chicken Sandwich	1	340	4
Hot Stuffed Potato, Plain	1	250	4
Hot Stuffed Potato, Bacon & Cheese	1	520	4
Hot Stuffed Potato, Broccoli & Cheese	1	400	3
Hot Stuffed Potato, Cheese	1	420	4
Hot Stuffed Potato, Chili & Cheese	1	500	5
Hot Stuffed Potato, Sour Cream & Chives	1	500	4
Jr. Bacon Cheeseburger	1	430	4

FOOD	PORTION	CALORIES	IRON
Jr. Cheeseburger	1	310	4
Jr. Hamburger	1	260	4
Jr. Swiss Deluxe	1	360	4
Kaiser Bun	1	200	2
Nuggets Sauce, Barbecue	1 pkg	50	1
Nuggets Sauce, Sweet & Sour	1 pkg	45	tr
Sandwich Bun	1	160	2
Single, Plain	1	340	5
Single w/ Everything	1	420	5
SALAD/SUPER BAR			
Bacon Bits	1 tbsp	40	tr
Breadsticks	2	30	tr
Broccoli	½ cup	12	tr
Cauliflower	½ cup	14	tr
Cheddar Chips	1 oz	160	tr
Cheese Tortellini in Spaghetti Sauce	2 oz	60	1
Chef Salad	1 (9 oz)	130	3
Chicken Salad	2 oz	120	tr
Chives	1 oz	71	5
Chow Mein Noodles	.5 oz	64	1
Croutons	.5 oz	60	1
Fettucini	2 oz	190	1
Flour Tortilla	1	110	tr
Garbanzo Beans	1 oz	46	1
Garden Salad	1 (8 oz)	70	1
Garlic Toast	1	70	tr
Green Peas	1 oz	21	tr
Lettuce, Iceberg	1 cup	8	tr

FOOD	PORTION	CALORIES	IRON
Lettuce, Romaine	1 cup	9	1
Olives, Black	1 oz	35	1
Pasta Medley	2 oz	60	1
Pasta Salad	¼ cup	35	tr
Pepperoni, Sliced	1 oz	140	tr
Picante Sauce	2 oz	18	tr
Pineapple Chunks	3 oz	60	1
Potato Salad	2 oz	125	1
Pudding, Butterscotch	2 oz	90	1
Pudding, Chocolate	2 oz	90	tr
Refried Beans	2 oz	70	1
Rotini	2 oz	90	1
Seafood Salad	2 oz	110	tr
Spaghetti Meat Sauce	2 oz	60	1
Spanish Rice	2 oz	70	2
Sunflower Seeds & Raisins	1 oz	140	2
Taco Chips	1.33 oz	260	1
Taco Meat	2 oz	110	2
Taco Salad	1 (17 oz)	530	5
Three Bean Salad	2 oz	60	tr
Tuna Salad	2 oz	100	tr
Turkey Ham	1 oz	35	1

PART III
Vitamin and Mineral Supplements

Iron Supplements

When a therapeutic dose of iron is needed to treat iron deficiency, ferrous sulfate is a good choice. It is absorbed well and is inexpensive. Other iron compounds are used as well. (*See* Types of Iron Supplements.)

The recommended therapeutic daily dose used to *treat iron deficiency* is 40 to 50 milligrams of iron. This is the amount that is usually absorbed from a 200- to 240-milligram iron supplement containing ferrous sulfate. Less is absorbed when the iron tablet is enteric coated or the iron is in a capsule form containing delayed-release granules.

Note: Iron supplements should be kept out of the reach of children. There are approximately 2,000 cases of iron poisoning each year in the United States. Most of these involve young children who swallow therapeutic iron supplements meant for adults. The lethal dose for a 2-year-old child is about three grams.

USING SUPPLEMENTS

The American Dietetic Association recently issued a statement on the use of vitamin and mineral supplements. It stressed that healthy children and adults should get their nutrients from foods. Eating a variety of foods, in moderation, reduces the risk for both nutrient deficiencies and excesses. It was noted that individual recommendations about supplement use should come from doctors and registered dietitians.

TYPES OF IRON SUPPLEMENTS

Elemental iron

Geritol Complete Tablets
Geritol Extend Caplets
One-a-Day Maximum Formula
One-a-Day Stressgard Formula
One-a-Day Women's Formula

Ferric ammonium citrate

Geritol Liquid
Geriplex-FS Liquid

Ferric pyrophosphate

Incremin With Iron Syrup
Troph-Iron

Ferrous fumarate

Allbee C-800 Plus Iron
Caltrate 600 + Iron & Vitamin D
Centrum
Femiron
Ferancee
Ferancee-HP
Ferro-Sequels
Gevral
Gevral T
Myadec
Os-Cal Fortified
Os-Cal Plus
Stresstabs + Iron
Stuartinic Tablets
The Stuart Formula
Theragran Stress Formula
Theragran-M
Unicap M
Unicap Plus Iron
Unicap Sr.
Unicap T
Vitron-C Tablets

Ferrous gluconate

Centrum Liquid
Fergon Elixir
Fergon Tablets
Gevrabon

Ferrous sulfate   Dayalets Plus Iron
                             Feosol Capsules
                             Feosol Elixir
                             Feosol Tablets
                             Geriplex-FS Kapseals
                             Optilets-M-500
                             Slow Fe
                             Surbex-750 With Iron

VITAMINS AND MINERALS

SUPPLEMENT	DOSE	MG IRON
Allbee C-800 Plus Iron Tablets	1	27
Caltrate 600 Tablets	1	18
Centrum Liquid	1 tbsp	9
Centrum Tablets	1	18
Centrum Silver Tablets	1	9
Dayalets Plus Iron Tablets	1	18
Femiron Tablets	1	20
Feosol Capsules	1	250
Feosol Elixir	1 tsp	220
Feosol Tablets	1	325
Ferancee Chewable	2	134
Ferancee-HP Tablets	1	110
Fergon Elixir	1 tsp	34
Fergon Tablets	1	36
Ferro-Sequels Tablets	1	150
Geriplex-FS Kapseals	1	6
Geriplex-FS Liquid	2 tbsp	15
Geritol Complete Tablets	1	50
Geritol Extend Tablets & Caplets	1	10

SUPPLEMENT	DOSE	MG IRON
Geritol Liquid	½ oz	50
Gevrabon Liquid	1 tsp	15
Gevral Tablets	1	18
Gevral T Tablets	1	27
Incremin Syrup	1 tsp	30
Myadec Tablets	1	30
One-a-Day Maximum Formula Tablets	1	18
One-a-Day Stressgard Formula Tablets	1	18
One-a-Day Women's Formula Tablets	1	27
Optilets-M-500 Tablets	1	20
Os-Cal Fortified Tablets	1	5
Os-Cal Plus Tablets	1	16.6
Slow Fe Tablets	1	50
Stresstabs + Iron Tablets	1	27
Stuartinic Tablets	1	100
Surbex-750 With Iron Tablets	1	27
The Stuart Formula Tablets	1	18
Theragran Stress Formula Tablets	1	27
Theragran-M Tablets	1	27
Troph-Iron Liquid	1 tsp	20
Unicap M Tablets	1	18
Unicap Plus Iron Tablets	1	22.5
Unicap Sr. Tablets	1	10
Unicap T Tablets	1	18
Vitron-C Tablets	1	200

APPENDIX 1

Interpreting Laboratory Values for Iron

There are common tests for iron deficiency. These include measurement of the number and size of red blood cells and the level of hemoglobin they contain. The transferrin saturation and total iron-binding capacity (TIBC) are more sensitive tests that will detect a developing iron deficiency. The ferritin levels measure the iron stores. In healthy people, when iron stores are high, transferrin saturation and serum ferritin are high, and total iron-binding capacity and serum transferrin are low.

Red Blood Cell Count (RBC): The number of red blood cells. In iron deficiency anemia, the RBC is low.

Hematocrit: The volume of packed red blood cells in a milliliter (ml) of blood.

Hemoglobin: The red pigment in blood cells that carries oxygen from the lungs through the bloodstream to body tissues.

Blood Cell Indices: When the mean corpuscular volume (MCV) and mean corpuscular hemoglobin concentration (MCHC) are reduced, this may indicate iron deficiency anemia.

Transferrin: Protein that carries iron throughout the body.

Total Iron-Binding Capacity: TIBC is increased in iron deficiency anemia.

Ferritin (serum): The most accurate measurement of total body stores. Blood-cell levels of ferritin parallel the amounts in other body cells. When these levels are reduced, iron stores are low.

Iron: The amount of iron in the blood

The ratio of iron to TIBC is frequently used to test for iron deficiency anemia. A ratio of less than 16 percent indicates iron deficiency.

Understanding the Numbers

Use this guide to help you interpret your own laboratory blood tests for iron. Don't be overwhelmed by the variety of tests or the number of measurement values used. You can compare the number on your lab report with the norm for that particular test.

The following table lists normal values for iron related laboratory tests.

TEST	NORMAL RANGE
FOR MEN	
Red Blood Cell Count (RBC)	4.3–5.6 million
Hemoglobin (Hg)	13.5–17.0 g/dl
Hematocrit (HCT)	40–51%
Ferritin	16–205 ng/ml
Transferrin	less than 200 mg/dl
Iron (Fe)	40–180 mcg/dl
Total Iron Binding Capacity (TIBC)	250–460 mcg/100 ml
Fe/TIBC	less than 16%
Mean Corpuscular Volume (MCV)	81–95 fl
Mean Corpuscular Hemoglobin Concentration (MCHC)	32.5–35.5 g/dl

TEST	NORMAL RANGE
FOR WOMEN	
Red Blood Cell Count (RBC)	3.8–5.0 million
Hemoglobin (Hg)	11.4–15.2 g/dl
Hematocrit (HCT)	34–46%
Ferritin	6–103 ng/ml
Transferrin	less than 200 mg/dl
Iron (Fe)	40–180 mcg/dl
Total Iron Binding Capacity (TIBC)	250–460 mcg/100 ml
Fe/TIBC	less than 16%
Mean Corpuscular Volume (MCV)	81–95 fl
Mean Corpuscular Hemoglobin Concentration (MCHC)	32.5–35.5 g/dl

gram (g)	=	⅕ of a teaspoon
milligram (mg)	=	one thousandth of a gram
microgram (mcg)	=	one millionth of a gram
nanogram (ng)	=	one billionth of a gram
deciliter (dl)	=	one tenth of a liter
fentoliter (fl)	=	one billionth of the microgram
milliliter (ml)	=	one thousandth of a liter

APPENDIX 2

Hemochromatosis

The first evidence of the harmful effects of too much iron was discovered when doctors treated people with a disease called *hemochromatosis*. People with hemochromatosis absorb too much iron. Hemochromatosis is a genetic disorder inherited in a recessive gene. This disorder is believed to affect about one in three hundred people, making it one of the most common genetic diseases in Western countries. In order to have a full-blown case of iron overload, it must be inherited from both parents. If the trait is inherited from only one parent, the condition is less severe.

It is estimated that one in ten people carries the gene for hemochromatosis. One percent of all marriages involve two carriers of the gene. It is estimated that 25 percent of their children will have hemochromatosis. Many people may have the condition but don't know it, and very few are ever diagnosed. What is especially alarming about hemochromatosis is that heart failure is often the earliest sign.

In hemochromatosis too much iron is absorbed from the intestines. This excess iron is deposited in and results in damage to body organs—especially the liver, pancreas, heart and pituitary gland. People with hemochromatosis have a total body iron content of 20 to 40 grams as compared with normal levels of only two or three. Most of the iron is deposited in the liver and pancreas. Liver enlargement, metallic gray skin color, shrinkage of the testicles, loss of body hair, joint disease, diabetes and heart failure are physical signs of iron overload.

To treat hemochromatosis one must lower the amount of iron stored in the body. Blood letting—regularly having some blood removed from the body—is the preferred treatment. There are also medications called *chelating agents*. These substances hook on to the iron and carry it out of the body. Many complications of the disease are improved when iron is removed from the body.

Besides hemochromatosis, iron overload is also seen in other diseases. Iron overload can be seen in liver disease, when people with normal iron stores take large amounts of iron supplements over a long time, or when repeated blood transfusions are needed to treat some types of anemia.

Annette B. Natow, Ph.D., R.D., and Jo-Ann Heslin, M.A., R.D., are the authors of fourteen books on nutrition, including *The Cholesterol Counter*, *The Fat Counter*, and *The Fat Attack Plan* (all available from Pocket Books). Both are former faculty members of Adelphi University and State University of New York, Downstate Medical Center. They are editors of the *Journal of Nutrition for the Elderly*, serve as editorial board members for the *Environmental Nutrition Newsletter*, and are frequent contributors to magazines and journals.

THE
CHOLESTEROL
COUNTER

NOW YOU CAN LOWER
YOUR CHOLESTEROL!

Cholesterol and Caloric Values
for 10,000 items - including
Fast Food, Take-Out, Packaged
and Processed Foods.

ALL NEW
THIRD EDITION
REVISED AND UPDATED

Annette Natow, Ph.D.,R.D.,
and Jo-Ann Heslin, M.A.,R.D.

POCKET BOOKS Available from Pocket Books

650

THE
SODIUM
COUNTER

Annette Natow, Ph.D.,R.D., and Jo-Ann Heslin, M.A.,R.D.

Bestselling Authors of
The Fat Counter and *The Cholesterol Counter*

POCKET BOOKS

Available from Pocket Books

731-01

THE
·FAT·
COUNTER

THE AVERAGE ADULT NEEDS
TO CUT DIETARY FAT BY
AT LEAST ONE THIRD! Now,
in one easy-to-use volume,
fat and calorie values for
OVER 10,000 FOODS.

ALL NEW
SECOND EDITION
REVISED AND UPDATED

Annette Natow, Ph.D.,R.D.,
and Jo-Ann Heslin, M.A.,R.D.